ANNUAL REVIEW OF NURSING RESEARCH: HEALTHCARE SIMULATION

VOLUME 39, 2021

ANNUAL REVIEW OF NURSING RESEARCH

Editors

Series Editor

Christine E. Kasper, PhD, RN, FAAN, FACSM

Dean and Professor
Crenshaw Endowed Chair
University of New Mexico College of Nursing
Albuquerque, New Mexico
and
Professor, Daniel K. Inouye
School of Nursing
Uniformed Services University of the Health Sciences
Bethesda, Maryland

Volume Editor

Tonya Andrade Schneidereith, PhD, CRNP, PPCNP-BC, CPNP-AC, CNE, CHSE-A, ANEF, FAAN

Associate Professor
University of Maryland School of Nursing
Baltimore, Maryland
and
Owner, CEO, and Managing Partner
SIMPL Simulation, LLC
Brooklandville, Maryland

Annual Review of Nursing Research: Healthcare Simulation

Volume 39, 2021

Series Editor

Christine E. Kasper, PhD, RN, FAAN, FACSM

Volume Editor

Tonya Andrade Schneidereith, PhD, CRNP, PPCNP-BC, CPNP-AC, CNE, CHSE-A, ANEF, FAAN

SPRINGER PUBLISHING

Springer Publishing Company, LLC
11 West 42nd Street, New York, NY 10036
www.springerpub.com
connect.springerpub.com/

Acquisitions Editor: Jaclyn Koshofer
Compositor: Exeter Premedia Services Private Ltd

ISSN: 0739-6686
ISBN: 978-0-8261-6633-3
e-book ISBN: 978-0-8261-6634-0
DOI: 10.1891/9780826166340

21 22 23 24 / 5 4 3 2 1

Printed in the United States of America.

This book is dedicated to the mentors who guide our way, the simulationists who tirelessly innovate, the learners who share their hearts and minds, the friends who listen, and the families who continually support our passion for healthcare simulation.

Contents

Part III—Simulation Practices, Operations, and Professional Development

Part IV—Technologies in Simulation

About the Volume Editor

Tonya Andrade Schneidereith, PhD, CRNP, PPCNP-BC, CPNP-AC, CNE, CHSE-A, ANEF, FAAN, is an innovative nurse educator, leader, and entrepreneur with over 30 years of pioneering work in healthcare and academic settings. She is an associate professor and full-time simulation educator in the University of Maryland School of Nursing's prestigious Debra L. Spunt Clinical Simulation Labs.

Dr. Schneidereith began her career as a pediatric nurse and was one of the country's first pediatric critical care nurse practitioners. She was selected for the National League for Nursing's (NLN) Leadership Development Program for Simulation Educators in 2015. Since then, Dr. Schneidereith has shared her expertise on projects for the NLN, the International Nursing Association for Clinical Simulation and Learning (INACSL), the Society for Simulation in Healthcare (SSH), the National Organization of Nurse Practitioner Faculties (NONPF), and the Global Network for Simulation in Healthcare. She served on the INACSL Standards of Best Practices Committee and chaired the INACSL Research Committee. She authored the *Thomas Sykes* unfolding cases for the NLN's Advancing Care Excellence-Pediatrics series and cocreated the NLN Vision Statement, *Integration of the Social Determinants of Health Into Nursing Education Curricula*. She is at the forefront of simulation in nurse practitioner (NP) education as an associate editor for NONPF's inaugural *NP Simulation Guidelines and Best Practices*. Her accomplishments and dedication to nursing have been recognized with awards and honors from the NLN, INACSL, SSH, and the Florida State University College of Nursing.

Dr. Schneidereith received her BSN from Florida State University, her MSN from the University of Pennsylvania, and her PhD from Johns Hopkins University. She holds certifications as a pediatric primary care and pediatric acute care nurse practitioner, nurse educator, and as one of a select few internationally designated healthcare simulation educators-advanced. Dr. Schneidereith is a fellow of the Academy of Nursing Education and the American Academy of Nursing.

Contributors

Michelle Aebersold, PhD, RN, CHSE, FAAN, Clinical Professor, School of Information, University of Michigan School of Nursing, Ann Arbor, Michigan

Sabrina Beroz, DNP, RN, CHSE-A, ANEF, Associate Director, School of Nursing, George Washington University, Ashburn, Virginia

Nicole Petsas Blodgett, PhD, RN, Assistant Professor, School of Nursing, Duke University, Durham, North Carolina

Kellie Bryant, DNP, WHNP, CHSE, Executive Director of Simulation, School of Nursing, Columbia University, New York, New York

Kimberly Budisalich, DNP, FNP-BC, Clinical Instructor, College of Nursing, The University of Alabama in Huntsville, Huntsville, Alabama

Dylan D. Cooper, MD, Professor of Clinical Emergency Medicine, Department of Emergency Medicine, Indiana University School of Medicine, Indianapolis, Indiana

Dawne-Marie Dunbar, MSN/Ed, RN, CNE, CHSE, Clinical Professor of Nursing/Director of Clinical Simulation, Westbrook College of Health Professions, University of New England, Portland and Biddeford, Maine

Crystel L. Farina, PhD(c), RN, CNE, CHSE, Director of Simulation and Experiential Learning, George Washington University School of Nursing, Ashburn, Virginia

Mary K. Fey, PhD, RN, CHSE-A, ANEF, FAAN, Senior Director, Harvard Medical School Department of Anesthesia, Massachusetts General Hospital, Boston, Massachusetts

Susan Gross Forneris, PhD, RN, CNE, CHSE-A, FAAN, Director, National League for Nursing, Center for Innovation in Education Excellence, Washington, DC

Ashley E. Franklin, PhD, RN, CNE, CHSE-A, Associate Professor, Harris College of Nursing & Health Sciences, Texas Christian University, Fort Worth, Texas

Katie Anne Haerling PhD, RN, CHSE, Associate Professor, School of Nursing and Healthcare Leadership, University of Washington Tacoma, Tacoma, Washington

Beth Fentress Hallmark, PhD, RN, CHSE-A, ANEF, Director of Simulation, College of Health Sciences and Nursing, Belmont University, Nashville, Tennessee

Lori Lioce, DNP, FNP-BC, CHSE-A, CHSOS, FAANP, FAAN, Clinical Professor, College of Nursing, The University of Alabama in Huntsville, Huntsville, Alabama

Kate J. Morse, PhD, MSN, RN, ACNP-Ret, Assistant Dean, College of Nursing & Health Professions, Drexel University, Philadelphia, Pennsylvania

Catherine Nicholas, EdD, MS, PA, Assistant Professor of Obstetrics and Gynecology, University of Vermont, Burlington, Vermont

Carla Nye, DNP, CPNP-PC, CNE, CHSE, Clinical Associate Professor, School of Nursing, Virginia Commonwealth University, Richmond, Virginia

Lori Podlinksi, EdD, MBA/MSN, RN, CHSE, Director of Simulation Education, Holy Name Medical Center, Teaneck, New Jersey

Julie A. Poore, DNP, RN, CHSE-A, Clinical Adjunct Associate Professor, Department of Community and Health Systems, Indiana University School of Nursing, Indianapolis, Indiana

Susan Prion, EdD, RN, CNE, CHSE, Associate Dean-Nursing and Professor, School of Nursing and Health Professions, University of San Francisco, San Francisco, California

Jill Sanko, PhD, APRN-BC, CHSE-A, FSSH, Assistant Professor, University of Miami, Coral Gables, Florida

Darlene A. Showalter, DNP, RN, CNS, Clinical Associate Professor, The University of Alabama in Huntsville College of Nursing, Huntsville, Alabama

J. Cedar Wang, MSN, RN, APN, GNP-BC, CHSE, Vice President of Nursing Operations, Holy Name Medical Center, Teaneck, New Jersey

Penni I. Watts, PhD, RN, CHSE-A, Associate Professor, School of Nursing, The University of Alabama at Birmingham School of Nursing, Birmingham, Alabama

Foreword

Simulation is the imitation of the operation of a real-world process or system over time (Banks et al., 2001). The use of the simulation of the clinical environment has provided nursing students the chance to practice their clinical and decision-making skills through various real-life experiences for the past 140 years. The dawn of simulation of patient care in nursing education originated in 1874 with the publication of the *Handbook for Hospital Sisters* by Florence S. Lees (Lees, 1874) where the use of an articulated skeleton for classroom instruction was suggested. In the early 1900s, the National League for Nursing Education advocated for classroom demonstrations and the use of anatomical models to enhance the learning experience for nursing students in their standard national curriculum (Nehring & Lashley, 2009). In the early years of professional nursing education, data were never published to support the effectiveness of these methods in instruction. Classroom instruction of clinical skill became popular and expanded rapidly to include variations of the life sized "Mrs. Chase" dolls first introduced in 1910 and were an early task trainer to develop proficiency in bathing patients, bandaging, IV needle insertion, and so on (Nehring & Lashley, 2009).

Through the years various forms of simulation as role-playing, games, computer-assisted instruction, standardized patients, virtual reality, and low-fidelity and high-fidelity manikins developed in concert with advancing technology. Fidelity refers to the ability of a simulation to mimic reality (Ventre et al., 2011). Currently sophisticated computer-controlled high-fidelity manikins can closely mimic various pathophysiological scenarios permitting close to real clinical practice in a controlled and safe simulation center environment (Bland et al., 2011).

As we go to press with this issue of the *Annual Review of Nursing Research*, a global pandemic of the SARS-CoV-2 virus has closed many clinical sites to nursing education. Schools of nursing around the world are needing to provide safe environments for the education of the future nursing workforce. Fortunately, many university-based schools of nursing have established sophisticated delivery of clinical education via both "online" Internet-delivered simulations, and, where possible, advanced clinical simulation centers equipped with the capacity for high-fidelity simulation of patient care. In these times of crisis, the use of sophisticated clinical simulation has permitted continued delivery of nursing education and the graduation of students to enter the workforce.

The research topics for the chapters were carefully chosen and compiled into this review of nursing research by Dr. Tonya Schneidereith, associate professor of nursing at the University of Maryland, Baltimore, who has served with distinction as the volume editor. She has long excelled as one of the leaders and innovators in the study of simulation for nursing education. As series editor, it is my hope that these topically based chapters will be used not only by those conducting research studies, but also as texts and supplements to nursing curricula for both the undergraduate and graduate students.

This issue comprises 11 chapters divided into topic areas of simulation in academia; hospital-based and interprofessional simulation; simulation practices, operations, and professional development; and technologies in simulation. These begin with Ashley E. Franklin and Nicole Petsas Blodgett reviewing simulation in undergraduate education in Chapter 1. In Chapter 2, Carla Nye reviews the state of simulation research in advanced practice nursing education. Catherine Nicholas and Jill Sanko, discuss human simulation in nursing education in Chapter 3, while J. Cedar Wang and Lori Podlinksi review the important study of hospital-based simulation in Chapter 4.

The issue continues with an in-depth review by Julie A. Poore and Dylan D. Cooper on the role of interprofessional simulation in both the classroom and clinical practice in Chapter 5. In Chapter 6, Kate J. Morse, Mary K. Fey, and Susan Gross Forneris review methods of evidence-based debriefing. In Chapter 7, Susan Prion and Katie Anne Haerling review research into the evaluation of simulation outcomes. In Chapter 8, Crystel L. Farina and Kellie Bryant reviews the research of simulation-based operations. In Chapter 9, Penni I. Watts, Beth Fentress Hallmark, and Sabrina Beroz investigate research into professional development for simulation education. Chapter 10 by Michelle Aebersold and Dawne-Marie Dunbar discusses virtual and augmented realities in nursing education. And, finally in Chapter 11, research into three-dimensional (3D) printing is reviewed by Lori Lioce, Kimberly Budisalich, and Darlene A. Showalter.

It is hoped that as our technology evolves it will inspire further innovations in the delivery of an enhanced nursing education through ever advancing forms of simulation.

Christine E. Kasper, PhD, RN, FAAN
Series Editor

REFERENCES

Banks, J., Carson, J. S. II., Nelson, B. L., & Nicol, D. M. (2001). *Discrete-event system simulation*. Pearson Education.

Bland, A. J., Topping, A., & Wood, B. (2011). A concept analysis of simulation as a learning strategy in the education of undergraduate nursing students. *Nurse Education Today*, *31*(7), 664–670. https://doi.org/10.1016/j.nedt.2010.10.013

Lees, F. S. (1874). *Handbook for hospital sisters*. W. Ibester & Co.

Nehring, W., & Lashley, F. (2009). Nursing simulation: A review of the past 40 years. *Simulation & Gaming*, *40*, 528–552. https://doi.org/10.1177/1046878109332282

Ventre, K. M., Collingridge, D. S., & DeCarlo, D. (2011). End-user evaluations of a personal computer-based pediatric advanced life support simulator. *Simulation in Healthcare*, 6(3), 134–142. https://doi.org/10.1097/SIH.0b013e318207241e

Preface

Never before has healthcare simulation been as important to nursing as it is now. When approached in early 2020 to create the 39th volume of *Annual Review of Nursing Research*, the COVID-19 pandemic had not yet hit the United States. Not long after, the seemingly overnight strains on hospitals and sudden shifts in academia left administrators, practitioners, faculty, and staff caught in a cyclone of unanticipated demands and unexpected change. There was an unprecedented reliance on healthcare simulation educators, spaces, and virtual trainings to solve every clinical need (Society for Simulation in Healthcare et al., 2020), including staff trainings to don and doff personal protective equipment (PPE; Dharamsi et al., 2020; Hughes et al., 2020), trial new respiratory techniques (Branecki et al., 2020; Trembley et al., 2020), and provide experiential learning opportunities to undergraduate (American Association of Colleges of Nursing, 2020; Hallmark, 2020; Morin, 2020) and graduate students (de Tantillo & Christopher, 2020; National Organization of Nurse Practitioner Faculties, 2020) who were no longer able to gain the hours demanded by accrediting bodies within the potentially virulent halls of clinical settings.

Although many of us have an idea of what "simulation" means in healthcare education, there is no singular definition. The Society for Simulation in Healthcare's Simulation Dictionary identifies six definitions with terms such as technique, strategy, pedagogy, application, and method (Lioce et al., 2020, p. 34). While it may seem obvious to those of us immersed in healthcare simulation, the techniques used to facilitate these quality experiences are a pedagogy unto themselves, grounded in the instructional continuity provided within simulated settings. The combinations of learning theories, teachings from organizational psychology, evidence derived from simulation research, and emerging technologies form the core of specialized knowledge used by simulation educators to create reflective, consistent, experiential learning opportunities.

The purpose of this edition is to provide a summary of the multiple facets that comprise and support healthcare simulation. It is my hope that those new to simulation will gain knowledge to champion small steps toward integration and, for those more seasoned, I hope to provide information that sparks new and exciting ways to reenvision simulation where you are. It is divided into four sections written by experts in their field: Simulation in Academia; Hospital-Based and Interprofessional Simulation; Simulation Practices, Operations, and Professional Development; and Technologies in Simulation. While you may be drawn to the chapters that most align with your current setting, I encourage you to read others as they contain history, methodology, and the state of the science that can be used to grow and improve your programs, operations, and personnel.

As we move into the "new normal" of healthcare practice and education, simulation is likely to provide increasingly more experiential learning opportunities. We must think differently but act purposefully. It is through the challenges brought about by the COVID-19 pandemic that we will see new possibilities and opportunities for creativity and out-of-the-box thinking, but all the while we must remember our obligation to enhance the science of simulation through meaningful data collection. Through simulation, we will improve, adapt, and overcome the current way of thinking, educating, and generating new knowledge for a stronger, smarter, and safer healthcare workforce.

Tonya Andrade Schneidereith, PhD, CRNP, PPCNP-BC, CPNP-AC, CNE, CHSE-A, ANEF, FAAN
Volume Editor

REFERENCES

American Association of Colleges of Nursing. (2020). *Considerations for COVID-19 preparedness and response in U.S. Schools of nursing.* https://www.aacnnursing.org/Portals/42/AcademicNursing/pdf/Considerations-for-COVID19-Nursing-Schools.pdf

Branecki, C. E., Jobeun, N. J., Ronnfeldt, T. J., Ash, M. A., Schulte, T. E., & Langenfeld, J. G. (2020). Novel barrier enclosure for both aerosol and droplet protection model. *Western Journal of Emergency Medicine: Integrating Emergency Care with Population Health, 21*(4), 790–794. https://doi.org/10.5811/westjem.2020.6.47834

de Tantillo, L., & Christopher, R. (2020). Transforming graduate nursing education during an era of social distancing: Tools from the field. *Nurse Education Today, 92*, 1–3. https://doi.org/10.1016/j.nedt.2020.104472

Dharamsi, A., Hayman, K., Yi, S., Chow, R., Yee, C., Gaylord, E., Tawadrous, D., Chartier, L. B., & Landes, M. (2020, August 1). Enhancing departmental preparedness for COVID-19 using rapid-cycle in-situ simulation. *Journal of Hospital Infection, 105*(4), 604–607. https://doi.org/10.1016/j.jhin.2020.06.020

Hallmark, B. F. ((2020). Summer). Replacing clinical with simulation amid the COVID-19 crisis. *Tennessee Nurse, 83*(2), 12. http://search.ebscohost.com/login.aspx?direct=true&AuthType=ip,shib&db=rzh&AN=143580518&site=ehost-live&scope=site&authtype=ip,shib&custid=s3555202

Hughes, P. G., Hughes, K. E., & Ahmed, R. A. (2020). Does my personal protective equipment really work? A simulation-based approach. *Medical Education*, *54*(8), 759–760. https://doi.org/10.1111/medu.14188

Lioce, L., Lopreiato, J., Downing, D., Chang, T. P., Robertson, J. M., Anderson, M., Diaz, D. A., Spain, A. E., & Terminology and Concepts Working Group. (2020). *Healthcare simulation dictionary* (2nd ed.). Agency for Healthcare Research and Quality. https://doi.org/10.23970/simulationv2

Morin, K. H. (2020). Nursing education after COVID-19: Same or different? *Journal of Clinical Nursing*, *29*(17–18), 3117–3119. https://doi.org/10.1111/jocn.15322

National Organization of Nurse Practitioner Faculties. (2020). *Statement regarding nurse practitioner students and direct care clinical hours*. https://cdn.ymaws.com/www.nonpf.org/resource/resmgr/board_resources/20200323_a_statement_on_np_s.pdf

Society for Simulation in Healthcare, International Nursing Association for Clinical Simulation and Learning, & Assocation for Standardized Patient Educators. (2020). *Combined statement on models & simulation and COVID-19*. https://www.inacsl.org/about/news/combined-statement-on-models-simulation-and-covid-19/

Trembley, L. L., Tobias, A. Z., Schillo, G., von Foerster, N., Singer, J., Pavelka, S. L., & Phrampus, P. (2020). A Multidisciplinary intubation algorithm for suspected COVID-19 patients in the emergency department. *Western Journal of Emergency Medicine: Integrating Emergency Care with Population Health*, *21*(4), 764–770. https://doi.org/10.5811/westjem.2020.5.47835

Part I

Simulation in Academia

CHAPTER 1

Simulation in Undergraduate Education

Ashley E. Franklin and Nicole Petsas Blodgett

ABSTRACT

Simulation is an integral component of undergraduate nursing education because it allows for a safe, timely, and prescriptive approach to meet learning objectives at the levels of individual simulations, courses, and academic programs. This review of the literature provides an overview of steps taken to move simulation forward in undergraduate nursing education, and it highlights educational theories, research, best practices, and policy statements underpinning modern nursing simulation. This chapter outlines simulation and curriculum integration approaches and provides examples of participant, course, and program outcomes.

Simulation, as an educational technique, may replace or amplify real experiences in traditional clinical settings with guided experiences that evoke and replicate substantial aspects of the real world in a fully interactive manner (Gaba, 2004; Lioce et al., 2020). Simulation is an integral component of undergraduate nursing education because it allows nursing students to develop and enhance their knowledge, skills, and attitudes, as well as analyze and independently respond to realistic situations (Morse et al., 2019; Pilcher et al., 2012). Educational leaders appreciate how simulation allows for robust, standardized, direct patient care

http://dx.doi.org/10.1891/0739-6686.39.3

experiences in a safe, open, nonthreatening environment while avoiding obstacles in traditional clinical experiences like downtime, workarounds, and low census (Aebersold, 2018; Richardson et al., 2014; Waxman et al., 2019). Faculty and learners appreciate both simulation technology and facilitation techniques that improve teaching–learning experiences (Howard et al., 2011; Starkweather & Kardong-Edgren, 2008).

While faculty utilize simulation to foster domain-specific skills in a controlled setting (Morse et al., 2019), it is important to recognize that simulation has moved beyond teaching psychomotor skills (Smiley, 2019; Waxman et al., 2019). For example, simulation can replicate clinical situations without risk to patient safety using a variety of modalities matched to components of nursing practice, including interactive manikins to practice physical assessment, standardized patients to practice communication, and virtual reality to practice clinical reasoning (Bradley et al., 2019; Pilcher et al., 2012). Simulation focuses on broad goals such as knowledge transfer, application, and skill development (Aebersold, 2016; Howard et al., 2011) while allowing learners to efficiently develop clinical reasoning skills and become competent patient care providers (Aebersold, 2018; Sullivan et al., 2019).

Surveys of the Boards of Nursing (BON) in the United States, the District of Columbia, and five nearby countries provide evidence of growth in adoption for simulation as a replacement for traditional clinical hours (Cipher et al., 2020; Smiley, 2019). In 2008, only 17 jurisdictions approved simulation (Nehring, 2008), while six years later 47 out of 61 jurisdictions allowed simulation to replace clinical hours in registered nurse programs (Hayden, Smiley, & Gross, 2014). Though jurisdictions allow simulation as a replacement for traditional clinical hours, the degree to which varies (Bradley et al., 2019, Breymier et al., 2015; Smiley, 2019).

The purpose of this chapter is to provide a summary of seminal documents and steps undertaken to move simulation forward in undergraduate nursing education, and it will highlight educational theories, research, best practices, and policy statements that underpin modern nursing simulation. This chapter will further outline curriculum integration models and provide examples of participant, course, and program outcomes.

EDUCATIONAL THEORIES UNDERPINNING SIMULATION

A variety of learning theories underpin simulation, and an emphasis on theory differentiates simulation from other technologies used in nursing education. In this section, we present a sample of learning theories frequently cited in simulation education and research.

Kolb's Experiential Learning Theory

Kolb (1984) describes a cognitive learning process where individuals have concrete experiences, followed by reflection, generation of abstract conceptualizations, and application of new knowledge to future practice (Figure 1.1). Kolb's theory resonates within simulation because active participation and guided reflection are hallmarks of modern simulation. Kolb's attention to reflective observation has also spurred a growing interest in the simulation community regarding the impact of the observer role on learning outcomes (Johnson, 2019; Zulkosky et al., 2016). According to Johnson (2019), observers in simulation show as much cognitive improvement as active simulation participants. Kolb articulates how learning is a connection between processing and perception, and different phases of learning may be preferred and different times (Howard et al., 2011; Lisko & O'Dell, 2010). For example, undergraduate nursing learners may prefer kinesthetic experiences and gravitate toward the "thinking and doing" phase of Kolb's learning cycle in simulation, where they can experiment with new ideas, practice problem-solving, and perform technical skills in a safe learning environment.

Kolb's experiential learning theory is frequently referenced in nursing literature (Aebersold, 2018; Howard et al., 2011; Morse, 2012; Poore et al., 2014; Victor Chmil et al., 2015). Nursing faculty draw connections between experiential learning theory and interprofessional simulation (Chapter 5), as well as in simulation with nursing students at the beginning of their curriculum (Poore et al., 2014; Victor Chmil et al., 2015). Poore et al. (2014) relate simulation to Kolb's concrete experience and point out that debriefing represents reflective observation. Through abstract conceptualization, learners consider the relevance of simulation to everyday practice, make plans to change their future behavior (Morse, 2012; Morse et al., 2019), and accommodate new knowledge into their mental model (Aebersold, 2018; Parker et al., 2015). Novice nurses solidify learning by active experimentation either in repeated simulations, future simulation, or traditional clinical experiences (Herrington & Schneidereith, 2017; Howard et al., 2011).

Cognitive Load Theory

Cognitive Load Theory contends that instructional design impacts information processing (Cabrera-Mino et al., 2019; Plass et al., 2010). Because knowledge acquisition depends upon available working memory during exposure to new material, learners use working memory to manipulate and understand new material. Working memory is limited in terms of capacity and is classified into three types, *intrinsic load*, *extraneous load*, and *germane load* (Pawar et al., 2018; Plass et al., 2010). *Intrinsic load* represents the difficulty of a learning task, *extraneous load* represents effort required to process a learning task as a negative consequence of

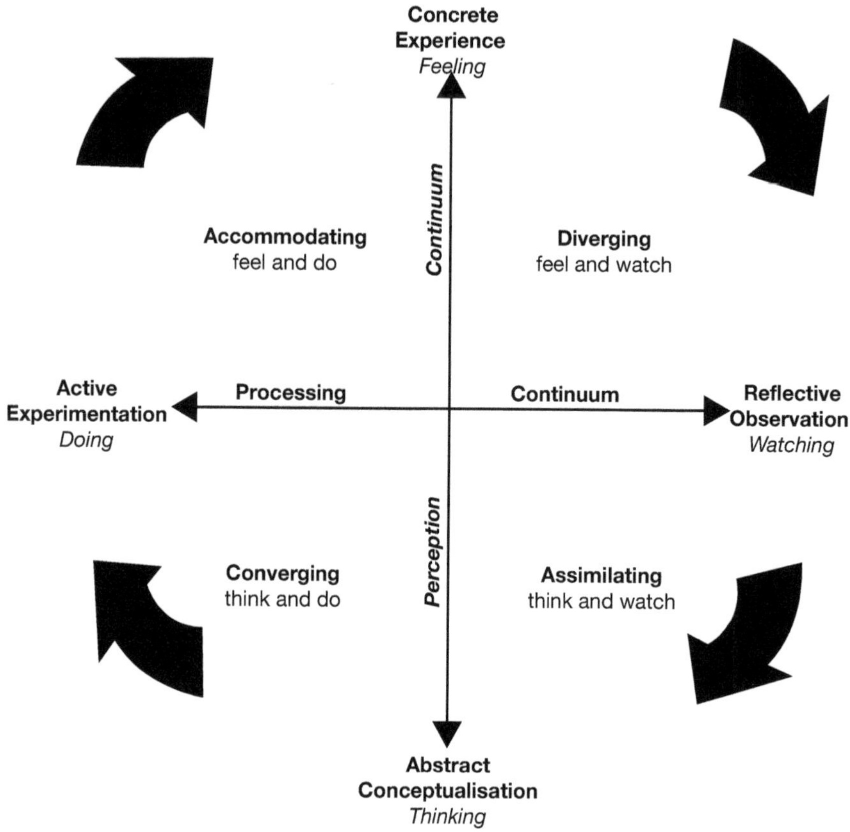

FIGURE 1.1 Kolb's experiential learning theory and learning style preferences.
Note. Used with permission from Don Clark (2014).

poor instructional design (Fraser et al., 2018; Schlairet et al., 2015), and *germane load* represents the effort involved in handling a learning task and incorporating it into working memory. The three types of cognitive load are additive, and learners become overwhelmed when cognitive load is out of balance with ability (Fraser et al., 2015; Plass et al., 2010).

Simulation learning outcomes have a parabolic relationship to cognitive load (Fraser et al., 2015), meaning that the greater the cognitive load, the less likely students are to achieve learning outcomes. It is common for nurse researchers to measure cognitive load in simulation alongside other learning outcomes (e.g., Cabrera-Mino et al., 2019; Josephsen, 2018; Pawar et al., 2018; Romero-Hall et al., 2016; Schlairet et al., 2015). As a result, educators pay a good deal of attention to simulation design elements that reduce extraneous load, such as prebriefing, consistent simulation preparation, and psychological safety (Fraser et al., 2015; Schlairet et al., 2015). Simulation can use quality simulation design to decrease extraneous load as learners practice at a level appropriate for their expertise and develop as many answers as possible to solve a problem (Reedy, 2015; van Merriënboer & Sweller, 2010). Organizing a curriculum of simulation to progress from simple to complex experiences with the appropriate cognitive load allows simulationists to maximize learning. Over time, learners can handle more realistic simulations and process tasks effectively in order to organize their knowledge into schemata that resembles actual clinical practice (Fraser et al., 2018; Reedy, 2015).

Deliberate Practice to Improve Cognitive and Psychomotor Skills

Ericsson's theory of deliberate practice (2004) asserts that superior performance develops gradually when individuals (a) have a specific goal, (b) receive detailed and immediate feedback about how to improve or what do next time to make performance better, and (c) take advantage of opportunities to practice similar tasks repeatedly. Following deliberate practice, this expert feedback on specific elements helps learners move toward meeting performance standards (Eppich et al., 2015; Fraser et al., 2018). Simulationists consider this type of feedback as "micro-debriefing," wherein the expert may stop a learner and briefly explore rationale for behavior (Gonzalez & Kardong-Edgren, 2017). Engaging in practice with the primary goal of improving a specific aspect of performance (e.g., diagnostic reasoning) is an integral part of deliberate practice; even those individuals considered to have natural gifts gradually attain superior performance by engaging in extended amounts of deliberate practice (Ericsson, 2004).

Simulationists use deliberate practice to enhance communication (Yeh et al., 2019) and psychomotor skills (Johnson et al., 2020). A meta-analysis of deliberate practice simulation favored simulation to support skill development (McGaghie et al., 2011). Several strengths of deliberate practice align with simulation, such as using preparation materials to organize a context for skill practice (Reedy, 2015), scaffolding to build on previous skill practice, peer coaching and feedback, and applying knowledge in a setting where learners hone their skills and improve their coordination over time while thinking on their feet, communicating with others, and performing skills simultaneously (Gonzalez & Kardong-Edgren, 2017; Ward et al., 2006).

NLN Jeffries Simulation Theory

The NLN Jeffries Simulation Theory illustrates the influence of context, background, and design on simulation experience and outcomes. Many simulationists also appreciate the theory's focus on facilitator–learner interactions, such as responding to learners, providing feedback, and debriefing (Aebersold, 2018; Jeffries et al., 2015b). Although nursing simulationists often focus on participant outcomes, including behavior, knowledge, skills, attitudes, and reactions (Jeffries et al., 2015b), this middle range theory aligns with recent calls to broaden evaluative methods that capture patient and systems-level outcomes (O'Donnell et al., 2014).

Educators and researchers recognize uniqueness in the blend of nursing practice and higher education best practices in simulation. Originally called the NLN Jeffries Simulation Framework (Jeffries, 2005), the educational practice's construct builds on Chickering and Gamson's (1987) principles to improve undergraduate education, including active learning, prompt feedback, student/faculty interaction, collaborative learning, high expectations, allowing diverse styles for learning, and time on task. The NLN Jeffries Simulation Theory has empirical support, including a systematic review (Adamson, 2015) and a state of the science project sponsored by the International Nursing Association for Clinical Simulation and Learning (INACSL; Ravert & McAfoos, 2014).

INFLUENCE OF BEST PRACTICE GUIDELINES, ORGANIZATIONS, AND RESEARCH

Three best practice guidelines (INACSL Standards Committee, 2016a) support simulation-based education, along with a series of publications sponsored by professional organizations (Lioce et al., 2020; Park et al., 2018; Society for Simulation in Healthcare [SSH], 2016). The most frequently cited are the INACSL Standards of Best Practice: Simulation^{SM}, first published in 2011. These peer-reviewed, living documents are cyclically updated as new evidence related to simulation design, implementation, debriefing, and evaluation becomes available (Sittner, 2016). The standards, updated in 2013 and again in 2016, address a broad range of topics including operations (INACSL Standards Committee, 2017), participant integrity (INACSL Standards Committee, 2016b), facilitation (INACSL Standards Committee, 2016c), and interprofessional simulation (INACSL Standards Committee, 2016d). The INACSL standards increase consistency of simulation and provide many simulation programs with a process for evaluating and improving operating procedures (Bradley et al., 2019; Waxman et al., 2019).

The SSH provides several resources to support simulation. The SSH accreditation standards (SSH, 2016) describe hallmark processes and outcomes of quality healthcare simulation in the areas of assessment, research, education, and systems integration. Simulation programs within academic institutions, hospitals, or stand-alone organizations may receive accreditation, and individuals may earn certification as a healthcare simulation educator from the SSH. The SSH Healthcare Simulationist Code of Ethics (Park et al., 2018) specifies six aspirational values to simulation: integrity, transparency, mutual respect, professionalism, accountability, and results orientation. Over 25 healthcare simulation organizations have adopted the code of ethics since its release in 2018. Also, the SSH Healthcare Simulation Dictionary (Lioce et al., 2020) offers standardized language and conceptual definitions for healthcare simulation. This language should be used by simulation scholars to create a cohesive body of literature from which standards of best practice can be formed. Simulationists recommend using standardized language to build the science of simulation and also to enhance communication and clarity.

The National League for Nursing (NLN) Vision Statement for Teaching with Simulation (NLN Board of Governors, 2015) provides recommendations to nursing deans and directors, faculty, and constituents to advance simulation. Collaboration is a major theme of the recommendations to link simulation faculty and foster partnerships between academic and clinical agencies. The NLN recognizes the importance of simulation faculty development and curricular integration with clear connections to desired learning outcomes.

The National Council of State Boards of Nursing (NCSBN) has Simulation Guidelines for Prelicensure Nursing Education Programs related to faculty preparation and program support. The guidelines were created by a panel of expert educators to assist BONs in developing simulation regulations for prelicensure programs (Alexander et al., 2015; Waxman et al., 2019). To effectively replace traditional clinical experiences with simulation, the guidelines recommend that simulation programs use a prescriptive methodology, including high-quality scenarios facilitated by faculty formally trained in simulation and theory-based debriefing (Alexander et al., 2015; Jeffries et al., 2015a).

The NCSBN National Simulation Study represents the most significant nursing simulation research to date. The large-scale, randomized controlled study determined that simulation is as effective, if not better, than traditional clinical experiences (Hayden, Smiley, Alexander et al., 2014). Between 2011 and 2014, researchers compared simulation delivered systematically at three doses (i.e., 10%, 25%, and 50% of traditional clinical hours were replaced with simulation) across a large sample of associate's degree and baccalaureate programs to examine nursing knowledge, clinical competency, and readiness for practice (Hayden, Smiley, & Gross, 2014; Haley, Smiley, Alexander et al., 2014). Findings demonstrated that up to 50% of clinical hours required in undergraduate curriculum could be replaced with simulation as long as high-quality simulations were facilitated by dedicated, trained faculty who follow the INACSL standards and use a theory-based debriefing model. These learners perceived they could synthesize new material, and standardized examination scores were comparable in pediatrics, maternal child, mental health, medical-surgical, and community health. Researchers also surveyed learners and their managers during their first six months of employment who found clinical competency and readiness for practice was consistent, even when simulation replaced 50% of traditional clinical hours (Hayden, Smiley, & Gross, 2014). This seminal work demonstrated that high-quality simulation could produce comparable end-of-program outcomes and new graduates who are ready for clinical practice.

STATE BOARD REGULATIONS FOR SIMULATION AS REPLACEMENT FOR TRADITIONAL CLINICAL EXPERIENCES

Each BON develops regulations for traditional clinical experiences and monitors learners' preparation (Bradley et al., 2019; Breymier et al., 2015; Smiley, 2019). Although there is increasing support for simulation learning outcomes and effectiveness, the challenge for individual BONs is to develop guidelines that safeguard the integrity of simulation as a replacement for traditional clinical experiences (Hayden, Smiley, & Gross, 2014; Spector et al., 2018). Traditional clinical experiences remain the gold standard of achieving nursing competence (Ironside & McNelis, 2010; Ironside et al., 2014), yet there is little evidence supporting that assumption. Research has demonstrated that learners experience many missed opportunities and considerable downtime while they wait for a clinical instructor or the patient during traditional clinical rotations. However, a benefit of high-quality simulation experiences, including purposeful debriefing and articulated outcomes, is little downtime during the scenario and few missed opportunities for learning (Bradley et al., 2019; Morse et al., 2019).

Acceptance of simulation for replacement of traditional clinical experiences is accelerating across nursing education (Bradley et al., 2019; Smiley, 2019). The INACSL Simulation Regulations Committee's (2020) website provides information on four criteria from each BON: percentage of clinical replacement hours, ratio of simulation to clinical hours, definition of simulation, and simulation educator requirements. Where available, the website provides each BON's dates of regulations updates, definition of simulation, and links to resources and regional simulation collaboratives. Some states have well-defined simulation criteria, while others are under development or nonexistent. Because simulation is the focus of many current BON conversations, it is prudent for educators to refer to their jurisdiction for the most up-to-date guidance. Thirty BONs have established simulation regulations (Bradley et al., 2019; Waxman et al., 2019). Currently, 17 BONs allow schools of nursing to utilize up to 50% simulation as a replacement for traditional clinical experiences and seven additional BONs allow for 25% to 30% replacement of clinical hours (INACSL Simulation Regulations Committee, 2020). Some states only allow additional simulation hours if academic institutions are accredited simulation programs (e.g., Colorado and North Carolina; Bradley et al., 2019; Waxman et al., 2019).

RATIO OF SIMULATION TO TRADITIONAL CLINICAL HOURS

Simulation can be used to supplement and replace traditional clinical hours (Hayden, Smiley, Alexander et al., 2014; Woda, Dreifuerst, & Garnier-Villareal, 2019), but replacement ratios are commonly debated. Since the 2014 National Simulation Study, simulationists have questioned the presumption that 1 hour in simulation is equivalent to 1 hour in traditional clinical experiences (Bradley et al., 2019; Breymier et al., 2015). The National Simulation Study used a 1-to-1 ratio (simulation:clinical) because, at that time, there was no evidence to support a higher ratio (Hayden, Smiley, & Gross, 2014). This trend continues as nearly 60% to 77% of nursing schools use a 1-to-1 ratio (Breymier et al., 2015; Smiley, 2019). Interestingly, 25 BONs do not define an equivalence ratio between simulation and traditional clinical experiences (Bradley et al., 2019). Emerging evidence from Sullivan et al. (2019) supports a 1-hour simulation-to-2-hour clinical equivalence ratio. Sullivan et al. (2019) found learners spend more time independently performing at higher levels of Miller's pyramid (e.g., application and analysis; Miller, 1990) in simulation compared to traditional clinical experiences.

Variation in the ratio of traditional clinical hours replaced with simulation continues at the course level. For example, Texas Christian University group simulations (averaging three students) use a 1-hour simulation-to-2-hour clinical ratio while individual simulations use 1-hour simulation-to-3-hour clinical. It is unclear why certain courses use a 1-to-1 ratio and others do not (Breymier et al., 2015). There is evidence that supports a 1-to-1 ratio (Meyer et al., 2011) and a 1-hour simulation-to-2-hour clinical ratio (Parker et al., 2011) in pediatric courses and a 1-hour simulation-to-2-hour clinical ratio in adult medical-surgical courses (Richardson et al., 2014; Zyniewicz, 2019). Lead course faculty (compared to individual faculty) often determine the ratio of simulation replacing traditional clinical hours at the course level (Breymier et al., 2015), and factors like clinical availability, clinical hours, facilitator-to-learner ratios, and faculty workload contribute to decision-making (Richardson et al., 2014). The decision to use a ratio of simulation replacement of traditional hours is more likely to be determined by administrators and curriculum committees without the guidance of the simulation center director (Breymier et al., 2015). Simulationists should guide the decision-making about the ratio of simulation replacement of clinical hours and curricular integration based on simulation design and institutional resource utilization.

There is not enough evidence in the literature that directly compares outcomes in simulation with traditional clinical experiences. As a result, educators have continued using the 1-to-1 ratio of simulation replacing traditional clinical hours. As discussed earlier, Sullivan et al. (2019) reported simulation learning outcomes and time-on-task compared to traditional clinical experiences in a multisite study and replicated gaps in traditional education reported by Ironside et al. (2014). These included a focus on clinical paperwork, and knowledge about medications and laboratory values rather than on students' overall understanding of a patient's condition, preferences, the implications for nursing care, and ways care could be improved. Educators have long highlighted the tension between task completion and learning in traditional clinical settings, so evidence for a 1-to-2 ratio of simulation to traditional clinical hours based on multisite data not only answers the question of simulation effectiveness, but also helps educators focus on learning outcomes and competency instead of time on task alone (Cipher et al., 2020; Ironside et al., 2014).

SIMULATION AND CURRICULAR INTEGRATION

Nurse educators have built an extensive body of literature that describes the process of developing individual simulation encounters. Simulation experiences that follow the INACSL Standards of Best Practice: Simulation^{SM} (INACSL Standards Committee, 2016a) provide rich learning opportunities that students might not otherwise have during their traditional clinical rotations. However, isolated simulation encounters that are not carefully integrated into an organized curriculum can result in an ineffective and inefficient use of time for both educators and learners (Herrington & Schneidereith, 2017; Howard et al., 2019; Leighton, 2018).

Although the National Simulation Study (Hayden, Smiley, Alexander et al., 2014) addressed curricular integration, there is a paucity of simulation integration effectiveness research and most evidence is descriptive in nature. There are various approaches to curricular simulation integration described in the literature (e.g., Howard et al., 2019; Leighton, 2018; Thomas et al., 2016). However, "curricular simulation integration" as a concept has not been well defined, so its meaning remains ambiguous. For the purpose of this article, curricular simulation integration is defined as the coordinated and purposeful use of simulation-based learning methods to meet predetermined learning goals within an approved curriculum. Factors shaping nursing curricular simulation integration include current trends, demographics of learners, and needs of the nursing profession.

In this section, current evidence to support curricular simulation integration is described, along with an overview of existing knowledge gaps and recommendations for future work. To facilitate curricular review and revision, a framework consistent with traditional curriculum design is used, including a needs assessment, curricular mapping, scaffolding, resource utilization, curricular planning, and evaluation.

Needs Assessment

Rather than adding individual simulation experiences to an already crowded undergraduate nursing curriculum, faculty should assess curricular needs and gaps (Aebersold, 2018; INACSL Standards Committee, 2016e). Needs assessments include the perspectives of learners, recent alumni, and educators, and they should encompass all courses. Additionally, needs assessments should include the faculty's perspective on willingness and readiness for curricular change and adjusting the amount, type, and scope of simulation. Failure to establish a critical mass of innovators or early simulation adopters could jeopardize the success of a simulation-related curricular change. A comprehensive needs assessment will help faculty evaluate the impact of curricular change, and gap analyses can identify differences between actual and desired performance (INACSL Standards Committee, 2016e; Leighton, 2018).

Required elements of a needs assessment may include the underlying cause of concern, organizational analysis, stakeholder survey, program outcome data, and a self-study comparing current practices to the INACSL standards (Aebersold, 2018; INACSL Standards Committee, 2016e; Thomas et al., 2016). The needs assessment may also reveal areas for improvement based on accreditation reports, standardized testing results (e.g., National Council Licensure Examination [NCLEX], Asssessment Technologies Institute® (ATI), Health Education Systems, Inc.® (HESI)), didactic examinations, feedback from clinical partners, access to clinical sites, low clinical performance, Quality and Safety Education in Nursing (QSEN) competencies, and others. Gathering objective data will create a transparent, defensible argument supporting curricular change. Finally, programs should assess learners' needs and learning style preferences related to technology (Howard et al., 2011). Products from the needs assessment and gap analysis should evolve into simulation program objectives.

Curricular Mapping

Educators should critically examine each course and clinical experience in order to determine how *content* (i.e., nursing knowledge) can be thoughtfully linked to *context* (i.e., patient care situations) both inside the classroom and in simulation (Waxman et al., 2019). Next, educators can add course-specific information to a curricular map to further explore areas needing improvement. Pinpointing vulnerable content and contexts allows faculty to design targeted simulation. Matching simulation to didactic content provides a nearly unparalleled strategy to enhance retention of material (Starkweather & Kardong-Edgren, 2008). Curricular mapping also prevents undesired duplication of content across several courses and guides faculty to design simulations that can have the most impact on learning and curricular effectiveness (Aebersold, 2018).

Curricular mapping requires input from faculty across the curriculum (e.g., didactic, traditional clinical settings, simulation labs). Each member of the curricular mapping work group brings a unique, germane perspective. For example, didactic educators can share topical outlines, classroom learning activities, and accreditation requirements, while clinical instructors can share common procedures, medical conditions, and policies from the clinical setting. When a simulation educator brings forward learning theories, simulation technologies, and resource availability, the work group is better able to bridge gaps identified in the needs assessment. Simulation faculty are indispensable members of the curricular mapping team. Table 1.1 provides an example of curricular mapping that can be used to achieve course objectives and end-of-program learning outcomes.

TABLE 1.1

Example of Scaffolding Objectives to Foster Program Outcomes

Sequence	Sample Course Objectives	Related Program Outcomes
Semester 1 Population: Adult Thread: Assessment	Psychomotor: Perform focused assessments using safe, competent, and compassionate approaches to gather subjective and objective data. Cognitive: Document assessment findings in electronic health record.	Meet complex health needs of individuals, families, populations, and communities. Use information systems and technology to provide care and optimize patient outcomes. Apply leadership and management principles to achieve safe, high-quality, person-centered care.
Semester 2 Population: Adult Threads: Safety, communication	Psychomotor: Demonstrate safe medication administration during formative assessments Cognitive: Describe appropriate communication techniques.	

TABLE 1.1

Example of Scaffolding Objectives to Foster Program Outcomes (Continued)

Sequence	Sample Course Objectives	Related Program Outcomes
Semester 3 Population: Adult, behavioral health Threads: Assessment, safety, clinical reasoning, communication	Psychomotor: Perform focused assessments on simulated medical-surgical and behavioral health patients. Psychomotor: Demonstrate safe medication administration during interactive group simulations. Cognitive: Describe clinical reasoning skills used in simulation. Affective: Use therapeutic communication to provide care for simulated patients and families.	
Semester 4 Population: Adult, maternal/family Threads: Assessment, safety, clinical reasoning, communication	Psychomotor: Perform focused assessments on simulated critical care and maternal/family patients. Psychomotor: Demonstrate safe medication administration skills during interactive group simulations. Cognitive: Apply the Clinical Judgment Model to interactive group simulations. Affective: Advocate for patient safety during interactive group simulations.	

(Continued)

TABLE 1.1

Example of Scaffolding Objectives to Foster Program Outcomes (Continued)

Sequence	Sample Course Objectives	Related Program Outcomes
Semester 5 Population: Adult Threads: Priority setting, assessment, safety, clinical reasoning, delegation	Cognitive: Prioritize focused assessments and safety checks for multiple simulation patients. Psychomotor: Demonstrate safe medication administration to multiple simulation patients. Cognitive: Utilize clinical reasoning skills to prioritize care for multiple simulation patients. Affective: Communicate with unlicensed assistive personnel in simulation in accordance with Nurse Practice Act.	

Source. Used with permission from Texas Christian University.

Scaffolding to Improve Learners' Understanding and Retention

A curricular map will allow faculty to scaffold simulation experiences and build on content and complexity from previous courses. Scaffolding, emerging from constructivism, posits that learning and retention occur when new knowledge is incorporated into existing knowledge (World Health Organization, 2018). Scaffolding allows learners to demonstrate knowledge, skills, and attitudes, add new knowledge, and apply new material. Scaffolding promotes learning efficiency (Thomas et al., 2016), but it requires that faculty understand curriculum organization, how simulation fits into course outcomes, and where concepts build in complexity over time (see Tables 1.1 and 1.2). Among undergraduate nursing learners, Shin et al. (2015) found that simulation had maximum benefit for upper levels, though it is hard to parse out whether the literature was biased toward simulation for upper-level learners or if simulation appeared to be more effective for learners who had concrete traditional clinical experiences to underpin simulation experiences. The timing of simulation events in relation to didactic content impacts what and how students learn. In a sample of nearly 200 learners

TABLE 1.2

Concept-Based Simulation Curriculum Exemplar

Content Area	Semester 1	Semester 2	Semester 3	Semester 4	Semester 5
Oxygenation	Respiratory assessment on healthy simulated patients	Oxygen administration using mid-fidelity manikins	Interactive group simulation with a simulated patient requiring oxygen, intravenous antibiotics, and patient teaching for pneumonia	Interactive group simulation with a newborn manikin patient who has apnea and requires ventilation with a bag valve mask and medication administration	Multiple patient simulation where two patients receive oxygen and one has underlying chronic obstructive pulmonary disease
Perfusion	Vital signs assessment on healthy simulated patients	Intravenous medication administration using bar code medication administration and task trainers	Interactive group simulation with a manikin heart failure patient receiving diuretics, oxygen, and intravenous fluids	Interactive group sepsis simulation with a manikin trauma patient and an embedded participant portraying a family member	Multiple patient simulation where two patients receive intravenous fluids and another experiences cardiac chest pain

Source. Used with permission from Texas Christian University.

working in interprofessional teams, Liaw et al. (2019) found a scaffolded learning approach with web-based instruction followed by virtual reality and/or simulation improved outcomes.

Faculty can build a content "scaffold" that gives depth to the curricular map by identifying layers of conceptual complexity. Scaffolding allows learners to pair new information with familiar concepts for enhanced learning (Coombs, 2018; Thomas et al., 2016). Since most concepts in nursing are not linear, it is unclear exactly which areas of nursing knowledge form the scaffold and which rest upon it. Moreover, nursing students have a wide range of preexisting cognitive scaffolds before entering the nursing curriculum, so knowing the starting level of complexity can be an enormous challenge. Herrington and Schneidereith (2017) proposed a scaffolded approach for professional nursing concepts (e.g., communication skills, scope of practice, priority setting, leadership) from the beginning to concluding stages of a nursing program, and acknowledged the endless possibilities for how nursing concepts could be arranged to promote scaffolded learning. Table 1.2 provides an example of scaffolding in sequential courses.

When planning for the placement of simulations in the curriculum, faculty should also ensure learners have an adequate technology scaffold upon which to build new knowledge. Technological scaffolding is conceptually defined as the provision of technology that helps support students as they engage in a learning task (Sharma & Hannafin, 2007, p. 29). While millennial learners are often thought to be experts at digital technology, evidence suggests that there is still a learning curve whenever new devices are introduced or when familiar devices are used for a different purpose. For example, students who are unfamiliar with the use of stethoscopes or expected physiologic sounds during a basic health assessment lab are likely to struggle when assessing a high-fidelity manikin with nonphysiological or mechanical sounds (e.g., squeaking plastic, air compressor). A student who is accustomed to using a smartphone to text or stream videos might be confused when asked to use the smartphone to call a provider during a simulation. In both of these cases, the student's lack of an adequate scaffold may prevent achievement of desired learning outcomes. Videos demonstrating appropriate use of equipment and orientation during prebriefing can support technology scaffolding in simulation.

When integrating simulation into a curriculum, faculty should be cognizant that simulation is both a tool for learning and a source of complexity in and of itself. Curricular needs and gaps that are mapped to a particular course should be classified according to their complexity across the curriculum (Leighton, 2018). Once this is completed, faculty must be sure to support a scaffold of conceptual and technological knowledge upon which learners can base clinical decisions and actions during simulation (Coombs, 2018). If nurse educators view learning as a building process upon a foundation of knowledge, with simulation as a mechanism for adding layers more efficiently than building one block at a time, then scaffolding directs learners to achieve new heights during their educational experience. Scaffolding helps faculty prioritize curricular integration of simulation with careful attention to learners' abilities. More empirical work related to scaffolding high-quality simulation across the nursing curriculum is needed.

Resource Utilization

Developing a feasible plan for curricular integration of simulation is key to success (Howard et al., 2019; Leighton, 2018). Although simulation can address curricular needs and gaps, oftentimes few resources are dedicated to simulation (e.g., one manikin, one room, or one trained faculty member). It takes a team of faculty to adopt the NCSBN Simulation Guidelines for Prelicensure Education Programs and incorporate simulation to foster success (Howard et al., 2019). Adequate resources are needed to provide high-quality simulation experiences, including support of other faculty, the curriculum committee, and administrators. Faculty should give careful consideration to cohort size, clinical hours, ratio of simulation to clinical hours, calendar logistics, faculty-to-learner ratios, setup and teardown, and simulation space (Blodgett et al., 2018). Flexibility in scheduling simulation events, room availability for debriefing, and trained faculty to facilitate debriefing are critical to an efficient simulation integration plan.

Budgeting operation costs for a simulation program is important for sustainability. The simulation experience should have maximum realism so that students do not expend cognitive energy understanding what is "real" and what must be imagined (Screws & Cason, 2019). High-fidelity simulation provides the greatest realism; however, high-fidelity simulation may be cost prohibitive or difficult for many programs to maintain (Peddle et al., 2020; Zamora et al., 2019). If simulation is used infrequently, administrators may be less likely to invest in simulation equipment, supplies, space, or personnel. However, a simulation program that is heavily used and fills curricular gaps of traditional clinical experiences or classroom activities is more likely to be funded. Therefore, faculty who are interested in curricular integration must base a clear business case on a strong return on investment (Hippe et al., 2020).

Planning Simulation Experiences Throughout the Curriculum

Several approaches to curricular simulation integration focus on nursing care for various illnesses, the nursing role within interprofessional teams, and evidence-based practice. Simulation integration can also be used to prioritize concepts, thread accreditation requirements, and address learners' performance gaps (see Table 1.2). When considering or designing simulation experiences, faculty are advised to include scenarios with patients demonstrating medical conditions likely encountered by learners (e.g., adults with hypertension) and common nursing procedures (e.g., assessment). In particular, faculty should provide ample opportunities to practice error-prone procedures in simulated clinical settings toward building competency, such as medication administration (Aebersold, 2018). Since learners are not guaranteed to provide independent care in traditional clinical settings, simulation practice ensures every learner has hands-on, independent practice with faculty feedback prior to graduation (Howard et al., 2011). Thoughtful curricular simulation integration reduces the undesired variability of clinical experiences and can ensure that students have a safe, standardized experience caring for patients with high-frequency conditions. In some specialty areas, faculty may include scenarios that are infrequently encountered in the clinical setting, but that provide essential opportunities to practice first aid or other lifesaving protocols that can help the learner gain familiarity with specific clinical concepts (e.g., postpartum hemorrhage, lethal cardiac dysrhythmias).

Availability of clinical sites and clinical faculty are also considerations when designing simulation experiences (Richardson et al., 2014; Zamora et al., 2019). Nursing programs often compete for clinical sites, including limited access to specialty areas (e.g., pediatrics, mental health, labor, and delivery), and many nursing programs integrate simulation to fill these gaps. For example, a birthing simulation allows learners to participate in a complete birthing process instead of potentially missing this learning opportunity in a traditional clinical setting.

Rather than spending laborious time developing and testing a new scenario, faculty may benefit from adapting peer-reviewed scenarios for their learners (see Table 1.3). Adapting scenarios saves a tremendous amount of planning time, but it is imperative that local simulation and clinical experts vet each scenario to ensure it aligns with course and program outcomes.

TABLE 1.3

Peer-Reviewed Simulations for Undergraduate Nursing

Organization	Examples of Validated Simulations
NLN Core & Complex Cases	https://www.laerdal.com/distributors/doc/236/NLN-Simulation-Scenarios
NLN Advancing Care Excellence (ACE) Scenarios	http://www.nln.org/professional-development-programs/advancing-care-excellence-series
vSim for Nursing	https://www.laerdal.com/us/vsim
NLN Integrating ACES and QSEN	http://www.nln.org/docs/default-source/professional-development-programs/sirc/supplemental-materials-for-integrating-qsen-and-aces.pdf?sfvrsn=2

Note. NLN = National League for Nursing.
ACE = Advancing Care Excellence for Seniors.
QSEN = Quality and Safety Education for Nurses.

Experts also recommend extending the simulation laboratory into classroom settings. Scalability, or the ability to make a small simulation-based learning experience available to a larger audience, has recently emerged in the literature. These experiences can include tag-team simulations (learners "tag in and out"), virtual reality, telesimulation, and a different role for observers (Kardong-Edgren et al., 2020). Classroom simulations increase the number of learners experiencing simulation in an efficient manner. For example, mental health simulations with embedded participants were facilitated in a large classroom and met affective learning outcomes related to mental illness (Aebersold, 2018). More research is needed, however, that compares learning outcomes in small group versus classroom simulation.

Faculty must also consider the level of fidelity for every simulation. Fidelity refers to the realism of simulation, and as the experience approaches reality, the fidelity increases (Lioce et al., 2020). Creating a high level of realism that mimics real life will aid learner achievement of desired learning objectives. However, there is not one level of fidelity that produces the best learning in all situations (Foronda et al., 2013). It is crucial to match the level of fidelity and the learners' level of experience (see Table 1.4) as different courses may have different simulation needs (Masters, 2014). Learner satisfaction improves with high-fidelity simulations (Mariani et al., 2013; Weaver, 2015) as do cognitive learning outcomes (Hayden, Smiley, Alexander et al., 2014). Therefore, it is important that the level of fidelity matches both scenario objectives and learners' needs.

Simulation Evaluation

There are several areas to consider when evaluating the integration of simulation across the undergraduate nursing curriculum, including evaluations of simulations, courses, and learners (see Chapter 7). Implementation of a comprehensive simulation program throughout the curriculum is a major undertaking that requires immense administrative, faculty, and staff support. Most importantly, the evaluation team must determine, based on qualitative and quantitative data, the degree to which the simulation addressed curricular needs and gaps. Data sources can include feedback from learner and faculty questionnaires, first-time NCLEX-RN pass rates, standardized test scores, and employer and alumni feedback. Because simulation is an element of the larger curriculum, data should be considered in aggregate. Changes in outcomes can likely relate to a combination of inputs such as didactic, clinical, and simulation experiences.

Another evaluation of simulation is at the course level. Faculty teams may use the needs assessment and curricular map as a starting point to determine how simulation impacted changes in each course. Data gathered from faculty

TABLE 1.4

Simulation Integration With Increasing Complexity Through Curriculum

Course	Simulation	Potential Technology (Level of Fidelity)
Health Assessment	Abnormal cardiac and respiratory assessment	Static manikin (low)
Medical-Surgical 1	Congestive heart failure with hypoglycemia	Interactive manikin (high)
Medical-Surgical 2	Cerebrovascular accident with family member present	Interactive manikin and embedded participant (high)
Care of Mother and Newborn	Postpartum magnesium sulfate toxicity with family member and newborn present	Two interactive manikins and an embedded participant (high)
Mental Health	Depression/suicide attempt with family member present	Two embedded participants (high)
Transition to Practice	Postoperative knee arthroplasty with acute pulmonary embolism	Interactive manikin (high)

Source. Adapted from Howard et al. (2011).

perspectives in end-of-year reports can be triangulated with learner perspectives from end-of-course evaluations. It may be appropriate to gather input from clinical partners about learners' performance in traditional clinical settings and alongside related simulation experiences. Course evaluations may also be used to provide feedback to simulation facilitators, including consistency and adherence to best practices for prebriefing and debriefing (INACSL Standards Committee, 2016c, 2016f). Valid and reliable tools like the Facilitator Competence Rubric (Leighton et al., 2018) may be helpful for course faculty to use for self-evaluation and to identify professional development needs. Many parts of evaluation start during the planning stages of a curricular change. For example, course faculty could decide a priori to have learners complete the Simulation Effectiveness Tool-Modified (Leighton et al., 2015) to capture perceptions of how well the simulation met their learning needs.

Evaluation of the learner, during simulation and debriefing, may be an early predictor of curricular outcomes. Kirkpatrick's (1994) four stages of evaluation are frequently used in simulation: (a) reacting immediately after training (e.g., satisfaction or self-confidence); (b) learning knowledge, skill, and attitudes about their profession; (c) changing behavior during simulation; and (d) transferring knowledge and behaviors to improve quality care and patient safety in traditional clinical experiences. Learners' reactions can be important early indicators of affective changes, but consensus from simulation experts maintains that satisfaction and self-confidence do not correlate to behavior changes either in simulation or traditional clinical experiences. Cognitive shifts that result in behavior changes need to be captured early in the curricular evaluation. Both formative and summative learner evaluations provide data on curricular effectiveness (INACSL, 2016g). For example, repeated disregard of a lowered side rail during separate simulations spread over a week raises questions about curricular inclusion of environmental safety. Faculty can use simulation observations to make recommendations on knowledge, skills, attitudes, and behaviors that impact patient outcomes (Morse et al., 2019). Real-time simulation observations can prevent negative patient outcomes by quickly informing faculty of the effectiveness of changes prior to full curricular implementation.

Simulation effectiveness should be the primary focus of learner, course, and curriculum evaluation (Harder, 2019). Howard et al. (2011) found high-fidelity simulation resulted in significantly higher standardized testing scores among undergraduate nursing students when compared to traditional case studies. The overall quality of a nursing program can be tied to the quality of the simulation program itself. Spector et al. (2020) found nursing programs with few simulation-related resources or out-of-date simulation equipment also had a tendency to underperform on accreditation benchmarks. Therefore, evaluating the quality of a simulation program, including curricular integration, facilitator competency, and resource utilization, is a wise use of departmental resources.

CONCLUSION

Simulation has changed the landscape of nursing education. It moves class content from faculty-centered and "let me show you and tell you" to learner-centered and "show me and tell me how you understand this" (Waxman et al., 2019). Since 2005, nurse educators have taken great strides to develop simulation best practices, implement simulation effectiveness research, and integrate simulation across the curriculum. Enthusiasm for simulation remains high across nursing programs, though many boards of nursing still await conclusive evidence to support the replacement of traditional clinical experiences with simulated experiences. In order to continue to move empirical evidence forward, visionary administrators will need to provide resources (e.g., staff, faculty, workload, equipment), encourage faculty buy-in, and pursue simulation training to develop innovative simulation approaches. Systematic reviews of simulation literature have helped educators understand the strengths and areas rich for future research (Cantrell et al., 2017; Doolen et al., 2016; Shin et al., 2015), including the equivalence ratio of simulation-to-clinical time, simulation dose, and curricular sequencing. These areas, specifically targeted to move simulation forward, are also part of the 2020–2023 INACSL Research Priorities (INACSL, 2020). It is essential that simulation experts advocate for teaching innovations through service to curriculum and evaluation committees and regional and state regulatory boards.

REFERENCES

Adamson, K. (2015). A systematic review of the literature related to the NLN/Jeffries simulation framework. *Nursing Education Perspectives*, *36*(5), 281–291. https://doi.org/10.5480/15-1655

Aebersold, M. (2016). The history of simulation and its impact on the future. *AACN Advanced Critical Care*, 27(1), 56–61. https://doi.org/10.4037/aacnacc2016436

Aebersold, M. (2018). Simulation-based learning: No longer a novelty in undergraduate education. *Online Journal of Issues in Nursing*, *23*(2). 1–13 https://doi.org/10.3912/OJIN.Vol23No02PPT39

Alexander, M., Durham, C. F., Hooper, J. L., & Jeffries, P. R. (2015). NCSBN simulation guidelines for prelicensure nursing programs. *Journal of Nursing Regulation*, *6*(3), 39–43. https://doi.org/10.1016/S2155-8256(15)3078303

Blodgett, N. P., Blodgett, T., & Kardong-Edgren, S. E. (2018). A proposed model for simulation faculty workload determination. *Clinical Simulation in Nursing*, *18*, 20–27. https://doi.org/10.1016/j.ecns.2018.01.003

Bradley, C. S., Johnson, B. K., Dreifuerst, K. T., White, P., Conde, S. K., Meakim, C. H., Curry-Lourenco, K., & Childress, R. M. (2019). Regulation of simulation use in United States prelicensure nursing programs. *Clinical Simulation in Nursing*, *33*, 17–25. https://doi.org/10.1016/j.ecns.2019.04.004

Breymier, T. L., Rutherford-Hemming, T., Horsley, T. L., Smith, L. G., & Connor, K. (2015). Substitution of clinical experiences with simulation in prelicensure nursing programs: A national survey in the United States. *Clinical Simulation in Nursing*, *11*(11), 472–478. https://doi.org/10.1016/j.ecns.2015.09.004

Cabrera-Mino, C.I., Shinnick, M. A., & Moya, S. (2019). Task-evoked pupillary responses in nursing simulation as an indicator of stress and cognitive load. *Clinical Simulation in Nursing*, *31*(c), 21–27. https://doi.org/10.1016/j.ecns.2019.03.009

Cantrell, M. A., Franklin, A. E., Leighton, K., & Carlson, A. (2017). The evidence in simulation-based learning experiences in nursing education: An umbrella review. *Clinical Simulation in Nursing*, *13*(12), 634–667. https://doi.org/10.1016/j.ecns.2017.08.004

Chickering, A. W., & Gamson, Z. F. (1987, March). Seven principles for good practice in undergraduate education. *AAHE Bulletin*, 3–7. https://files.eric.ed.gov/fulltext/ED282491.pdf

Cipher, D. J., LeFlore, J., Urban, R. W., & Mancini, M. E. (2020). Variability of clinical hours in prelicensure nursing programs: Time for a reevaluation. *Teaching and Learning in Nursing*, *23*, 41–46. https://doi.org/10.1016/j.teln.2020.05.005

Clark, D. (2014). *Kolb's learning styles and experiential learning model*. http://nwlink.com/~donclark/hrd/styles/kolb.html

Coombs, N. M. (2018). Educational scaffolding: Back to basics for nursing education in the 21st century. *Nursing Education Today*, *68*, 190–200. https://doi.org/10.1016/j.nedt.2018.06.007

Doolen, J., Mariani, B., Atz, T., Horsley, T. L., O'Rourke, A., McAffee, K., & Cross, C. L. (2016). High-fidelity simulation in undergraduate nursing education: A review of simulation reviews. *Clinical Simulation in Nursing*, *12*(7), 290–302. https://doi.org/10.1016/j.ecns.2016.01.009

Eppich, W. J., Hunt, E. A., Duval-Arnold, J. M., Siddall, V. J., & Cheng, A. (2015). Structuring feedback and debriefing to achieve mastery learning goals. *Academic Medicine*, *90*(11), 1501–1508. https://doi.org/10.1097/ACM.0000000000000934

Ericsson, K. A. (2004). Deliberate practice and the acquisition and maintenance of expert performance in medicine and related domains. *Academic Medicine*, *79*(10), S70–S81. https://doi.org/10.1097/00001888-200410001-00022

Foronda, C., Liu, S., & Bauman, E. B. (2013). Evaluation of simulation in undergraduate nurse education: An integrative review. Clinical Simulation in Nursing, 9(10), e409-e416. http://dx.doi.org/ 10.1016/j.ecns.2012.11.003

Fraser, K., Ayres, P., & Sweller, J. (2015). Cognitive load theory for the design of medical simulations. *Simulation in Healthcare*, *10*(5), 295–307. https://doi.org/10.1097/SIH.0000000000000097

Fraser, K., Meguerdichian, M. J., Haws, J. T., Grant, V. J., Bajaj, K., & Cheng, A. (2018). Cognitive load theory for debriefing simulations: Implications for faculty development. *Advances in Simulation*, *3*, 28. https://doi.org/10.1186/s41077-018-0086-1

Gaba, D. M. (2004). The future vision of simulation in health care. *BMJ Quality and Safety in Healthcare*, *13*(Supp. 1), i2–i10. https://doi.org/10/1136/qshc/2004.009878

Gonzalez, L., & Kardong-Edgren, S. (2017). Deliberate practice for mastery learning in nursing. *Clinical Simulation in Nursing*, *13*(1), 10–14. http://doi.org/10.1016/j.ecns.2016.10.005

Harder, N. (2019). Simulation and patient safety: Continuing to provide evidence. *Clinical Simulation in Nursing*, *29*, 38–39. https://doi.org/10.1016/j.ecns.2019.03.006

Hayden, J. K., Smiley, R. A., Alexander, M. A. Kardong-Edgren., S, & Jeffries, P. R. (2014). The NCSBN National Simulation Study: A longitudinal, randomized, controlled study replacing clinical hours with simulation in pre-licensure nursing education. *Journal of Nursing Regulation*, *5*(Suppl.), s3–s40. https://doi.org/10.1016/S2155-8256(15)30062-4

Hayden, J. K., Smiley, R. A., & Gross, L. (2014). Simulation in nursing education: Current regulations and practices. *Journal of Nursing Regulation*, *5*(2), 25–30. https://doi.org/10.1016/S2155-8256(15)30084-3

Herrington, A., & Schneidereith, T. (2017). Scaffolding and sequencing core concepts to develop a simulation-integrated nursing curriculum. *Nurse Educator*, *42*, 204–207. https://doi.org/10.1097/NNE.0000000000000358

Hippe, D. S., Umoren, R. A., McGee, A., Bucher, S. L., & Bresnahan, B. W. (2020). A targeted systematic review of cost analyses for implementation of simulation-based education in healthcare. *SAGE Open Medicine*, *8*, 2050312120913451. https://doi.org/10.1177/2050312120913451

Howard, V. M., Englert, N., Kameg, K., & Perrozi, K. (2011). Integration of simulation across the undergraduate curriculum: Student and faculty perspectives. *Clinical Simulation in Nursing*, *7*(1), e1–e10. https://doi.org/10.1016/j.ecns.2009.10.004

Howard, V. M., Leighton, K., & Gore, T. (2019). Simulation in healthcare education. In R. Nelson & N. Staggers (Eds.), *Health informatics: An interprofessional approach* (2nd ed., pp. 454–471). Elsevier.

INACSL Standards Committee. (2017). INACSL standards of best practice: Simulation SM: Operations. Clinical Simulation in Nursing, 13(12), 681-687. https://doi.org/10.1016/j.ecns.2017.10.005

INACSL Simulation Regulations Committee. (2020). *INACSL Simulation regulation map*. https://www.inacsl.org/simulation-regulations/

INACSL Standards Committee. (2016a). INACSL standards of best practice: Simulation[SM]: Simulation. *Clinical Simulation in Nursing*, *12*, S5–S50. https://doi.org/10.1016/j.ecns.2016.09.009

INACSL Standards Committee. (2016b). INACSL standards of best practice: Simulation[SM]: Professional integrity. *Clinical Simulation in Nursing*, *12*, S30–S33. http://doi.org/10.1016/%20.%20j.ecns.2016.09.010

INACSL Standards Committee. (2016c). INACSL standards of best practice: Simulation[SM]: Facilitation. *Clinical Simulation in Nursing*, *12*, S16–S20. https://doi.org/10.1016/j.ecns.2016.09.007

INACSL Standards Committee. (2016d). INACSL standards of best practice: Simulation[SM]: Simulation-Enhanced Interprofessional Education (Sim-IPE). *Clinical Simulation in Nursing*, *12*, S34–S38. https://doi.org/10.1016/j.ecns.2016.09.011

INACSL Standards Committee. (2016e). INACSL standards of best practice: Simulation[SM]: Simulation design. *Clinical Simulation in Nursing*, *12*, S5–S12. https://doi.org/10.1016/j.ecns.2016.09.005

INACSL Standards Committee. (2016f). INACSL standards of best practice: Simulation[SM]: Debriefing. *Clinical Simulation in Nursing*, *12*, S21–S25. http://doi.org/10.1016/%20.%20j.ecns.2016.09.008

INACSL Standards Committee. (2016g, December). INACSL standards of best practice: Simulation[SM]: Participant evaluation. *Clinical Simulation in Nursing*, *12*, S26–S29. http://doi.org/10.1016/%20.%20j.ecns.2016.09.009

International Nursing Association for Clinical Simulation and Learning. (2020). *Research priorities*. https://www.inacsl.org/about/research-priorities/

Ironside, P. M., & McNelis, A. M. (2010). Clinical education in prelicensure nursing programs: Findings from a national survey. *Nursing Education Perspectives*, *31*(4), 264–265.

Ironside, P. M., McNelis, A. M., & Ebright, P. (2014). Clinical education in nursing: Rethinking learning in practice settings. *Nursing Outlook*, *62*(3), 185–191. https://doi.org/10.1016/j.outlook.2013.12.004

Jeffries, P. R. (2005). A framework for designing, implementing, and evaluating simulations used as teaching strategies in nursing. *Nursing Education Perspectives*, *26*(2), 96–103.

Jeffries, P. R., Dreifuerst, K. T., Kardong-Edgren, S., & Hayden, J. (2015a). Faculty development when initiating simulation programs: Lessons learned from the National Simulation Study. *Journal of Nursing Regulation*, *5*(4), 17–23. https://doi.org/10.1016/S2155-8256(15)30037-5

Jeffries, P. R., Rodgers, B., & Adamson, K. (2015b). NLN Jeffries simulation theory: Brief narrative description. *Nursing Education Perspectives*, *36*(5), 292–293. https://doi.org/10.5480/1536-5026-36.5.292

Johnson, B. K. (2019). Simulation observers learn the same as participants: The evidence. *Clinical Simulation in Nursing*, *33*, 26–34. https://doi.org/10.1016/j.ecns.2019.04.006

Johnson, C. E., Kimble, L. P., Gunby, S. S., & Davis, A. H. (2020). Using deliberate practice and simulation for psychomotor skill competency acquisition and retention. *Nurse Educator*, *45*(3), 150–154. https://doi.org/10.1097/NNE.0000000000000713

Josephsen, J. (2018). Cognitive load measurement, worked-out modeling, and simulation. *Clinical Simulation in Nursing*, *23*(10), 10–15. https://doi.org/10.1016/j.ecns.2018.07.004

Kardong-Edgren, S., Swoboda, S., & Sullivan, N. (2020). Simulation as clinical replacement: Contemporary approaches in healthcare professional education. In D. Nestel, G. Reedy, L. McKenna, & S. Gough (Eds.), *Clinical education for the health professions*. Springer Publishing. https://doi.org/10.1007/978-981-13-6106-7_44-1

Kirkpatrick, D. L. (1994). *Evaluating training programs: The four levels*. Berrett-Koehler.

Kolb, D. A. (1984). *Experiential learning: Experience as the source of learning and development*. Prentice-Hall.

Leighton, K. (2018). Curriculum development in nursing simulation programs. In C. Foisy-Doll & K. Leighton (Eds.), *Simulation champions: Fostering courage, caring, and connection* (pp. 397–428). Wolters Kuwer.

Leighton, K., Mudra, V., & Gilbert, G. E. (2018). Development and psychometric evaluation of the facilitator competency rubric. *Nursing Education Perspectives*, *39*(6), E3–E9. https://doi.org/10.1097/01.NEP.0000000000000409

Leighton, K., Ravert, P., Mudra, V., & Macintosh, C. (2015). *Simulation effectiveness tool-modified*. https://sites.google.com/view/evaluatinghealthcaresimulation/set-m

Liaw, S. Y., Tan, K. K., Wu, L. T., Tan, S. C., Choo, H., Yap, J. Lim., M, S., Wong, L., & Ignacio, J. (2019). Finding the right blend of technologically enhanced learning environments: Randomized controlled study of the effect of instructional sequences on interprofessional learning. *Journal of Medical Internet Research*, *21*(5), e12537. https://doi.org/10.2196/12537

Lioce, L., Lopreiato, J., Downing, D., Chang, T. P., Robertson, J. M., Anderson, M., Diaz, D. A., Spain, A. E., & the Terminology and Concepts Working Group. (2020). *Healthcare simulation dictionary* (2nd ed.). Agency for Healthcare Research and Quality. AHRQ Publication No. 20-0019. https://doi.org/10.23970/simulationv2

Lisko, S. A., & O'Dell, V. (2010). Integration of theory and practice: Experiential learning theory and nursing education. *Nursing Education Perspectives*, *31*, 106–108. https://doi.org/10.1043/1536-5026-31.2.106

Mariani, B., Cantrell, M. A., Meakim, C., Prieto, P., & Dreifuerst, K. T. (2013). Structured debriefing and students' clinical judgment abilities in simulation. *Clinical Simulation in Nursing*, *9*(5), e147–e155. https://doi.org/10.1016/j.ecns.2011.11.009

Masters, K. (2014). Journey toward integration of simulation in a baccalaureate nursing curriculum. *Journal of Nursing Education*, *53*(2), 102–104. https://doi.org/10.3928/01484834-20131209-03

McGaghie, W. C., Issenberg, B., Cohen, E. R., Barsuk, J. H., & Wayne, D. B. (2011). Does simulation-based medical education with deliberate practice yield better results that traditional clinical education? A meta-analytic comparative review of the evidence. *Academic Medicine*, *86*(6), 706–711. https://doi.org/10.1097/ACM.0b013e318217e119

Meyer, M. N., Connors, H., Hou, Q., & Gajewski, B. (2011). The effect of simulation on clinical performance: A junior nursing student clinical comparison study. *Simulation in Healthcare*, *6*(5), 269–277. https://doi.org/10.1097/SIB.0b013e8233a048

Miller, G. E. (1990). The assessment of clinical skills/competence/performance. *Academic Medicine*, *65*(9), s63–s67. https://doi.org/10.1097/00001888-199009000-00045

Morse, C. J. (2012). Debriefing after simulated patient experience. In L. Wilson & L. Rockstraw (Eds.), *Human simulation for nursing and health professions* (pp. 58–68). Springer Publishing.

Morse, C. J., Fey, M., Kardong-Edgren, S., Mullen, A., Barlow, M., & Barwick, S. (2019). The changing landscape of simulation-based education. *American Journal of Nursing*, *119*(8), 42–48. https://doi.org/10.1097/01.naj.0000577436.23986.81

National League for Nursing Board of Governors. (2015). *A vision statement for teaching with simulation*. http://www.nln.org/docs/default-source/about/nln-vision-series-(position-statements)/vision-statement-a-vision-for-teaching-with-simulation.pdf?sfvrsn=2

Nehring, W. M. (2008). U.S. boards of nursing and the use of high-fidelity patient simulators in nursing education. *Journal of Professional Nursing*, *24*(2), 109–117. https://doi.org/10.1016/j.profnurs.2007.06.027

O'Donnell, J. M., Decker, S., Howard, V., Levett-Jones, T., & Miller, C. W. (2014). NLN/Jeffries simulation framework state of the science project: Simulation learning outcomes. *Clinical Simulation in Nursing*, *10*(7), 373–382. https://doi.org/10.1016/j.ecns.2014.06.004

Park, C. S., Murphy, T. F., & the Code of Ethics Working Group. (2018). *Healthcare simulationist code of ethics*. https://www.ssih.org/Code-of-Ethics

Parker, R. A., McNeill, J., & Howard, J. (2015). Comparing pediatric simulation and traditional clinical experience: Student perceptions, learning outcomes, and lessons for faculty. *Clinical Simulation in Nursing*, *11*(3), 188–193. https://doi.org/10.1016/j.ecns.2015.01.002

Pawar, S., Jacques, T., Deshpande, K., Pusapati, R. R., & Meguerdichian, M. J. (2018). Evaluation of cognitive load and emotional states during multidisciplinary critical care simulation sessions. *BMJ Simulation & Technology Enhanced Learning*, *4*(2), 87–91. https://doi.org/10.1136/bmjstel-2017-000225

Peddle, M., Livesay, K., & Marshall, S. (2020). Preliminary report of a simulation community of practice needs analysis. *Advances in Simulation*, *5*, 11. https://doi.org/10.1186/s41077-020-00130-4

Pilcher, J., Goodall, H., Jensen, C., Huwe, V., Cordelia, J., Reynolds, R., & Karlsen, K. A. (2012). Special focus on simulation: Educational strategies in the NICU: Simulation-based learning: It's not just for NRP. *Neonatal Network*, *31*(5), 281–287. https://doi.org/10.1891/0730-0832.31.5.281

Plass, J. L., Moreno, R., & Brunken, R. (2010). *Cognitive load theory*. Cambridge University Press.

Poore, J. A., Cullen, D. L., & Schaar, G. L. (2014). Simulation-based interprofessional education guided by Kolb's experiential learning theory. *Clinical Simulation in Nursing*, *10*(5), e241–e247. https://doi.org/10.1016/j.ecns.2014.01.004

Ravert, P., & McAfoos, J. (2014). NLN/Jeffries simulation framework: State of the science summary. *Clinical Simulation in Nursing*, *10*(7), 335–336. https://doi.org/10.1016/j.ecns.2013.06.002

Reedy, G. B. (2015). Using cognitive load theory to inform simulation design and practice. *Clinical Simulation in Nursing*, *11*(8), 355–360. https://doi.org/10.1016/j.ecns.2015.05.004

Richardson, H., Goldsamt, L. A., Simmons, J., Gilmartin, M., & Jeffries, P. R. (2014). Increasing faculty capacity: Findings from an evaluation of simulation clinical teaching. *Nursing Education Perspectives*, *35*(4), 308–314. https://doi.org/10.5480/13-1384

Romero-Hall, E., Watson, G. S., Adcock, A., Bliss, J., & Adams Tufts, K. (2016). Simulated environments with animated agents: Effects on visual attention, emotion, performance, and perception. *Journal of Computer Assisted Learning*, *32*(4), 360–373. https://doi.org/10.1111/jcal.12138

Schlairet, M. C., Schlairet, T. J., Sauls, D. H., & Bellflowers, L. (2015). Cognitive load, emotion, and performance in high-fidelity simulation among beginning nursing students: A pilot study. *Journal of Nursing Education*, *54*(3), s5–s11. https://doi.org/10.3928/01484834-20150218-10

Screws, S., & Cason, M. (2019). Mass casualty incident simulation for a small space with limited resources. *Nursing Education Perspectives*, *41*(9), E52–E53. https://doi.org/10.1097/01.NEP.0000000000000600

Sharma, P., & Hannafin, M. J. (2007). Scaffolding in technology-enhanced learning environments. *Interactive Learning Environments*, *15*(1), 27–46. https://doi.org/10.1080/10494820600996972

Shin, S., Park, J. H., & Kim, J. H. (2015). Effectiveness of patient simulation in nursing education: Meta-analysis. *Nurse Education Today*, *35*, 176–182. https://doi.org/10.1016/j.nedt.2014.09.009

Sittner, B. S. (2016). Extra! Extra! Read all about it! INACSL standards of best practice: Simulation^{SM} have been revised! *Clinical Simulation in Nursing*, *12*, S1–S2. https://doi.org/10.1016/j.ecns.2016.10.002

Smiley, R. A. (2019). Survey of simulation use in prelicensure nursing programs: Changes and advancements, 2010 – 2017. *Journal of Nursing Regulation*, *9*(4), 48–61. https://doi.org/10.1016/S2155-8256(19)30016-X

Society for Simulation in Healthcare. (2016). *Accreditation standards*. https://www.ssih.org/Credentialing/Accreditation/Full-Accreditation

Spector, N., Hooper, J., Silvestre, J., & Qian, H. (2018). Board of nursing programs: Changes and advancements, 2010 – 2017. *Journal of Nursing Regulation*, *8*(4), 22–23. http://doi.org/10.1016/S2155-8256(19)30016-X

Spector, N., Silvestre, J., Alexander, M., Martin, B., Hooper, J. I., Squires, A., & Ojemeni, M. (2020). NCSBN regulatory guidelines and evidence-based quality indicators for nursing education programs. *Journal of Nursing Regulation*, *11*(2), S1–S64. https://www.journalofnursingregulation.com/article/S2155-8256(20)30075-2/pdf

Starkweather, A., & Kardong-Edgren, S. (2008). Diffusion of innovation: Embedding simulation into nursing curricula. *International Journal of Nursing Education Scholarship*, *5*(1). 1–12. https://doi.org/10.2202/1548-923X.1567

Sullivan, N., Swoboda, S. M. Breymier., T, Lucas., L, Sarasnick., J, Rutherford-Hemming., T, Budhathoki., C, & Kardong-Edgren, S. (2019). Emerging evidence toward a 2: 1 clinical to simulation ratio: A study comparing the traditional clinical and simulation settings. *Clinical Simulation in Nursing*, *30*, 34–41. https://doi.org/10.1016/j.ecns/2019.03.003

Thomas, P. A., Kern, D. E., Hughes, M. T., & Chen, B. Y. (Eds.). (2016). *Curriculum development for medical education: A six-step approach* (3rd ed.). John Hopkins University Press.

van Merriënboer, J. J. G., & Sweller, J. (2010). Cognitive load theory in health professional education: Design principles and strategies. *Medical Education*, *44*, 85–93. https://doi.org/10.1111/j.1365-2923.2009.03498.x

Victor Chmil, J., Turk, M., Adamson, K., & Larew, C. (2015). Effects of an experiential learning simulation design on clinical nursing judgment development. *Nurse Educator*, *40*(5), 228–232. https://doi.org/10.1097/NNE.0000000000000159

Ward, P., Williams, A. M., & Hancock, P. A. (2006). Simulation for performance and training. In K. A. Ericsson, N. Charness, P. J. Feltovich, & R. R. Hoffman (Eds.), *The Cambridge handbook of expertise and expert performance*. Cambridge University Press.

Waxman, K. T., Bowler, F., Forneris, S. G., Kardong-Edgren, S., & Rizzolo, M. A. (2019). Simulation as a nursing education disrupter. *Nursing Administration Quarterly*, *43*(4), 300–305. https://doi.org/10.1097/NAQ.0000000000000369

Weaver, A. (2015). The effect of a model demonstration during debriefing on students' clinical judgment, self-confidence, and satisfaction during a simulated learning experience. *Clinical Simulation in Nursing*, *11*(1), 20–26. http://doi.org/10.1016/j.ecns.2014.10.009

Woda, A., Dreifuerst, K. T., & Garnier-Villareal, M. (2019). The impact of supplemental simulation on newly licensed registered nurses. *Clinical Simulation in Nursing*, *28*, 1–5. https://doi.org/10.1016/j.ecns.2018.12.002

World Health Organization. (2018). *Simulation in nursing and midwifery education*. https://www.euro.who.int/__data/assets/pdf_file/0011/383807/snme-report-eng.pdf?ua=1

Yeh, V. J.-H., Sherwood, G., Durham, C. F., Kardong-Edgren, S., Schwartz, T. A., & Beeber, L. S. (2019). Online simulation-based mastery learning with deliberate practice: Developing interprofessional communication skill. *Clinical Simulation in Nursing*, *32*, 27–38. https://doi.org/10.1016/j.ecns.2019.04.005

Zamora, Z., Shedd, J., & Kittipha, P. (2019). Budget friendly simulation for clinical nursing education: Putting it all together. *Nursing Education Perspectives*, *40*(2), 123–124. https://doi.org/10.1097/01.NEP.0000000000000357

Zulkosky, K. D., White, K. A., & Price, A. L. (2016). Effect of simulation role on clinical decision-making accuracy. *Clinical Simulation in Nursing*, *12*(3), 98–106. https://doi.org/10.1016/j.ecns.2016.01.007

Zyniewicz, T. (2019). Simulation as replacement for traditional clinical in pre-licensure nursing education: Outcomes of different ratios of replacement time for traditional clinical with simulation. *Dissertation*. https://aquila.usm.edu/dissertations/1662

CHAPTER 2

State of Simulation Research in Advanced Practice Nursing Education

Carla Nye

ABSTRACT

Simulation is used in advanced practice nursing education for both formative learning experiences and summative competency testing. However, there has been a lack of cohesive data to support the use of simulation as a replacement for direct patient care hours. This chapter presents an overview of research designs and the leveled Kirkpatrick framework used in simulation research. Research articles evaluating the effect of simulation on advanced practice learners are presented by research design and Kirkpatrick level. There is evidence that simulation has a positive impact on Kirkpatrick Level 1 (Reactions) and Kirkpatrick Level 2 (Changes in Knowledge, Skills, and Attitudes). However, there is a tremendous need for evidence that simulation can impact Kirkpatrick Level 3 (Behavior) and Level 4 (Results and Outcomes).

http://dx.doi.org/10.1891/0739-6686.39.33

INTRODUCTION

Simulation is a pedagogy widely used in advanced practice nursing (APN) education (Hawkins-Walsh et al., 2011; National Organization of Nurse Practitioner Faculties [NONPF], 2013; Nye et al., 2019), and anecdotal support for APN simulation abounds in the academic simulation community (Nye et al., 2020). However, wide use and support does not equate to generations of best evidence and implementation of best practices in education. The overarching question to be addressed is: Do the data support simulation as an effective pedagogy in the education of APN students? Additional related questions include:

- What do the data mean in relation to the current methods of teaching and evaluating APN students?
- What is the best way to teach content to APN students?
- Does learning in simulation transfer to clinical practice?
- Can simulation be substituted for direct patient care?

Obtaining clear and unequivocal answers to these questions is imperative. APN education is facing a series of challenges and growth opportunities where solutions may be met through the delivery of quality simulations (American Association of Colleges of Nursing [AACN], 2015; Coppa et al., 2018; National League for Nursing, 2018; Nye et al., 2020; Rutherford-Hemming, et al., 2016; Schneidereith & Daniels, 2019; Warren et al., 2016).

Using simulation to provide a safe environment for formative practice of the knowledge, skills, and attitudes requisite for a safe and competent APN is a frequent practice. It is also common to use objective structured clinical examinations (OSCEs) at the end of a course, such as health assessment to determine if the student can demonstrate identified competencies in a simulated environment (Clark, 2015; Day et al., 2018; Nye et al., 2019; Prettyman et al., 2018). The movement toward competency-based curriculum frameworks has created another opportunity for evaluation (Giddens et al., 2014; Hodges et al., 2019). The AACN published a vision statement on the future of nursing education, which includes a transition toward competency-based education and assessment (AACN, 2019). Competency assessment is the future of nursing education and the evidence exists to support the use of simulation in assessing APN competency (Kesten et al., 2015; Starkweather et al., 2017).

Two systematic reviews were published on the use of simulation in APN education in 2016. Warren et al. (2016) reviewed research on the use of high-fidelity simulation in APN education from 2007 to 2014. This review found an overall increase in student knowledge, confidence, and satisfaction when learning incorporated high-fidelity simulation. Rutherford-Hemming et al. (2016)

reviewed APN-related simulation research published between 2010 and 2015. This review included both manikin and standardized patient (SP) simulations and found that simulation generally had a positive impact on satisfaction, confidence, and knowledge. However, there were minimal studies that evaluated changes in student behavior or performance. While these studies support the positive impact that simulation has on students, they do not identify whether key lessons learned in simulation are: (a) incorporated into the student's mental framework and (b) transferred to patient care.

There have been recent calls to revisit the discussion on use of simulation as a replacement for clinical hours in APN education (Anderson et al., 2019; Jeffries et al., 2019). The NONPF and the National Task Force (NTF) on Quality Nurse Practitioner Education support the use of simulation as an educational pedagogy for any hours above the minimum requirement of 500 direct patient care hours (NONPF, 2020; NTF, 2016). However, the lack of strong evidence on the efficacy of simulation as a replacement for clinical hours has limited the support needed to incorporate simulation hours within the minimum 500-hour direct patient care requirement (Jeffries et al., 2019; NONPF, 2013, 2020).

This chapter reviews research published on simulation in APN education from 2015 to 2020 and those studies prior to 2015 that measured the impact of simulation on the transfer of knowledge and skills to patient care. There is also a short review of simulation pedagogy, leveled educational outcomes using the Kirkpatrick framework (Kirkpatrick & Kirkpatrick, 2009), and an overview of educational research designs related to Kirkpatrick's framework.

SIMULATION PEDAGOGY

For many years, the goal of nursing education has been to craft an APN curriculum that facilitates the incorporation of vast and often disparate information into a cohesive and functioning whole (Benner et al., 2010). Lectures provided on overheads or PowerPoints provided lists of items to remember, including diseases, risk factors, signs and symptoms, treatments, and outcomes. Faculty would sometimes include an anecdote to help students combine components of the various lists to place a patient's health situation in context. Lab experiences included health assessments on each other, and each skill was conducted in isolation with limited connection to the patient and their lived experience. This type of education provided memorizable facts, but offered minimal assistance that helped students bridge the theory–practice gap so often experienced by nursing and nurse practitioner (NP) students (Onda, 2012).

Benner et al. (2010) advised that creating contextually based learning experiences is a powerful and effective tool that can be used to create associations between concepts and also develop critical thinking skills. The situated cognition learning theory, or learning in a realistic context, provides strong support for simulation to bridge the theory–practice gap in nursing education (Brown et al., 1989; Onda, 2012). Simulation is a pedagogy that provides this realistic framing of a patient in a situated context so that students are forced to coalesce multiple aspects of knowledge, skills, and attitudes (KSAs) and apply them in a realistic situation (INACSL Standards Committee, 2016). Becker and Reisman (2007) found that simulation produced a greater gain in critical thinking than the same content taught in a classroom setting. To a simulationist, the anecdotal evidence supporting simulation is collected daily from facilitating and observing deeper levels of learning (Nye et al., 2020). However, the nursing profession requires more than anecdotal data. The ethos of using best practices is incorporated into the professional documents guiding simulation, and it is imperative to incorporate evidence into decision-making regarding the use of simulation in APN education.

KIRKPATRICK LEVELS

There is a strong need in APN education to explore simulation's impact on building the critical KSAs required for a practice-ready APN graduate. Simulation is a tool and a resource, but it can also be costly in terms of time, equipment, and expense (Nye et al., 2020; Peddle et al., 2020). It is important when building a simulation program to be able to determine the value and return on investment for stakeholders. Anecdotal evidence of avid simulationists cannot serve as the only source to advocate for the use of simulation in APN programs. Determining key characteristics of published work can help identify evidence that is substantial enough to change policies, including outcome measures and research design.

The four levels of outcomes within the Kirkpatrick model are widely used in educational research (Kirkpatrick & Kirkpatrick, 2009). Table 2.1 provides a description of each level and examples of how these levels can be evaluated in APN education.

EDUCATIONAL RESEARCH DESIGNS

A second characteristic for consideration when evaluating evidence is the study design, including the research methodology, measurement tools, and results. The quality of the evaluation tools is a major limiting factor in many studies (Burt & Corbridge, 2018; Jarding et al., 2018). Measurement tools without reliability and validity testing should be interpreted with caution, and the lack of measurement tools with strong psychometric support is frequently mentioned as an issue when gathering APN simulation data (Anderson et al., 2019; Jeffries et al., 2019).

TABLE 2.1
Kirkpatrick Outcome Levels With Examples

Level	Focus	Desired Outcomes	Simulation Examples
Level 1	Reaction	Was the training satisfying, relevant, engaging?	Postsimulation surveys are conducted to determine if learners were satisfied with and engaged by the simulation.
Level 2a	Attitudes/ perceptions	Did the perceptions or attitudes of the participants change due to the simulation?	Students complete a pre- and posttest on their perceived level of confidence and comfort with managing a patient with a simulation-specific disease process.
Level 2b	Knowledge/ skills	Did the learners acquire knowledge or skills due to the simulation?	Students complete a pre- and posttest knowledge quiz regarding simulation-specific disease knowledge or management plans.
Level 3	Behavior	Do the learners transfer the learning to workplace, clinical, or future simulations?	Baseline simulation assessments are compared to preceptor evaluations or future simulation assessments. Baseline student clinical performance is compared to postsimulation clinical performance.
Level 4a	Results	Is there a change in system outcomes due to the training?	This is difficult to do in relation to a program-based simulation. This data is gathered in workplace simulations.
Level 4b	Patient outcomes	Is there a change in patient outcomes related to the training?	This is difficult to do in relation to a program based simulation. This data is gathered in workplace simulations.

Source. Kirkpatrick and Kirkpatrick (2009); Yardley and Dornan (2012).

This section provides a broad overview of common educational research designs used in simulation: cross-sectional, pre- and posttest, quasiexperimental, qualitative, and experimental. The relationship between design and Kirkpatrick levels will also be discussed, but it is not intended for this section to be a primary reference for research design, limitations, or potential biases. There are many sources for more detailed information that are beyond the scope of this chapter.

Cross-Sectional Design

In a cross-sectional design, researchers gather data at a single point in time (Mangold & Adler, 2019; Spector, 2019). A survey that is completed after an educational intervention is a cross-sectional study and, in educational evaluation, this type of design is often used to gather reactions to an educational experience. Frequently measured variables in simulation are satisfaction, knowledge, and self-assessed confidence or sense of competence. Because the survey occurs after the educational experience, there are no baseline measurements of the study variables, and it is therefore difficult to attribute outcomes to the specific educational intervention. For example, a simulation to enhance APN learners' knowledge on the care of a patient with hypertension was implemented and a knowledge test was given immediately after the simulation. This would be a measure of the learner's knowledge at this moment in time, but it would be impossible to determine if the postsimulation knowledge score was related to the simulation or to the amount of knowledge or experience that the learner had upon entering the simulation. A common postsimulation satisfaction survey, which measures a learner's reaction to the simulation, is Kirkpatrick Level 1. While it is important for educators to gather this information to assess an educational strategy, this data cannot discern whether the change in understanding or performance is a result of participation in the simulation (Mangold & Adler, 2019).

Pre- and Posttest Research Design

This design is commonly used when introducing a new simulation or a new method of teaching content to a cohort of learners (Marsden & Torgerson, 2012). All learners have the same experience whereby a pretest is given, the educational intervention is conducted, then a posttest is given. Often the pretest and posttests are given using the same tool. Pre-and posttest data are compared, and changes in KSAs can be attributed to the educational intervention. This type of evaluation is helpful in determining the immediate impact of an educational strategy and can inform educators on the extent to which their strategy impacted student learning (Eccles et al., 2003). However, long-term data on the effect of the simulation, the impact of the simulation, or knowledge or skill transfer to other settings are not possible to determine with this research design (Marsden & Torgerson, 2012).

Quasiexperimental Design

Quasiexperimental designs are similar to experimental designs but lack randomized assignments to either the control or experimental groups (Mangold & Adler, 2019). This design is common in educational research as it improves the research rigor through addition of one or more elements to a pretest/posttest research design (Mangold & Adler, 2019). Adding a control group is one method to create a quasiexperimental design, but the control group is often one of convenience and the participants are not randomized (Eccles et al., 2003). For example, a new simulation is being planned for the following semester and faculty gather data on a current group of students. The following semester the new simulation is added to the curriculum. Data from the initial group who did not have the simulation (the control group) is compared to the data from the group who did have the simulation (the experimental group). While there is a control group, the two groups were not randomly selected.

Increasing the number of pre- and posttest measurements is a second method of creating a quasiexperimental design. In a simple pre- and posttest design, a knowledge survey is given before and after a simulation. In a quasiexperimental design, there may be additional variables that are measured before and after the simulation such as roles played, attitudinal surveys, or preceptor feedback surveys.

Qualitative Design

The purpose of a qualitative design is to explore the meaning of, or gain a better understanding of, the lived experience of individuals or groups of individuals (Astalin, 2013; Bearman, 2019). The goal is understanding how the participants perceive their situation and how this perception influences their behavior or decision-making. Qualitative studies can be conducted as personal interviews, focus groups, or through written data from participants. The data is read for themes and patterns until a new understanding emerges.

Experimental Design

Experimental designs are used to examine the differences between two groups while controlling for additional variables. There are several key elements to an experimental design. There must be a control group that does not receive the intervention so there can be a direct comparison in outcomes between the group that received the intervention and the group that did not receive the intervention. Second, the participants in the study must be randomly assigned to either the control or intervention group, and there must also be enough participants to ensure quality statistical analyses. Quality experimental outcomes are the hallmark required for evidence-based practice changes, however, experimental designs are complicated to conduct in the midst of active educational delivery (Eccles et al., 2003; Issenberg et al., 2005).

REVIEW OF NURSE PRACTITIONER SIMULATION RESEARCH (2015–2020)

This literature review on the use of simulations in APN education from 2015 to 2020 will also provide a more detailed examination of APN simulation studies from 2009 to 2014 that investigated Kirkpatrick Level 3 (Changes in Behavior). A systematic search for English-language literature identified 135 articles published on the use of simulation in APN education. PubMed/MEDLINE and the Cumulative Index to Nursing and Allied Health Literature (CINAHL) were searched-for articles published between January 2015 and July 30, 2020. The search used a combination of keywords and controlled vocabulary for the concepts "nurse practitioner," "advanced practice nurse," "graduate nurse," "education," and "simulation."

Kirkpatrick Level 1: APN Reaction to Simulation

Most APN simulation studies published between 2015 and 2020 used a cross-sectional design focused on satisfaction. The published articles often provide detailed information about the simulation and methodology used to implement the simulations but did not provide specific evidence relating simulation and acquisition of content-specific KSAs.

Published work during 2015 to 2020 reported high student satisfaction and highly beneficial simulations. These reports included studies of on-call simulations (Griffith et al., 2019; Kelly et al., 2019; Woroch et al., 2018); acute care simulations (Keiser & Turkelson, 2019); health assessment simulations (Ndiwane et al., 2017); virtual clinical simulations (Bryant et al., 2015); and interprofessional-related simulations (IPEs; Iverson et al., 2018; Tankimovich et al., 2020).

Many of the studies used a researcher-developed tool and several studies used tools that have psychometric support. Included were *The National League for Nursing Student Satisfaction and Confidence in Learning Scale* (Bryant et al., 2015; Keiser & Turkelson, 2019); the *Student Perceptions of Interprofessional Clinical Education-Revised (SPICE-R)* (Iverson et al., 2018); and the *Student Satisfaction Survey* (Ndiwane).

Kirkpatrick Level 2: APN Learning: KSA

Studies with Kirkpatrick Level 2 outcome measures were conducted using either a cross-sectional or a pre- and posttest design. There was an almost universal use of researcher-developed measurement tools (Drake et al., 2020; Gatewood, 2019; Phillips et al., 2020; Woroch et al., 2020).

Cross-Sectional Design: Perceived Competence/Confidence

Woroch et al. (2020) used a cross-sectional design to measure perceived competence. This group reported that learners felt more confident and prepared to begin clinical after completing four primary care simulations of patients with high-frequency primary care diagnoses.

Cross-Sectional Design: Perceived Skills

Gatewood (2019) created a didactic and simulation experience to prepare preclinical NP students to communicate their clinical learning objectives with interprofessional preceptors. Surveys were sent to both preceptors and students after the students started clinical. Both students and preceptors reported that the students were prepared to discuss their learning objectives and were prepared for clinical. No specific data on the outcome measures were provided.

Pre- and Posttest Design: Knowledge Changes

The following studies compared learner knowledge levels before and after a simulation. These studies reported significant gains in knowledge regarding telehealth simulations (Phillips et al., 2020); forensic knowledge (Drake et al., 2020); and cultural humility (Ndiwane et al., 2017). Ndiwane et al. used the *Cultural Assessment Survey* which has published psychometrics.

Pre- and Posttest Design: Perceived Competence/Confidence

Pre- and posttest design studies that measured learner self-reported confidence included simulation on forensic management of a trauma patient (Drake et al., 2020), IPE teamwork simulation (Tankimovich et al., 2020), IPE primary care on-call simulation (Conelius et al., 2019), IPE breast and cervical cancer screening (Weston et al., 2018), and on-call acute care simulation (Griffith et al., 2019). All studies used researcher-developed tools and reported an increase in self-confidence scores from pre- to posttest. Drake et al. (2020), Conelius et al. (2019), and Weston et al. (2018) provided statistical analysis and reported significant improvement in confidence ratings from pre- to posttest.

Pre- and Posttest Design: Perceived Skills

Only one study explored students' changed perceptions of perceived professional skills needed to conduct an on-call patient encounter. Prior to the simulation, Griffith et al. (2019) reported that students rated the top three skills needed to provide on-call primary care patient management as clear communication (93%), critical thinking (86%), and self-confidence (44%). Following the simulation, the top three included critical thinking (97%), self-confidence (55%), and access to resources (34%).

Qualitative Design

Schwindt and McNelis (2015) conducted a qualitative analysis of a reflective assignment related to an initial intake interview simulation for psych-mental health NP learners. Themes that emerged included the importance of feedback from both the SPs and the faculty on learning, the deep insight that was gained from completing the reflection paper, and the increased confidence in the ability to function in the professional role. Sisler et al. (2019) compared the impact of health-related screening tools presimulation training to no health-related screening tools pretraining. The cohort with training identified more patient health issues than the cohort without training. Themes that emerged from data analysis included considering the root of the problem, balancing patient and clinician priorities, developing interpersonal skills, being mindful, and "If we don't ask, they often will not share" (Sisler et al., 2019, p. 527).

Experimental Design

In a randomized controlled trial of 472 healthcare trainees, including 27 NP students, participants were randomized into a control group who received the usual education on palliative care communication skills or the experimental group engaged in Codetalk. Codetalk is a simulation-based workshop to educate healthcare trainees on palliative care communication skills. The intervention group had a significant increase in self-assessed palliative care communication compared to the control group ($p < .001$). The significant improvement was in three of the four specific communication indicators: expressing empathy, discussing spiritual issues, and eliciting goals of care (Brown et al., 2016).

Kirkpatrick Level 3: APN Behavioral Change (2009–2015)

Level 3 behavioral changes include demonstration of critical thinking, organization, and communication (Kirkpatrick & Kirkpatrick, 2009). Studies that measure quantifiable changes in learner behavior provide evidence that a simulation has an impact with strong educational relevance. To determine if a simulation has engendered a change in behavior, a quasiexperimental or experimental design is preferred. In quasiexperimental designs there should be a baseline measurement of learner behavior before the intervention, and then a measurement of behavior after the intervention. This measurement can be the lone variable or can be combined with additional measurements on a learner's reaction and changes in content-specific KSAs. In an experimental design, learners are recruited and randomized to a control or intervention group, with baseline and postintervention measurements for comparison. This study design provides the most reliable data to support changes in evidence-based education.

In a pre- and posttest design, Bays et al. (2014), used video-recorded communication simulations to measure communication performance before and after a series of palliative care communication training sessions. There was significant improvement in 8 of the 11 outcome measures from the pretraining simulation to the posttraining simulation ($p < .05$).

Paige et al. (2014) measured changes in team and individual performance of nursing students, nurse anesthesia students, and medical students through two operating room simulations. There was an overall improvement in mean team performance score and two subscales showed significant improvement: shared mental model ($p < .001$) and adaptive communication and response ($p < .001$). The team-based behavior subscale of the individual performance measure also showed a significant improvement ($p < .001$).

In a study of teaching methodology on the performance of ultrasound-guided regional anesthesia, Gasko et al. (2012) found that the performance of nurse anesthesia students was significantly better 2 months posttraining when students were taught with a combination of virtual CD-ROM and simulation training compared to simulation only or virtual CD-ROM training only ($p < .05$).

Fleming et al. (2009) compared virtual reality simulation and SP simulation on alcohol screening and brief intervention skills. Interprofessional participants were randomized into either the virtual reality simulation intervention group or the SP-only education control group. All participants completed three SP scenarios to gather baseline data. The intervention group trained with the computer-based virtual reality intervention. Six months postbaseline, students repeated the simulations with the SPs. The intervention group demonstrated significantly improved screening ($p < .001$) and brief intervention ($p < .04$) performance than the control group at 6 months.

Bryant et al. (2015) used a convenience sample of family nurse practitioner (FNP) online learners to investigate the use of virtual clinical simulations in a health assessment course. Learners were randomly assigned to an intervention group of virtual clinical simulations or the control group with standard course activities. Participation in the intervention group was voluntary. There were no significant differences between groups on health assessment skills in an on-campus simulation at the end of the course.

Nippita et al. (2018) reported the impact of two simulators used to train intrauterine contraception (IUC) insertion skills in a randomized controlled trial of NP and interns. Learners were randomized to either the high-fidelity simulator group or the low-fidelity coaster pelvic model group. Both groups received identical computer-based didactic instruction followed by practice on the assigned model. Learners completed a knowledge, perceived comfort, and competence survey before didactic instruction, after didactic instruction, and 3 months postinstruction. There was no significant difference in knowledge, self-perceived comfort, and competence at baseline, or skill performance immediately postinstruction or 3 months postinstruction. There was a significant improvement in comfort and confidence from baseline to 3 months posttraining for those students who had the opportunity to insert IUCs in the clinical environment.

Kirkpatrick Level 4: Professional Change

Rutherford-Hemming's (2012) quasiexperimental investigation into the impact of simulation on clinical performance suggests that behavior in the simulated environment is positively correlated to behavior in the clinical environment, including significant changes in the domains of physical examination ($p < .01$), history of present illness ($p < .01$), and facilitating skills ($p < .05$). In a randomized controlled trial, Curtis et al. (2013) assessed the impact of a simulation-based palliative care communication training with internal medicine residents and NP students on family or patient perceptions of quality of communication. Learners were randomized to the simulation-based intervention or usual training. There were no significant differences in patient or family scoring of quality of communication or quality of end-of-life communication from before to after the intervention. However, patients who communicated with the intervention group showed significantly higher depression scores.

DISCUSSION OF FINDINGS

The literature from 2015 to 2020 finds similar outcomes to the work of Rutherford-Hemming et al. (2016) and Warren et al. (2016). There is growing data to support simulation to improve student's self-reported confidence and competence, increase knowledge, and provide a methodology of education that is satisfying and beneficial to students. These findings support the power of contextually based learning to enhance the learner's belief in their ability to manage patient care scenarios.

Rutherford-Hemming (2012) found strong positive correlations between behavior in the simulation environment and behavior in the clinical area. This supports the concept that simulation can not only be a measure of learning transfer, but also used to measure competency. The report by Kesten et al. (2015) also used simulation to measure competency and the results further support the movement toward competency-based education.

There are studies that show the potential of simulation to change behavior. Fleming et al. (2009) found that virtual reality simulation resulted in significantly improved alcohol screening and brief intervention skills 6 months postintervention. Gasko et al. (2012) found students who were trained with simulation and traditional education methods had significantly higher performance scores than students who had education or simulation only. Paige et al. (2014) reported significant improvement in operating room team performance after two simulations. A recent systematic review and meta-analysis that combined data from undergraduate and postgraduate nursing students found that high-fidelity patient simulations demonstrated significantly larger effect sizes in both knowledge and performance when compared to other teaching methods (La Cerra et al., 2019). These reports are promising; however, the APN literature is missing an abundance of clear and unambiguous findings to demonstrate simulation's ability to change behavior. This does not mean that the effect does not exist, but more studies are needed to demonstrate the impact of simulation on behavior in the APN population.

A series of well-planned quasiexperimental or experimental studies that investigate the effect of APN simulations on Kirkpatrick Level 3 and Level 4 outcomes are needed. An important starting point is psychometric testing to develop reliable clinical and simulation evaluation tools. Studies in APN education should include a comparison between groups with simulation and those with usual education. There should be baseline and postintervention behavioral measurements. Ideally, studies will be conducted that measure the impact of simulation on performance postgraduation. Moving the outcomes to Kirkpatrick Level 3 will fill the missing gaps in the literature.

CONCLUSION

This chapter began with a discussion of the upcoming changes in APN education. There will be a continued need for growth of APN programs. There will be continued issues with finding appropriate clinical placements. There will be a move toward competency-based education. There will be more pressure for "practice-ready" graduates. High-quality simulation, done strategically, may be the pedagogical answer to all.

REFERENCES

American Association of Colleges of Nursing. (2015). *Re-envisioning the clinical education of advanced practice registered nurses [white paper]*. https://www.aacnnursing.org/Portals/42/News/White-Papers/APRN-Clinical-Education.pdf

American Association of Colleges of Nursing. (2019, January). *AACN's vision for academic nursing*. https://www.aacnnursing.org/Portals/42/News/White-Papers/Vision-Academic-Nursing.pdf

Anderson, M., Campbell, S., Nye, C., Diaz, D., & Boyd, T. (2019). Simulation in Advanced practice education: Let's dialogue! *Clinical Simulation in Nursing*, *26*, 81–85. https://doi.org/10.1016/j.ecns.2018.10.011

Astalin, P. K. (2013). Qualitative research designs: A conceptual framework. *International Journal of Social Science and Interdisciplinary Research*, 2(1), 118–124.

Bays, A. M., Engelberg, R. A., Back, A. L., Ford, D. W., Downey, L., Shannon, S. E., Curtis, J. R. (2014). Interprofessional communication skills training for serious illness: Evaluation of a small-group, simulated patient intervention. Journal of Palliative Medicine, 17(2), 159-166.

Bearman, M. (2019). Key concepts in qualitative research design. In D. Nestel, J. Hui, K. Kunkler, M. W. Scerbo, & A. W. Calhoun (Eds.), *Healthcare simulation research* (pp. 169–174). Springer Publishing. https://doi.org/10.1007/978-3-030-26837-4_23

Becker, D. E., & Reisman, F. K. (2007). *The effect of patient simulation on the critical thinking of advanced practice nursing students*. Doctoral dissertation, Drexel University. Islandora Repository http://hdl.handle.net/1860/1758

Benner, P., Sutphen, M., Leonard, V., & Day, L. (2010). *Educating nurses: A call for radical transformation. The Carnegie Foundation.*

Brown, C. E., Back, A. L., Ford, D. W., Kross, E. K., Downey, L., Shannon, S. E., Curtis, J. R., & Engelberg, R. A. (2016). Self-assessment scores improve after simulation-based palliative care communication skill workshops. *American Journal of Hospice & Palliative Medicine*, *35*(1), 45–51. https://doi.org/10.1177/1049909116681972

Brown, J. S., Collins, A., & Duguid, P. (1989). Situated cognition and the culture of learning. *Educational Researcher*, *18*(1), 32–42. https://doi.org/10.2307/1176008

Bryant, R., Miller, C. L., & Henderson, D. (2015). Virtual clinical simulations in an online advanced health appraisal course. *Clinical Simulation in Nursing*, *11*(10), 437–444. https://doi.org/10.1016/j.ecns.2015.08.002

Burt, L., & Corbridge, S. (2018). Teaching diagnostic reasoning: A review of evidence-based interventions. *International Journal of Nursing Education and Scholarship*, *15*(1). 1–14 https://doi.org/10.1515/ijnes-2018-0003

Clark, C. A. (2015). Evaluating nurse practitioner students through objective structured clinical examination. *Nursing Education Perspectives*, *36*(1), 53–54. https://doi.org/10.5480/13-1078.1

Conelius, J. P., Grossman, S. P., & Becht, L. G. (2019). Interprofessional "on-call" e-learning for family nurse practitioner students: Preparing for primary care across the life span. *Journal of the American Association of Nurse Practitioners*, *31*(2), 104–109. https://doi.org/10.1097/JXX.0000000000000120

Coppa, D., Schneidereith, T., & Farina, C. L. (2018). Simulated home-based health care scenarios for nurse practitioner students. *Clinical Simulation in Nursing*, *26*, 38–43. https://doi.org/10.1016/j.ecns.2018.10.002

Curtis, J. R., Back, A. L., Ford, D. W., Downey, L., Shannon, S. E., Doorenbos, A. Z., Kross, E. K., Reinke, L. F., Feemster, L. C., Edlund, B., Arnold, R. W., O'Connor, K., & Engelberg, R. A. (2013). Effect of communication skills training for residents and nurse practitioners on quality of communication with patients with serious illness: A randomized trial. *JAMA*, *310*(21), 2271–2281. https://doi.org/10.1001/jama.2013.282081

Day, C., Barker, C., Bell, E., Sefcik, E., & Flournoy, D. (2018). Flipping the objective structured clinical examination: A teaching innovation in graduate nursing education. *Nurse Educator*, *43*(2), 83–86. https://doi.org/10.1097/NNE.0000000000000421

Delaney, K. R., Swartwout, K., Livesay, S. L., & Bavis, M. P. (2019). Establishing nurse practitioner clinical practicums: Addressing fiscal realities. *Journal of the American Association of Nurse Practitioners*, *31*(11), 657–662. https://doi.org/10.1097/JXX.0000000000000333

Doherty, C. L., Fogg, L., Bigley, M. B., Todd, B., & O'Sullivan, A. L. (2020). Nurse practitioner student clinical placement processes: A national survey of nurse practitioner programs. *Nursing Outlook*, *68*(1), 55–61. https://doi.org/10.1016/j.outlook.2019.07.005

Drake, S. A., Godwin, K. M., Wolf, D. A., & Gallagher, M. (2020). Evaluation of fundamental forensic knowledge and perceived ability in emergency nurse practitioner education via forensic simulation. *Journal of Forensic Nursing*, *16*(1), 22–28. https://doi.org/10.1097/JFN.0000000000000277

Eccles, M., Grimshaw, J., Campbell, M., & Ramsay, C. (2003). Research designs for studies evaluating the effectiveness of change and improvement strategies. *Quality & Safety in Health Care*, *12*(1), 47–52. https://doi.org/10.1136/qhc.12.1.47

Fleming, M., Olsen, D., Stathes, H., Boteler, L., Grossberg, P., Pfeifer, J., Schiro, S., Banning, J., & Skochelak, S. (2009). Virtual reality skills training for health care professionals in alcohol screening and brief intervention. *Journal of the American Board of Family Medicine*, 22(4), 387–398. https://doi.org/10.3122/jabfm.2009.04.080208

Gasko, J., Johnson, A., Sherner, J., Craig, J., Gegel, B., Burgert, J., Sama, S., & Franzen, T. (2012). Effects of using simulation versus CD-ROM in the performance of ultrasound-guided regional anesthesia. *AANA Journal*, *80*(Suppl. 4), S56–S59.

Gatewood, E. (2019). Use of simulation to increase self-directed learning for nurse practitioner students. *The Journal of Nursing Education*, *58*(2), 102–106. https://doi.org/10.3928/01484834-20190122-07

Giddens, J. F., Lauzon-Clabo, L., Morton, P. G., Jeffries, P., Mcquade-Jones, B., & Ryan, S. (2014). Re-envisioning clinical education for nurse practitioner programs: Themes from a national leaders' dialogue. *Journal of Professional Nursing*, *30*, 273–278. https://doi.org/10.1016/j.profnurs.2014.03.002

Griffith, P. B., Kelly, M. M., & Becker, D. (2019, December). On-call simulation for adult gerontology acute care nurse practitioner students: A comparative descriptive study. *Journal of the American Association of Nurse Practitioners*. 1–12 Advance online publication. https://doi.org/10.1097/JXX.0000000000000355

Hawkins-Walsh, E., Berg, M., Docherty, S., Lindeke, L. Gaylord., N, & Osborne, K. (2011). A national survey of the primary and acute care pediatric nurse practitioner educational preparation. *Journal of Pediatric Healthcare, 25*(1), 5–16. https://doi.org/10.1016/j.pedhc.2010.06.005

Hodges, A. L., Konicki, A. J., Talley, M. H., Bordelon, C. J., Holland, A. C., & Galin, F. S. (2019). Competency-based education in transitioning nurse practitioner students from education into practice. *Journal of the American Association of Nurse Practitioners, 31*(11), 675–682. https://doi.org/10.1097/JXX.0000000000000327

INACSL Standards Committee. (2016, December). INACSL standards of best practice: Simulation[SM] Simulation glossary. *Clinical Simulation in Nursing, 12*, S39–S47. http://doi.org/10.1016/j.ecns.2016.09.012

Issenberg, S. B., Mcgaghie, W. C., Petrusa, E. R., Gordon, D. L., & Scalese, R. J. (2005). Features and uses of high-fidelity medical simulations that lead to effective learning: A BEME systematic review. *Medical Teacher, 27*(1), 10–28. https://doi.org/10.1080/01421590500046924

Iverson, L., Bredenkamp, N., Carrico, C., Connelly, S., Hawkins, K., Monaghan, M. S., & Malesker, M. (2018). Development and assessment of an interprofessional education simulation to promote collaborative learning and practice. *Journal of Nursing Education, 57*(7), 426–429. https://doi.org/10.3928/01484834-20180618-08

Jarding, L., Hogden, L. A., Messier, S. E., Kozmenko, V., Simanton, E., Bjornson, K., & Ortman Brockmueller, C. (2018). Development and validation of simulation-based procedural checklists for evaluation of neonatal nurse practitioner performance. *Advances in Neonatal Care, 18*(5), 386–392. https://doi.org/10.1097/ANC.0000000000000520

Jeffries, P. R., Bigley, M. B., McNelis, A. M., Cartier, J. M., Pintz, C., Slaven-Lee, P. W., & Zychowicz, M. E. (2019). A call to action: Building evidence for use of simulation in nurse practitioner education. *Journal of the American Association of Nurse Practitioners, 31*(11), 627–632. https://doi.org/10.1097/JXX.0000000000000335

Keiser, M. M., & Turkelson, C. (2019). Using simulation to evaluate clinical performance and reasoning in adult-geriatric acute care nurse practitioner students. *Journal of Nursing Education, 58*(10), 599–603. https://doi.org/10.3928/01484834-20190923-08

Kelly, M. M., Blunt, E., & Nestor, K. (2019). After-hours/on-call simulation in primary care nurse practitioner education. *Clinical Simulation in Nursing, 26*, 49–53. https://doi.org/10.1016/j.ecns.2018.05.002

Kesten, K. S., Brown, H. F., & Meeker, M. C. (2015). Assessment of APRN student competency using simulation: A pilot study. *Nursing Education Perspectives, 36*(5), 332–334. https://doi.org/10.5480/15-1649

Kirkpatrick, J., & Kirkpatrick, W. (2009). *Kirkpatrick, then and now: A strong foundation for the future*. Kirkpatrick Partners.

La Cerra, C., Dante, A., Caponnetto, V., Franconi, I., Gaxhja, E., Petrucci, C., Alfes, M. C., & Lancia, L. (2019). Effects of high-fidelity simulation based on life-threatening clinical condition scenarios on learning outcomes of undergraduate and postgraduate nursing students: A systematic review and meta-analysis. *BMJ Open*, *9*(2), e025306. https://doi.org/10.1136/bmjopen-2018-025306

Mangold, K., & Adler, M. (2019). Designing quantitative research studies. In D. Nestel, J. Hui, K. Kunkler, M. W. Scerbo, & A. W. Calhoun (Eds.), *Healthcare simulation research* (pp. 169–174). Springer Publishing. https://doi.org/10.1007/978-3-030-26837-4_23

Marsden, E., & Torgerson, C. J. (2012). Single group, pre- and post-test research designs: Some methodological concerns. *Oxford Review of Education*, *38*(5), 583–616. https://doi.org/10.1080/03054985.2012.731208

National League for Nursing. (2018). *Findings from the 2018 NLN biennial survey of schools of nursing academic year 2017–2018 executive summary*. http://www.nln.org/newsroom/nursing-education-statistics/biennial-survey-of-schools-of-nursing-academic-year-2017-2018

National Organization of Nurse Practitioner Faculties. (2013, November). *NP education today, NP education tomorrow*. Executive summary. http://c.ymcdn.com/sites/nonpf.site-ym.com/resource/resmgr/Docs/Executive_SummaryNov2013.pdf?hhSearchTerms=

National Organization of Nurse Practitioner Faculties. (2020, March 23). *Statement regarding nurse practitioner students and direct care clinical hours*. https://cdn.ymaws.com/www.nonpf.org/resource/resmgr/board_resources/20200323_a_statement_on_np_s.pdf

National Task Force on Quality Nurse Practitioner Education. (2016). *Criteria for evaluation of nurse practitioner programs* (5th ed.). Washington DC: National Organization of Nurse Practitioner Faculties.

Ndiwane, A. N., Baker, N. C., Makosky, A., Reidy, P., & Guarino, A. J. (2017). Use of simulation to integrate cultural humility into advanced health assessment for nurse practitioner students. *Journal of Nursing Education*, *56*(9), 567–571. https://doi.org/10.3928/01484834-20170817-11

Nippita, S., Haviland, M. J., Voit, S. F., Perez-Peralta, J., Hacker, M. R., & Paul, M. E. (2018). Randomized trial of high- and low-fidelity simulation to teach intrauterine contraception placement. *American Journal of Obstetrics and Gynecology*, *218*(2), 258.e1–258.e11. https://doi.org/10.1016/j.ajog.2017.11.553

Nye, C., Campbell, S.H., Fancher, S., Short, C., & Thomas, M. (2019). The use of simulation in advanced practice nursing programs: A North American perspective. *Clinical Simulation in Nursing*, *26*, 3–10. https://doi.org/10.1016/j.ecns.2018.09.005

Nye, C., Campbell, S.H., Fancher, S., Short, C., & Thomas, M. (2020). *The use of simulation in advanced practice nursing programs: A qualitative examination* [Manuscript in Preparation]. School of Nursing, Virginia Commonwealth University.

Onda, E. L. (2012). Situated cognition: its relationship to simulation in nursing education. *Clinical Simulation in Nursing*, *8*(7), e273–e280. https://doi.org/10.1016/j.ecns.2010.11.004

Paige, J. T., Garbee, D. D., Kozmenko, V., Yu, Q., Kozmenko, L., Yang, T., Bonanno, L., & Swartz, W. (2014). Getting a head start: High-fidelity, simulation-based operating room team training of interprofessional students. *Journal of the American College of Surgeons*, *218*(1), 140–149. https://doi.org/10.1016/j.jamcollsurg.2013.09.006

Peddle, M., Livesay, K., & Marshall, S. (2020). Preliminary report of a simulation community of practice needs analysis. *Advances in Simulation*, *5*, 11. https://doi.org/10.1186/s41077-020-00130-4

Phillips, T. A., Munn, A. C., & George, T. P. (2020). Assessing the impact of telehealth objective structured clinical examinations in graduate nursing education. *Nurse Educator*, *45*(3), 169–172. https://doi.org/10.1097/NNE.0000000000000729

Prettyman, A. V., Knight, E. P., & Allison, T. E. (2018). Objective structured clinical examination from virtually anywhere. *The Journal for Nurse Practitioners*, *14*(8), e157–e163. https://doi.org/10.1016/j.nurpra.2018.05.007

Rutherford-Hemming, T. (2012). Learning in simulated environments: effect on learning transfer and clinical skill acquisition in nurse practitioner students. *Journal of Nursing Education*, *51*(7), 403–406. https://doi.org/10.3928/01484834-20120427-04

Rutherford-Hemming, T., Nye, C., & Coram, C. (2016). Using simulation for clinical practice hours in nurse practitioner education in the United States: A systematic review. *Nurse Education Today*, *37*, 128–135. https://doi.org/10.1016/j.nedt.2015.11.006

Schneidereith, T., & Daniels, A. (2019). Integration of simulation to prepare adult-gerontology acute care nurse practitioners. *Clinical Simulation in Nursing*, *26*(1), 18–23. http://doi.org/10.1016/j.ecns.2018.10.009

Schwindt, R., & McNelis, A. (2015). Integrating simulation into a reflection-centered graduate psychiatric/mental health nursing curriculum. *Nursing Education Perspectives*, *36*(5), 326–328. https://doi.org/10.5480/15-1614

Sisler, S. M., Schapiro, N. A., Stephan, L., Mejia, J., & Wallace, A. S. (2019). Consider the root of the problem: increasing trainee skills at assessing and addressing social determinants of health. *Translational Behavioral Medicine*, *9*(3), 523–532. https://doi.org/10.1093/tbm/ibz046

Spector, P. E. (2019). Do not cross me: Optimizing the use of cross-sectional designs. *Journal of Business and Psychology*, *34*, 125–137. https://doi.org/10.1007/s10869-018-09613-8

Starkweather, A. R., Sargent, L., Nye, C., Albrecht, T., Cloutier, R., & Foster, A. (2017). Progressive Assessment and Competency Evaluation (PACE) framework for integrating simulation in nurse practitioner education. *The Journal for Nurse Practitioners*, *13*(7), e301–e310. https://doi.org/10.1016/j.nurpra.2017.04.012

Tankimovich, M., Swails, J., & Hamburger, M. (2020). Nurse practitioner and medical students' perceptions of teamwork before and after a standardized patient pilot simulation. *Nursing Education Perspectives*, *41*(3), 171–173. https://doi.org/10.1097/01.NEP.0000000000000503

Warren, J. N., Luctkar-Flude, M., Godfrey, C., & Lukewich, J. (2016). A systematic review of the effectiveness of simulation-based education on satisfaction and learning outcomes in nurse practitioner programs. *Nurse Education Today*, *46*, 99–108. https://doi.org/10.1016/j.nedt.2016.08.023

Weston, C., Akinlotan, M., Lichorad, A., McClellan, D., Helduser, J., Ojinnaka, C., Holland, B., & Bolin, J. N. (2018). The impact of interprofessional education on family nurse practitioner students' and family medicine residents' knowledge and confidence in screening for breast and cervical cancer. *Journal of the American Association of Nurse Practitioners*, *30*(9), 511–518. https://doi.org/10.1097/JXX.0000000000000072

Woroch, R. A., Alvarez, D. V., Yingling, C. T., & Handrup, C. T. (2018). Family nurse practitioner/psychiatric mental health nurse practitioner collaboration in drug-seeking telephone triage simulation in an advanced practice registered nurse curriculum. *Clinical Simulation in Nursing*, *18*, 14–19. https://doi.org/10.1016/j.ecns.2018.01.002

Woroch, R. A., Sefton, M. G., & Yingling, C. T. (2020). Using simulation to prepare for clinicals in front-loaded FNP curricula. *Clinical Simulation in Nursing*, *39*, 45–50. https://doi.org/10.1016/j.ecns.2019.11.002

Yardley, S., & Dornan, T. (2012). Kirkpatrick's levels and education 'evidence'. *Medical Education*, *46*, 97–106. https://doi.org/10.1111/j.1365-2923.2011.04076.x

CHAPTER 3

Human Simulation in Nursing Education

Catherine Nicholas and Jill S. Sanko

ABSTRACT

Although, human simulation methodology has its origins in medical education, nursing education has increased its use of simulated patient (SP) methodology to improve the education of nursing students across the curricula. This chapter will review the history of human simulation, introduce the human simulation continuum, and review different applications of SP methodology in undergraduate and graduate nursing education.

HISTORY OF HUMAN SIMULATION

Definitions and Terminology

> Human simulation involves human roles players interacting with learners in a wide range of experiential learning and assessment contexts. (Lewis et al., 2017, p. 1)

From simulated patient to standardized patient to simulated participant, different terms have been used to describe humans in simulation over the 50-year history of the methodology. The terms tend to be used interchangeably in the literature, which can cause confusion to those educators/researchers responsible for developing human simulation activities (Beigzadeh et al., 2016; Churchouse & McCafferty, 2012; Sanko et al., 2020).

http://dx.doi.org/10.1891/0739-6686.39.53

Simulated patient (SP) refers to a person "who has been carefully coached to simulate an actual patient so accurately that the simulation cannot be detected by a skilled clinician" (Barrows, 1993, p. 444). They can portray an asymptomatic or normal patient, can have abnormal findings on physical exam (PE), and/or can simulate abnormal findings (Box 3.1). Because they experience an encounter from the patient point of view and can feel if a PE maneuver is done correctly, they can be more accurate in their feedback than faculty observations (Swanson & Stillman, 1990).

Box 3.1: *Advantages of SP Methodology*

1. SPs are trained to have learner's practice their skills repeatedly.
2. SPs are trained in best practices and can provide standardized feedback to all learners.
3. Learners can practice difficult communication topics (giving bad/sad news, disclosure, and apologies, etc.) in a safe, supported environment where mistakes are part of the learning process and patients are not harmed.
4. All learners can be assured of seeing the same level of difficulty and the same series of problems instead of relying on time and chance in the clinical setting.
5. SPs are trained to provide standardized assessment to enable faculty to compare students within the same curriculum.

(Barrows, 1968, p. 674)

Educators soon realized that the method could be used for testing performance and the term standardized patient was developed. Canadian psychometrician Geoffrey Norman used this term to describe someone who is trained to portray a specific condition in a realistic, standardized, and repeatable way (Wallace, 1997). The portrayal /presentation varies based only on the learner's performance. Between 1992 and 2004, the strict standardization of portrayal allowed the development of licensing examinations using standardized patient methodology to assess knowledge, skills, and attitudes in Canada and the United States.

As the use of human simulation expands, people are now portraying customers, family members, lawyer/judges, social workers, teachers/students, and healthcare professionals. Subsequently, new terms emerged, such as confederates or embedded participant for "an individual other than the patient who is scripted in a simulation to provide realism, additional challenges, or information for the learner e.g. paramedic, receptionist, family member technician"(Lioce et

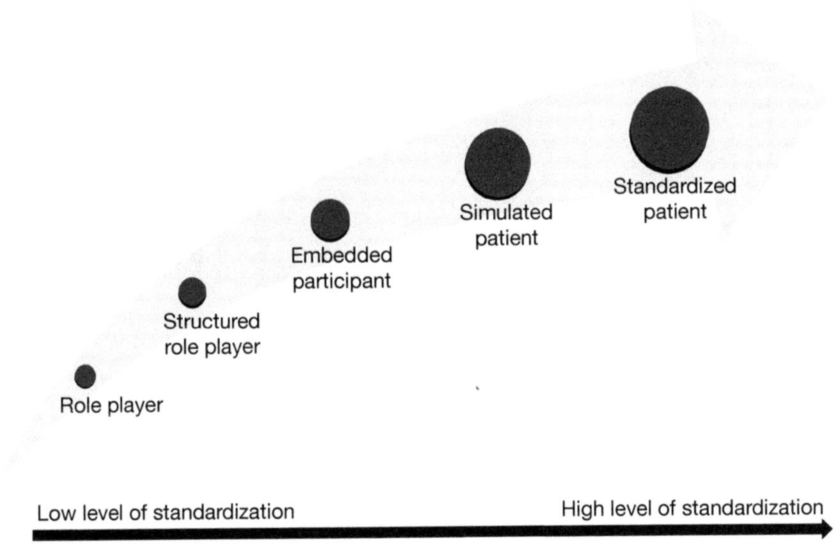

FIGURE 3.1 Human simulation continuum model.

al., 2020, p. 12). The term simulated participant is considered by the Association of Standardized Patient Educators (ASPE) "as a more inclusive term" (Lewis et al., 2017, p.2) to refer to all humans in any simulation activity.

Throughout this chapter the authors use SP as an umbrella term. Additionally, a recent study by Sanko et al. (2020) found the term SP to be widely understood as the person who plays a patient in a simulation encounter and also provides feedback to learners. In fact, this study uncovered the common problem of inconsistent terminology in the community of practice. Given the variability of terms used throughout the simulation community, the authors of this chapter use terms and definitions from the SSH dictionary and other credible sources. Later in the chapter, a framework (Figure 3.1) and table of terms and definitions (Table 3.1) are presented with corresponding sourcing information so that readers are not confused by terms that may differ from ones currently in use or found in other written material.

As members of the larger simulation community, the issue around terminology usage needs work and represents an opportunity for leaders to take a role in shaping single terms with single definitions for the purposes of communicating through a common language. Coalescing around agreed-upon terms will help in the continued evolution of this field. Simulation is not the first discipline to grapple with this issue, nor will it be the last. There is important work needed to move these efforts forward. To have a deeper understanding of the evolution of

TABLE 3.1
Human Simulation Roles, Training, and Uses

	Term	Definition	SPE	SP	Uses
Low level of standardization	Role player	A person who imagines being themselves or another person in a particular situation (improvisation).	Provides the broad outline of the simulation. Clarifies role.	Interprets as they see fit.	Learning activities. No standardization needed.
	Structured role player	Improvisation meets structure.	Provides specific objectives. Trains SP to a prepared script on a limited aspect of a situation. Clarifies role.	Works from script. Interprets as they see fit.	Learning activities. Some standardization needed.
High level of standardization	Embedded participant /confederate	A person who is trained and scripted to play a role in a simulation in order to guide the simulation.	Provides specific objectives. Trains SPs to a prepared script. Trains SP how to guide the learners and avoid unintended cuing.	Often has the background of the embedded participant (nurse, MD, etc.). Requires knowledge of the healthcare team dynamics and culture.	Learning and low stakes assessment. Standardization required.

(*Continued*)

TABLE 3.1

Human Simulation Roles, Training, and Uses (Continued)

Term	Definition	SPE	SP	Uses
Simulated patients	Trained to relevant clinical information. Able to respond flexibly to the needs of individual learners. Can use their own history or experiences.	Provides specific objectives and relevant clinical information. Provides parameters so SP does not mislead the learner.	Follows the objectives. Knows the clinical information. Respects the parameters provided.	Learning and low stakes assessment. Some standardization required.
Standardized Patients	Carefully trained SP who portrays a patient with a specific condition in a realistic, standardized, and repeatable way. Variation is based on the learner's performance.	Provides specific objectives. Trains to all background and clinical information. Trains SP to portrayal and use of assessment tool and method of feedback.	Follows all aspects of the case at all times; portrayal is reproducible and standardized. Uses checklist to assess learner and provide feedback.	Learning and low stakes and high stakes assessment including licensure. High degree of standardization among SPs and across sites.

human simulation, the originators of the method are described in the following section.

PIONEERS AND EARLY INNOVATORS

Dr. Howard Barrows

In 1963, after observing a neurological patient "switch" his sensory loss from the affected side to the healthy side during a neurology board exam, Dr. Howard Barrows conceived the concept of the "programmed patient" (Barrows, 1971; Barrows & Abrahamson, 1964). Dr. Barrows realized he could train healthy lay people to present signs and symptoms of a specific problem consistently and accurately to the point where a trained clinician could not tell the difference.

> We encourage the SPs not to learn the patient's role as in intellectual scripts but to understand what it is like to be the actual patient with the feelings and problems the patient has. (Barrows, 1993, p. 445)

He renamed the programmed patient to simulated patient. Working with the simulated patients, he not only trained them to present PE findings, but also trained them to assess and provide feedback to the learner using a case-specific checklist.

Dr. Robert Kretzchmar

Inspired by Barrows, Dr. Robert Kretzchmar, an obstetrician/gynecologist, recruited and trained lay women to teach the breast and pelvic examinations using their own bodies. These were the first gynecology teaching assistant (GTA), created in 1968.

> The qualities she brings to the instructional system include sensitivity as a woman, educational skill in pelvic examination instruction, knowledge of female pelvic anatomy and physiology, and, most important, sophisticated interpersonal skills to help medical students learn in a nonthreatening environment. (Kretzschmar, 1978, p. 367)

Dr. Paula Stillman

In the mid-1970s. Dr. Paula Stillman, a pediatric clerkship director, created a program to teach students interviewing skills by training lay women as "simulated mothers" to offer presentations of common pediatric complaints for the purposes of honing skills. To provide the learners with consistent feedback, she developed the first behaviorally anchored Likert Scale of interviewing skills. The scale was called the Arizona Clinical Interview Rating (ACIR) Scale (Stillman et al., 1997;

Stillman et al., 1983; Stillman et al., 1976; Stillman et al., 1977). Seeing the success of the simulated interviewing course, Dr. Stillman created a physical diagnosis course to teach PE skills. She trained SPs to become "patient instructors" or PIs to teach and assess over 200 PE skills on their own bodies using detailed description designed by clinicians. Physical Exam Teaching Associates (PETA/PTA) are trained to teach, assess, and provide feedback to learners about the complete PE.

> Not only did they know what it felt like when each maneuver was done correctly, but they know how to teach the student to do it properly. (Wallace, 1997, p. 12)

Josiah Macy Jr. Foundation

The Josiah Macy Jr. Foundation, a philanthropic foundation, was founded in the 1930s to improve health by advancing education and training of health professionals and by fostering innovation in clinical learning environments (Josiah Macy Jr. Foundation, n.d.). In 1984, they hosted a number of conferences focused on standardized patient methodology. The organization continued to promote this learning and assessment methodology by supporting other conferences, offering innovation grants, and supporting the formation of six consortia for medical schools to collaborate and study the impact of standardized patient methodology on learning and assessment.

The Association of Medical Colleges, Liaison Committee on Medical Education, and The United States Licensing Examination

In 1992, The Association of American Medical Colleges (AAMC), an not-for-profit association dedicated to transforming healthcare through innovative medical education, patient care, and groundbreaking medical research, sponsored and published the proceedings from a consensus conference on the use of standardized patient methodology in the teaching and evaluation of clinical skills (Anderson, 1993; AAMC, 2020). The research studies that followed, along with the call to ensure medical student clinical competency, led to the creation of standardized patient programs within the majority of medical schools (Liaison Committee on Medical Education, 2020).

In 1993 and 1994 respectively, Canada and the United States implemented a national standardized patient-based performance assessment as part of the licensure process. The United States Medical Licensing Examination Step 2 Clinical Skills exam is a 12-station SP-based assessment that tests medical students on "their ability to be patient-centered, to address diagnostic challenges posed, to prepare the patient for the next steps document the encounter appropriately" (United States Medical Licensing Examination, 2019, p.3). This approach, while beginning in North America, quickly spread around the world (Abe et al., 2009;

Cleland et al., 2009; Harden & Gleeson, 1979; Kaplonyi et al., 2017; Kneebone et al., 2006; Nestel & Bearman, 2014; Newble, 2004; van der Vleuten & Swanson, 1990).

Birth of a New Profession: The Standardized Patient Educator

As SP methodology grew in use and understanding, a new profession of the standardized patient educator (SPE) was growing along with it (Lewis et al., 2017)). The term SPE refers to "those who work to develop expertise in SP methodology and are responsible for training and/or administering SP-based simulation". Some may be trainers who exclusively work with SPs while others may be faculty or healthcare professionals who work with SPs as part of their clinical and/or academic role" (Lewis et al., 2017, p. 3). Since the early 1990s, individuals who were developing expertise in writing case materials, training SPs, and implementing SP activities began to collaborate and share what they were learning. Out of these early collaborations emerged a community of practice. Early meetings of SPEs were part of the AAMC annual meetings. Eventually, SPEs began to offer their own conferences to share innovations for education and to develop mechanisms for professional development of SPEs. These efforts led to the formation of The Association of Standardized Patient Educators or ASPE in 2001. ASPE's mission is to promote best practices (Box 3.2) in SP methodology, foster dissemination of research and scholarship, and advance the professional development of the SPE and faculty who engage in human simulation (ASPE, n.d.).

Box 3.2: ASPE Standards of Best Practices

1. Safe Work Environment
2. Case Development
3. Training SPs
4. Program Management
5. Professional Development

To that end, ASPE published the Standards of Best Practices (SOBPs) to "ensure the growth and integrity of SP-based endeavors" (Lewis et al., 2017, p.3). The document is the result of 10 years of work and is based on evidence and methods reflective of the perspectives of many cultures and fields of practices (Lewis et al., 2017). The SOPBs are for implementation when working with any human in simulation, alongside the International Nursing Association for Clinical Simulation and Learning (INASCL) Standards of Best Practice: Simulation^{SM} (Sittner et al., 2015).

The SOBPs are divided into five domains (Box 3.2) based on five values: safety, quality, professionalism, accountability, and collaboration (Gliva-McConvey et al., 2020). A significant contribution to the SPE/SP community of practice is the first domain: Safe Work Environment. Safety is crucial to ensure an optimal experience for learners, faculty, staff, and SPs. The SOBPs outline the ethical responsibility of SPEs that ensures the safety of SPs, including consideration of the activity's design, management of faculty/client expectations, and identification and mitigation of safety threats through SP debriefing/de-rolling. Multiple studies examining SPs' perspectives revealed that a socially supporting environment and the role of the SPE in setting clear guidelines regarding their physical, cognitive, and psychological safety were very important to SPs engagement, effort, motivation, satisfaction, and retention (Pritchard et al., 2017; Pritchard et al., 2020; Schlegel et al., 2016; Simmenroth-Nayda et al., 2016).

The first step in creating a safe work environment is an understanding that the SP methodology is the tool, and the individual SP is the human co-collaborator and educational team member. Moving from the phrase "using SPs" to "engaging SPs or using SP methodology reminds team members of the true value and contributions made by SPs" (McNaughton & Anderson, 2017).

> Because SPs are actual humans, the phrase "using SPs" engenders a notion of SPs as inert tools, like hammers that can be picked up and put down without thought to the effect its "use" may have had on it. In our conversations with fellow SP educators, we are hearing this language increasingly critiqued. Those of us actively engaged with SPs in the field believe that although SPs are a dynamic educational resource, they are more than just "fleshy manikins." (McNaughton, 2012, p. 127)

SP METHODOLOGY

Human Simulation Continuum Model

> The context in which SPs are working determines the degree of repeatability or standardization of their behavior, both within an individual SP's performance and between SPs portraying the same role. The behavior can be seen as part of a continuum. (Lewis et al., 2017, p. 3)

Gliva-McConvey et al. (2020) provide a framework (Figure 3.1) in which all the different terms associated with the SP are defined by the training techniques used and the role of the SP.

The figure shows that, as a high level of standardization is approached, the degree of preparation and reproducibility increases. SPEs are important as trainer and coach at all levels to ensure that the SP is fully prepared to meet the goals and objectives of the event or purpose of the assessment (see Table 3.1). Not all

SPs may possess the qualities required at every level, so careful selection when recruiting is required (Gliva-McConvey et al., 2020).

Human Simulation in Nursing Education

The use of SP methodology as part of nursing education does not have the longevity or historic precedent compared to medical education. However, there is an increased use of SP-based education aimed to improve the education of nursing students across the curricula. According to Becker et al. (2006), SP problem-based learning was considered a new pedagogical method in nursing education that was used to enhance curricular objectives, augment learning, and evaluate competence of students. It is not surprising that a more contemporary beginning to utilization has limited the ubiquitous and substantial role of SP-based learning opportunities across various nursing programs. Its current use is more often in graduate nursing programs, mostly through nurse practitioner education (Becker et al., 2006).

Anecdotally, the use of SP-based simulation to augment educational practice has significant support; however an examination of the research demonstrates that the impacts of SP-based simulation in nursing has mixed results (Rutherford-Hemming et al., 2019). There appear to be more positive findings related to the use of SP-based simulation in medical education than nursing. One example of such is a study by Swiggart et al. (2012), who showed the positive impact of SP-based simulation in safety education of medical students related to controlled substance prescribing. This literature may speak more to the limited use of SP-based simulation in nursing education than its actual impact as an appropriate and useful educational modality for nursing. Another reason there are fewer studies of SP-based simulation in nursing may be related to the lack of simulation practices (immersive manikin-based, SP-based, or otherwise) needed to evaluate competency and mastery in the same way as medical education. The use of simulation in nursing education remains primarily one that is seated in formative assessment over summative assessment, however, this is shifting (Zitzelsberger, et al., 2017). Despite these current realities, SP methodology in nursing education has promise and advantages, including the ability to improve clinical reasoning skills and decrease anxiety prior to starting clinical rotations (Sarmasoglu et al., 2016).

Undergraduate Nursing

With clinical sites becoming more difficult to secure, there is an increased need for simulation-based education and SP-based simulation to fully prepare safe and effective nursing graduates. SP-based simulation is currently used to bolster fundamental skills and lessen student anxiety related to the newness of the clinical environment, fear of harming patients, and uncertainty of skills (Yoo & Yoo, 2003). In this section, the literature on the most common uses of SP-based simulation in undergraduate nursing education is briefly summarized.

Psychiatric

A 2017 review of the literature on SP methodology in psychiatric nursing education showed insufficient evidence regarding effectiveness (Goodman & Winter, 2017). The article noted that the use of SP methodology to augment education and assess skills in the area of psychiatric / mental health (PMH) was gaining popularity (Goodman & Winter, 2017). Among the studies, only one was a randomized control design and the results of the study demonstrated no significant difference in the groups on a knowledge pretest/posttest. The students in the study (Becker et al., 2006) articulated through open-ended qualitative questions a positive overall experience through the SP encounter, stating that it afforded them the opportunity to critically think and practice various interviewing approaches. Given the dearth of proof regarding the role of SPs in learning, coupled with a juxtaposition of learner opinion, it is incumbent upon educators to study the impacts while simultaneously prioritizing the importance of hard evidence on perceptions of learning.

Skills

Technical. Many technical skills can be sharpened with the use of SP methodology, human patient simulators (aka high-fidelity simulators), task trainers, or a combination of these modalities. However, for many nursing skills, SPs offer advantages that may provide a greater platform for learning and mastery. A literature search yielded increasing evidence on the use of SP methodology in teaching and practice of technical skills. Tuzer et al. (2016) compared the effects of using high-fidelity simulators or SP-based activities on the thoracic examination skills of undergraduate nursing students and found both modalities improved knowledge and performance scores, but those who worked with SPs had significantly higher knowledge scores than those only exposed to high-fidelity simulators. Additionally, clinical competence in fundamental nursing skills has been shown to be enhanced through teaching with SP methodology over traditional methods (Yoo & Yoo, 2003). Self-reported levels of confidence in completing health histories was found to be improved using SPs (Andrea & Kotowski, 2017). Furthermore, the use of SPs to develop students' psychomotor skills has been shown to be effective (Sarmasoglu et al., 2016). Finally, Basak et al. (2019) demonstrated the effectiveness of using SPs for hand hygiene over the use of a low-fidelity manikin. This finding is interesting due to the fact that the skill of hand washing does not appear to need the use of an SP to master, yet their randomized control trial demonstrated otherwise.

Nontechnical. Nontechnical skills include communication, teamwork, decision-making, leadership, and situational awareness (Gordon et al., 2017). Using SP-based education and simulation as a whole has been successful in developing these important skills.

Communication. SP methodology to teach therapeutic communication is gaining momentum in undergraduate nursing. A recent integrated review of 19 studies found that SP-based activities bolstered skills related to various patient and family communication challenges, including hearing-impaired patients, depressed patients, suicide prevention and other psychiatric disorders, dying patients and their families, cancer patients, and communication skills in general (MacLean et al., 2017). From this review, and as also suggested by its authors, the current use of SP methodology to teach communications skills in nursing is narrow and demonstrates significant potential for expansion. Areas for expansion include team communication, communication of safety concerns and discoveries, as well as communication with other specific groups (i.e., children, elderly, intellectually challenged), and the use of an interpreter when speaking with patients and families who speak a different language.

End-of-life, spiritual, and palliative care. SP-based education can offer a richer learning experience when teaching end-of-life, spiritual, and palliative care. A recent article by Kenny et al. (2016) outlined an approach to improve and validate pediatric nurses' communication skills with SPs. This study specifically looked at whether clinical communication skills acquired through 3 years of training could transfer to end-of-life scenarios. Findings demonstrated that participants experienced a range of emotions from anxiety and fear to empowerment related to participating in an end-of-life scenario. Participants also noted the "realness" of the experience as demonstrated through the quote: "I then forgot it was role play and it felt quite natural" (Kenny et al., 2016, p. 150). The study concluded that the approach gave participants the opportunity to utilize and transfer their generic communication skills to a novel situation.

Other work showed that the use of SP methodology, coupled with the inclusion of clergy, helped students develop a better understanding of the role of teamwork in end-of-life care (Lewis-Pierre et al., 2020). Additionally, a comparison of SP end-of-life simulation coupled with online modules demonstrated that simulation improved students' attitudes toward dying over traditional didactic methods (Lewis-Pierre et al., 2019).

Graduate and Specialized Programs

SP methodology in graduate-level nursing education occurs more frequently than in undergraduate nursing education. This may be related to the predominate educational model used in graduate nursing. Undergraduate nursing education uses a nursing-centric model, whereas graduate nursing programs often align more closely with medical models. This difference in graduate education may relate to: (a) professional work requirements and expected levels of independence and (b) the need to develop different clinical skills that more closely mirror physicians. Given the wide use of SP methodology in medical education, it makes sense that a nursing program that requires individuals with similar clinical skills would utilize a similar pedagogical approach (Vessy & Huss, 2002). One key difference in graduate nursing programs compared to medical education is the use of SP-based encounters for summative or formative assessments. The commonality in each of these programs is leading the way for development of formative and summative evaluation of graduate nursing students through SP encounters (Becker et al., 2006; Vessy & Huss, 2002).

Despite the increased frequency of SPs in graduate nursing educational programs, undergraduate nursing programs and graduate nursing programs often use SP methodology to teach similar concepts and skills. These include communication, cultural competence (Ndiwane et al., 2014), end-of-life and palliative care (Shawler, 2011), psychiatric-mental health applications (Shawler, 2008), and various technical and nontechnical skills. Unique uses in graduate nursing education include hybrid simulation for teaching emergency births in midwifery education (Miller et al., 2015), emergency responses (Ballman et al., 2016; Davis, 2017), distance learning (Ballman et al., 2016), and quality and safety education (Schlegel et al., 2016; Webster, 2013). Given the versatility of the approach, the only limiting factor in using SP methodology may be resources and imagination.

Because of the difficulties securing appropriate clinical rotations for nurse practitioner and other graduate nursing students, many expect an increase in the use of SP-based simulation (Barber & Schuessler, 2018). Fortunately, research on the impacts of SPs in graduate nursing programs has demonstrated promise as an effective teaching strategy (Ballman et al., 2016; Barber & Schuessler, 2018). Moreover, faculty opinions on the usefulness of SP-based education demonstrates effectiveness from the perspective of the educator (Vessy & Huss, 2017) as well as overall satisfaction from the perspective of the student (Becker et al., 2006).

Interprofessional Education

Interprofessional education (IPE) is now a requirement of most healthcare professions educational programs (see Chapter 5). Simulation-based education is one of the most powerful ways to educate students about the core competencies for successful interprofessional work. The use of standardized patients within IPE offers a rich opportunity to develop teamwork, communication, skills, knowledge, ethics, and respect for role differences. The literature is rich with examples of the creative ways in which educators are using SP methodology to enhance IPE encounters. Examples include using older adults as SPs (Davis, 2017), pharmacology education for nurse practitioner and pharmacy students (Koo et al., 2014), end-of-life care (Gannon et al., 2017), infection control (Luctkar-Flude et al., 2016), large audience SP IPE encounters (J. Sanko, personal communication, January, 2020), teamwork, and patient safety, as well as numerous other examples from various combinations of disciplines.

Other Considerations When Selecting Modalities and Approaches

Studies have shown that when given the choice, many learners prefer SPs over high-fidelity simulators for topics where either could be used (Sanko et al., 2012; Wisborg et al., 2009). Additionally, realism is an important factor in learning for some, therefore, learner needs should be considered when selecting a modality. One study found that SPs and manikins were both effective in teaching response to a decompensating patient, but SP encounters scored higher in overall realism and on posttest assessments (Alsaad et al., 2017).

EMERGING USES

Virtual Standardized Patients

The definition of virtual patients is vague by design and meant to be inclusive of the any patient within computer-based simulations. Terms used for virtual patient also include human-based simulation online and avatar-based virtual patients. Human-based simulation online (discussed further in the Telesimulation section) can include a live SP portrayed through a virtual meeting space (e.g., Zoom, WebEx) and is not significantly different from SP in-person simulations (Gliva-McConvey et al., 2020).

The avatar-based virtual patients, also referred to as virtual standardized patients (VSPs), can include those with and without artificial intelligence. VSPs were created to address gaps found in the delivery of healthcare simulation and offer an additional interactive approach for assessing and teaching critical skills to healthcare professions in situations with limited human resources (Talbot et al., 2012). VSPs can repeatedly provide both clinical variations and an entirely standardized experience (Cendan & Lok, 2012), while offering increased accessibility and limited faculty oversight. VSPs also offer a more scalable solution for increasing curricular demands with a more cost-effective solution to augment traditional SP-based education, but may also have the limitation of a narrow range of questions to which the "patient" can respond (Feldman et al., 2006).

The inability of these to reliably produce appropriate interactions and responses to substantially replicate human interactions demonstrates that there is still work to be done (Bond et al., 2019; Talbot et al., 2012). The technology that drives these sophisticated computer-based avatars is evolving rapidly with new products and companies emerging each year.

Augmented Reality

Augmented reality (AR; Chapter 10) is no longer a futuristic possibility. It can be found in everyday applications, such as holograms that provide directions in airports and in children's games, so it is no surprise that it is being explored for educational uses. AR has now found its way into SP-based education, albeit not quite as widespread or mainstream. One example is the use of augmented overlays via a specially equipped stethoscope that simulates abnormal heart and lung sounds when placed on the correct anatomical location of an SP (Mckenzie et al., 2004). As the technology improves and becomes less expensive and more accessible, more uses are sure to follow.

Telesimulation Education

The coronavirus pandemic pushed educators to provide creative, high-quality simulations while maintaining social distancing (Chick et al., 2020; Loeb et al., 2020; Zhou et al., 2020). One way this was accomplished was through deployment of SP-based education via a telesimulation encounter (see Chapter 4). Programs hired SPs for videoconferencing, experiential learning opportunities that now replaced face-to-face human interactions. Simulationists who conducted these encounters attest to the powerful learning during these exchanges and discovered a lot about what was possible through technology and creativity. After the pandemic, many will see this successful marriage of teleconferencing and simulation continue to be used in new and interesting ways.

Addressing Health Inequities and Impact of Systemic Racism

SP-enhanced curricula that addresses racial and ethnic differences is gaining momentum in nursing education (Ndiwane et al., 2014). This use of SP methodology is timely given the projections that by 2060, nearly one of every five Americans will be born outside the United States, and by 2044, more than half will belong to a minority (any group other than non-Hispanic White; Colby & Ortman, 2015). Most SP cases focus on elements of cultural competency/humility where understanding, sensitivity, and empathy are important. (Aeder et al., 2007;

Buenconsejo-Lum & Maskarinec, 2004; Foronda et al., 2018; Guiton et al., 2004; Lau et al., 2016; San, 2015). These areas include substance abuse, elder abuse, religious and faith-based diversity, sexual identity and LGBTQ+, poverty, victims of gang-related behavior, disability, mental illness, intimate partner violence, issues facing military families, and homelessness (Bahreman & Swoboda, 2016).

While inroads have been made to address diversity, there is still much work to be done. Conigliaro et al. (2020) and Foronda et al. (2020) identified a White-dominant narrative throughout simulation, including an underrepresentation of racial diversity in manikins, body parts/task trainers, SPs, and simulation staff and faculty. Simulationists can play a role in the dominant narrative and create what Truglio et al. (2020) refer to as anti-racist clinical skills curriculum. Anti-racism is an active and consistent process of change to eliminate individual, institutional, and systemic racism and redistribute power and privilege (National Museum of African American History & Culture, n.d.).

SP methodology was started from an activist stance. Activism is described as "intentional action with the goal of bringing about positive change" (McIntosh, 2020, p.1). Drs. Howard Barrows and Paula Stillman saw an opportunity to change training and evaluation of healthcare professionals and students regarding patient-centered care. Their ideas and innovations were not readily accepted, yet they recognized the power in the methodology and knew that by working together, they could advance the profession and have a greater impact on transforming professionals through human interaction (Wallace, 1997). The formation of ASPE ensured the growth, integrity, and safe use of SP methodology and, after more than a decade of work, the ASPE SOBPs were published. For the first time, safe work practices for SPs were elucidated and support was provided for ethnically and linguistically diverse cohorts of SPs (Lewis et al., 2017).

The pandemic of 2020 uncovered structural and scientific racism that many believe resulted in gross social and health inequities for Black, Indigenous, and People of Color (BIPOC; Oppel et al., 2020). Structural racism is based on a doctrine of White supremacy; economic, political, social, and cultural structures and actions and beliefs that systematize and perpetuate an unequal distribution of privileges, resources, and power (Gee & Ford, 2011). Scientific racism stems from a belief in biological evidence of race and racial inferiority/superiority, including biological differences and inferiority of Black people to White people (deShazo, 2020). Addressing health inequity takes organizational and individual efforts and simulation can provide opportunities to care for underserved/unserved patient populations in a safe, supporting learning environment (Hellman et al., 2018; Holm et al., 2017; Kumagai & Lypson, 2009; Tervalon & Murray-Garcia, 1998). A few examples include the health inequity of people living with disabilities, the negative impacts of social determinants of health and systemic racism, and opportunities to provide respectful/informed LGBTQA care (Good et al., 2005; Weinick et al., 2011; Wilkerson et al., 2010). Simulationists can contribute to the cultural and structural humility of learners, faculty, and staff by integrating nonnormative presentations of love, gender, race, religion, and health concerns into all SP case development (Benn-John, 2019; Nicholas et al., 2020). Simulation can also help learners gain skills needed to counteract the microaggressions and bias they may face daily from patients, colleagues, and faculty while learning how individual biases can affect clinical practice (Chang et al., 2012; Isaacson, 2014). It is also important to consider the impact of learner bias on culturally and linguistically diverse SPs in simulated settings and prepare to protect the SPs, psychological safety as well (Lewis et al., 2017).

To create a psychologically and physically safe work and learning space (Kolbe et al., 2020) for racially diverse groups, Foldy et al. (2009) cautions us "that power inequities drive dynamics in racially diverse teams, often leading to conflict, withdrawal or assimilation—all of which an impede team learning" (p. 25). To create a safe space, attend to identity safety (Davies et al., 2005) by openly acknowledging social and racial identities in the group.

> Creating identity safe environments involves assuring individuals that their social identities are not a barrier- that they are welcome, supported and valued. Identity safe spaces challenge the validity, relevance or acceptance of negative stereotypes linked to certain identities. Identity safe spaces embrace diversity. (Davies et al., 2005, p. 278)

To establish a safe space when there is an inherent imbalance of power built into the system involves creation of what Arao and Clemens (2013) refer to as brave spaces. Brave spaces contain five main elements:

1. Controversy with civility where varying opinions are accepted.
2. Owning intentions and impacts; acknowledging and discussing the impact of these on the emotional well-being of another person.
3. Challenge by choice, where individuals have an option to step in and out of challenging conversations.
4. Respect for one another's basic personhood.
5. Agreement to not intentionally inflict harm on one another.

Considerations for how to assure identity safety and creation of brave spaces will be key to success in the recruitment and retention of culturally and linguistically diverse SPs, staff, and simulation faculty.

CONCLUSION

From the time that simulation became widely used in nursing education, it had been touted as a method to provide a safe learning environment where errors could be learned from and reflected upon. Currently, use of SP methodology for formative experiences may be more common than its use for summative evaluation of skill competence. Additionally, high-stakes skill-based exams are not yet a part of the nursing licensing exams, therefore there is no real incentive to incorporate SP-based summative evaluation into the whole of nursing education. This utilization furthers the notion that simulation should only be used in formative applications, however, many applications of simulation for demonstrating competence mastery exist. The authors feel that failing to utilize simulation, but more specifically SP-based simulation, in a capacity to evaluate skill mastery is shortsighted. In a discipline that depends upon the acquisition, incorporation, and application of knowledge and skills, awarding a practice license subsequent to a single knowledge-based assessment falls short of ensuring that nurses can practice fully and safely. The authors also argue that there is a real benefit as demonstrated in the literature in using simulation to evaluate nursing practice readiness and competence. Opponents of this idea may fear that shifting to using simulation experiences as part of summative assessments will degrade the learning potential that simulation encounters afford because it could create reluctance of students to be vulnerable during formative encounters thus muting the possibility of learning from mistakes. Additionally, opponents of using simulation for summative evaluation as part of nursing education cite the issues around problematic validity and reliability of tools, and potential errors related to the interpretation of passing or failing. While each of these issues are valid concerns, nursing can learn from medical colleagues, as they have been successful in utilizing SPs and simulation for these purposes for decades.

ACKNOWLEDGMENTS

Thank you to Gayle Gliva-McConvey for her review on the virtual patient and Emma Vick for her review of the section on health inequities.

REFERENCES

Abe, K., Suzuki, T., Fujisaki, K., & Ban, N. (2009). A national survey to explore the willingness of Japanese standardized patients to participate in teaching physical examination skills to undergraduate medical students. *Teaching and Learning in Medicine*, *21*(3), 240–247. https://doi.org/10.1080/10401330903018567

Aeder, L., Altshuler, L., Kachur, E., Barrett, S., Hilfer, A., Koepfer, S., & Shelov, S. P. (2007). The "Culture OSCE"-Introducing a formative assessment into a postgraduate program. *Education for Health*, *20*(1), 11.

Alsaad, A. A., Davuluri, S., Bhide, V. Y., Lannen, A. M., & Maniaci, M. J. (2017). Assessing the performance and satisfaction of medical residents utilizing standardized patient versus manikin-simulated training. *Advances in Medical Education and Practice*, *8*, 481–486. https://doi.org/10.2147/AMEP.S134235

Anderson, M. B. Proceedings of the AAMC's consensus conference on the use of standardized patients in the teaching and evaluation of clinical skills. *Academic Medicine*, *68*, 437–484. https://doi.org/10.1097/00001888-199306000-00001

Andrea, J. A., & Kotowski, P. (2017). Using standardized patients in an undergraduate nursing health assessment class. *Clinical Simulation in Nursing*, *13*(7), 309–313. https://doi.org/10.1016/j.ecns.2017.05.003

Arao, B., & Clemens, K. (2013). From safe spaces to brave spaces, in LM Landreman (ed) in *The art of effective Facilitation* (pp. 135–150). Sterling Virginia: Stylus Publishing.

ASPE: The Global Network for Human Simulation Education. (n.d.). https://www.aspeducators.org/

Association of American Medical Colleges. (2020). https://www.aamc.org/

Bahreman, N., & Swoboda, S. (2016). Honoring diversity: Developing culturally competent communication skills through simulation. *The Journal of Nursing Education*, *55*(2), 105–108. https://doi.org/10.3928/01484834-20160114-09

Ballman, K., Garritano, N., & Beery, T. (2016). Broadening the reach of standardized patients in nurse practitioner education to include the distance learner. *Nurse Educator*, *41*, 230–233. https://doi.org/10.1097/NNE.0000000000000260

Barber, L. A. M., & Schuessler, J. B. (2018). Standardized patient simulation for a graduate nursing program. *The Journal for Nurse Practitioners*, *14*(1), e5–e11. https://doi.org/10.1016/j.nurpra.2017.09.017

Barrows, H. S. (1968). Simulated patients in medical teaching. *Canadian Medical Association Journal*, *98*(14), 674–676.

Barrows, H, S. (1971). *Introduction, simulated patients (Programmed Patients)*. Charles C Thomas.

Barrows, H. S. (1993). An overview of the uses of standardized patients for teaching and evaluating clinical skills. *Academic Medicine*, *68*, 443–443. https://doi.org/10.1097/00001888-199306000-00002

Barrows, H. S., & Abrahamson, S. (1964). The programmed patient: A technique for appraising student performance in clinical neurology. *Academic Medicine*, *39*(8), 802–805.

Basak, T., Aciksoz, S., Unver, V., & Aslan, O. (2019). Using standardized patients to improve the hygiene care skills of first-year nursing students: A randomized controlled trial. *Collegian*, *26*(1), 49–54. https://doi.org/10.1016/j.colegn.2018.03.005

Becker, K. L., Rose, L. E., Berg, J. B., Park, H., & Shatzer, J. H. (2006). The teaching effectiveness of standardized patients. *Journal of Nursing Education*, *45*(4), 103–111. https://doi.org/10.3928/01484834-20060401-03

Beigzadeh, A., Bahmanbijri, B., Sharifpoor, E., & Rahimi, M. (2016). Standardized patients versus simulated patients in medical education: Are they the same or different.

Journal of Emergency Practice and Trauma, *2*(1), 25–28. https://doi.org/10.15171/jept.2015.05

Benn-John, J. (2019). Decolonizing western medicine and systems of care: Implications for education. In N. N. Wane, M. S. Todorova, & K. L. Todd (Eds.), *Decolonizing the spirit in education and beyond: Resistance and solidarity*. Springer Nature.

Bond, W. F., Lynch, T. J., Mischler, M. J., Fish, J. L., McGarvey, J. S., Taylor, J. T., Kumar, D. M., Mou, K. M., Ebert-Allen, R. A., Mahale, D. N., Talbot, T. B., & Aiyer, M. (2019). Virtual standardized patient simulation: Case development and pilot application to high-value care. *Simulation in Healthcare: Journal of the Society for Simulation in Healthcare*, *14*(4), 241–250. https://doi.org/10.1097/SIH.0000000000000373

Buenconsejo-Lum, L. E., & Maskarinec, G. G. (2004). Using standardized patients to enhance cross-cultural sensitivity. *Asia Pacific Family Medicine*, *3*.

Cendan, J., & Lok, B. (2012). The use of virtual patients in medical school curricula. *Advances in Physiology Education*, *36*(1), 48–53. https://doi.org/10.1152/advan.00054.2011

Chang, E. S., Simon, M., & Dong, X. Q. (2012). Integrating cultural humility into health care professional education and training. *Advances in Health Sciences Education*, *17*(2), 269–278. https://doi.org/10.1007/s10459-010-9264-1

Chick, R. C., Clifton, G. T., Peace, K. M., Propper, B. W., Hale, D. F., Alseidi, A. A., & Vreeland, T. J. (2020). Using technology to maintain the education of residents during the COVID-19 pandemic. *Journal of Surgical Education*, *77*(4), 729–732. https://doi.org/10.1016/j.jsurg.2020.03.018

Cleland, J. A., Abe, K., & Rethans, J. J. (2009). The use of simulated patients in medical education: AMEE Guide No 42. *Medical Teacher*, *31*(6), 477–486. https://doi.org/10.1080/01421590903002821

Colby, S. L., & Ortman, J. M. (2015). *Projections of the size and composition of the U.S. population 2014–2060*. Census.gov. www.census.gov/population/projections/data/national/2014.html

Churchouse, C., & McCafferty, C. (2012). Standardized patients versus simulated patients: is there a difference? *Clinical Simulation in Nursing*, *8*(8), e363–e365. https://doi.org/10.1016/j.ecns.2011.04.008

Conigliaro, R. L., Peterson, K. D., & Stratton, T. D. (2020). Lack of diversity in simulation technology. *Simulation in Healthcare*, *15*(2), 112–114. https://doi.org/10.1097/SIH.0000000000000405

Davies, P. G., Spencer, S. J., & Steele, C. M. (2005). Clearing the air: Identity safety moderates the effects of stereotype threat on women's leadership aspirations. *Journal of Personality and Social Psychology*, *88*(2), 276–287. https://psycnet.apa.org/doi/10.1037/0022-3514.88.2.276

Davis, K. (2017). Activities in geriatrics and gerontology education and research. *Age in Action*, *32*(2), 1–7.

deShazo, R. D. (2020). How American medicine got to this place. *The American Journal of the Medical Sciences*, *359*(2), 63–66. https://doi.org/10.1016/j.amjms.2019.11.003

Feldman, T. M., Kalet, A. L., Sabar, S., & Kachur, E. K. (2006). A randomized trial of teaching clinical skills using virtual and live standardized patients. *Journal of General Internal Medicine*, *21*(5), 424–429. https://doi.org/10.1111/j.1525-1497.2006.00421.x

Foldy, E. G., Rivard, P., & Buckley, T. R. (2009). Power, safety, and learning in racially diverse groups. *Academy of Management Learning & Education*, *8*(1), 25–41. https://doi.org/10.5465/amle.2009.37012177

Foronda, C. L., Baptiste, D. L., Pfaff, T., Velez, R., Reinholdt, M., Sanchez, M., & Hudson, K. W. (2018). Cultural competency and cultural humility in simulation-based education: An integrative review. *Clinical Simulation in Nursing*, *15*, 42–60. https://doi.org/10.1016/j.ecns.2017.09.006

Foronda, C. L., Prather, S. L., Baptiste, D., Townsend-Chambers, C., Mays, L., & Graham, C. (2020). Underrepresentation of racial diversity in simulation: An international study. *Nursing Education Perspectives*, *41*(3), 152–156. https://doi.org/10.1097/01.NEP.0000000000000511

Gannon, J., Motycka, C., Egelund, E., Kraemer, D., Smith, W., & Solomon, K. (2017). Teaching end-of-life care using interprofessional simulation. *Journal of Nursing Education*, *56*(4), 205–210. https://doi.org/10.3928/01484834-20170323-03

Gee, G. C., & Ford, C. L. (2011). Structural racism and health inequities: Old issues, New Directions1. *Du Bois Review: Social Science Research on Race*, *8*(1), 115. https://dx.doi.org/10.1017%2FS1742058X11000130

Gliva-McConvey, G., Nicholas, C., & Clark, L (Eds.). (2020). *Comprehensive healthcare simulation: Implementing best practices in standardized patient methodology*. Springer Publishing.

Good, M. D., James, C., Good, B. J., & Becker, A. F. (2005). The culture of medicine and racial, ethnic, and class disparities in healthcare. In *The blackwell companion to social inequalities* (pp. 396–423). Malden, MA: Blackwell Publishing, Ltd.

Goodman, J. H., & Winter, S. G. (2017). Review of use of standardized patients in psychiatric nursing education. *Journal of the American Psychiatric Nurses Association*, *23*(5), 360–374. https://doi.org/10.1177%2F1078390317712697

Gordon, M., Fell, C. W. R., Bos, H., Farrell, M., & Stewart, A. (2017). Learning health 'safety' within non-technical skills interprofessional simulation education: A qualitative study. *Medical Education Online*, *22*(1), 1272838. https://doi.org/10.1080/10872981.2017.1272838

Guiton, G., Hodgson, C. S., May, W., Elliott, D., & Wilkerson, L. (2004, April 12). Assessing medical students' cross-cultural skills in an objective structured clinical examination. https://escholarship.org/uc/item/71z975w3

Harden, R. M., & Gleeson, F. A. (1979). Assessment of clinical competence using an objective structured clinical examination (OSCE). *Medical Education*, *13*(1), 39–54. https://doi.org/10.1111/j.1365-2923.1979.tb00918.x

Hellman, A. N., Cass, C., Cathey, H., Smith, S. L., & Hurley, S. (2018). Understanding poverty: Teaching social justice in undergraduate nursing education. *Journal of Forensic Nursing*, *14*(1), 11–17. 10.1097/JFN.0000000000000182

Holm, A. L., Gorosh, M. R., Brady, M., & White-Perkins, D. (2017). Recognizing privilege and bias: an interactive exercise to expand health care providers' personal awareness. *Academic Medicine*, *92*(3), 360–364. https://doi.org/10.1097/ACM.0000000000001290

Isaacson, M. (2014). Clarifying concepts: Cultural humility or competency. *Journal of Professional Nursing*, *30*(3), 251–258. https://doi.org/10.1016/j.profnurs.2013.09.011

Josiah Macy, Jr. (n.d.). *Foundation*. https://macyfoundation.org

Kaplonyi, J., Bowles, K. A., Nestel, D., Kiegaldie, D., Maloney, S., Haines, T., & Williams, C. (2017). Understanding the impact of simulated patients on health care learners' communication skills: A systematic review. *Medical Education*, *51*(12), 1209–1219. https://doi.org/10.1111/medu.13387

Kenny, G., Cargil, J., Hamilton, C., & Sales, R. (2016). Improving and validating children's nurses' communication skills with standardized patients in end of life care. *Journal of Child Health Care*, *20*(2), 145–152. https://doi.org/10.1177%2F1367493514555588

Kneebone, R., Nestel, D., Wetzel, C., Black, S., Jacklin, R., Aggarwal, R., & Darzi, A. (2006). The human face of simulation: Patient-focused simulation training. *Academic Medicine*, *81*(10), 919–924. https://doi.org/10.1097/01.ACM.0000238323.73623.c2

Kolbe, M., Eppich, W., Rudolph, J., Meguerdichian, M., Catena, H., Cripps, A., & Cheng, A. (2020). Managing psychological safety in debriefings: A dynamic balancing act. *BMJ Simulation and Technology Enhanced Learning*, *6*(3). http://dx.doi.org/10.1136/bmjstel-2019-000470

Koo, L., Layson-Wolf, C., Brandt, N., Hammersla, M., Idzik, S., Rocafort, P., & Windemuth, B. (2014). Qualitative evaluation of a standardized patient clinical simulation for nurse practitioner and pharmacy students. *Nurse Education in Practice*, *14*(6), 740–746. https://doi.org/10.1016/j.nepr.2014.10.005

Kretzschmar, R. M. (1978). Evolution of the gynecology teaching associate: An education specialist. *American Journal of Obstetrics and Gynecology*, *131*(4), 367–373. https://doi.org/10.1016/0002-9378(78)90409-X

Kumagai, A. K., & Lypson, M. L. (2009). Beyond cultural competence: Critical consciousness, social justice, and multicultural education. *Academic Medicine*, *84*(6), 782–787. https://doi.org/10.1097/ACM.0b013e3181a42398

Lau, P. M. Y., Woodward-Kron, R., Livesay, K., Elliott, K., & Nicholson, P. (2016). Cultural respect encompassing simulation training: Being heard about health through broadband. *Journal of Public Health Research*, *5*(1). pp. 36–42. https://doi.org/10.4081/jphr.2016.657

Lewis, K. L., Bohnert, C. A., Gammon, W. L., Hölzer, H., Lyman, L., Smith, C., & Gliva-McConvey, G. (2017). The association of standardized patient educators (ASPE) standards of best practice (SOBP). *Advances in. Simulation*, *2*(1), 1–8. https://doi.org/10.1186/s41077-017-0043-4

Lewis-Pierre, M., & Sanko, J. (2020). Sigma 31st International Nursing Research Congress). *Exploring the impact of chaplains in interprofessional end-of-life simulation with undergraduate nursing students*. To be Presented at Sigma 31st International Nursing Research Congress Virtual Conference.

Lewis-Pierre, L., Mckay, M., Sanko, J., Gattamorta, K., & Azaiza, K. (2019). Comparing online module with simulation on Attitudes toward the dying. *Journal of Palliative Care*, *34*(4), 218–223. https://doi.org/10.1177/0825859719829491

Lewis-Pierre, M., & Sanko,J.(2020). *Exploring the impact of chaplains in interprofessional end-of-life simulation with undergraduate nursing students*. Sigma 31st International Nursing Research Congress Virtual Conference.sigma.nursingrepository.org.

Liaison Committee on Medical Education http://lcme.org/

Lioce, L., Lopreiato, J., Downing, D., Chang, T. P., Robertson, J. M., Anderson, M., Diaz, D. A., Spain, A. E., & the Terminology and Concepts Working Group. (2020). *Healthcare simulation dictionary–Second Edition*. Agency for Healthcare Research and Quality. AHRQ Publication No. 20-0019

Loeb, A. E., Rao, S. S., Ficke, J. R., Morris, C. D., Riley, L. H., & Levin, A. S. (2020). Departmental experience and lessons learned with accelerated introduction of telemedicine during the COVID-19 crisis. *The Journal of the American Academy of Orthopaedic Surgeons*, e469–e476. https://doi.org/10.5435/JAAOS-D-20-00380

Lopreiato, J., Downing, D., & Gammon, W. *Terminology & concepts working group. healthcare simulation dictionary*. 2016file:///C:/Users/Paul%20Prior/Downloads/Sim-Dictionary%20(1).pdf

Luctkar-Flude, M., Hopkins-Rosseel, D., Jones-Hiscock, C., Pulling, C., Gauthier, J., Knapp, A., & Brown, C. (2016). Interprofessional infection control education using standardized patients for nursing, medical and physiotherapy students. *Journal of Interprofessional Education & Practice*, 2, 25–31. https://doi.org/10.1016/j.xjep.2016.03.004

MacLean, S., Kelly, M., Geddes, F., & Della, P. (2017). Use of simulated patients to develop communication skills in nursing education: An integrative review. *Nurse Education Today*, *48*, 90–98. https://doi.org/10.1016/j.nedt.2016.09.018

McIntosh, M. L. (2020). From ally to activist: Embracing activism as an essential component of social justice educational leadership to combat injustice in American schools. *Journal for Leadership, Equity, and Research*, *6*(2), 1–14.

Mckenzie, F. D., Garcia, H. M., Castelino, R. J., Hubbard, T. W., Ullian, J. A., & Gliva, G. A. (2004). *Augmented standardized patients now virtually a reality*. Third IEEE and ACM International Symposium on Mixed and Augmented Reality. (pp. 270–271). https://doi.org/10.1109/ISMAR.2004.18

McNaughton, N. (2012). *A theoretical analysis of the field of human simulation and the role of emotion and affect in the work of standardized patients*. Unpublished, Doctoral Degree, University of Toronto. http://hdl.handle.net/1807/32770

McNaughton, N., & Anderson, M. (2017). Standardized patients: It's all in the words. *Clinical Simulation in Nursing*, *13*(7), 293–294. https://doi.org/10.1016/j.ecns.2017.05.014

Miller, J. L., Avery, M. D., Larson, K., Woll, A., Vonachen, A., & Mortenson, A. (2015). Emergency birth hybrid simulation with standardized patients in midwifery education: Implementation and evaluation. *Journal of Midwifery & Women's Health, 60*(3), 298–303. https://doi.org/10.1111/jmwh.12276

National Museum of African American History & Culture. (n.d). *Talking about race*. https://nmaahc.si.edu/learn/talking-about-race/topics/being-antiracist

Ndiwane, A., Koul, O., & Theroux, R. (2014). Implementing standardized patients to teach cultural competency to graduate nursing students. *Clinical Simulation in Nursing, 10*(2), E87–E94. https://doi.org/10.1016/j.ecns.2013.07.002

Nestel, D., & Bearman, M. (2014). *Simulated patient methodology: Theory, evidence and practice*. John Wiley & Sons.

Newble, D. (2004). Techniques for measuring clinical competence: Objective structured clinical examinations. *Medical Education, 38*(2), 199–203. https://doi.org/10.1111/j.1365-2923.2004.01755.x

Nicholas, C., Cohen-Tigor, D., LaMarra, D., Smith, C., Gliva-McConvey, G., & Chapin, A. (2020). Chapter 10 standardized/simulated patient program management and administration- spinning plates. In G. Gliva-McConvey, C. Nicholas, & L. Clark (Eds.), *Comprehensive healthcare simulation: Implementing best practices in standardized patient methodology*. Springer Publishing.

Oppel, R. A., Gebeloff, R., Rebeca Lai, K. K., Wright, W., & Smith, M. (2020, July 5). The fullest look yet at the racial inequity of coronavirus. *New York Times*. https://www.nytimes.com/interactive/2020/07/05/us/coronavirus-latinos-african-americans-cdc-data.html

Pritchard, S. A., Blackstock, F. C., Keating, J. L., & Nestel, D. (2017). The pillars of well-constructed simulated patient programs: A qualitative study with experienced educators. *Medical Teacher, 39*(11), 1159–1167. https://doi.org/10.1080/0142159X.2017.1369015

Pritchard, S. A., Denning, T., Keating, J. L., Blackstock, F. C., & Nestel, D. (2020). "It's not an acting Job… Don't underestimate what a simulated patient does": A qualitative study exploring the perspectives of simulated patients in health professions education. *Simulation in Healthcare, 15*(1), 21–29. https://doi.org/10.1097/SIH.0000000000000400

Rutherford-Hemming, T., Alfes, C. M., & Breymier, T. L. (2019). A systematic review of the use of standardized patients as a simulation modality in nursing education. *Nursing Education Perspectives, 40*(2), E1–E2. https://doi.org/10.1097/01.NEP.0000000000000401

San, E. O. (2015). Using clinical simulation to enhance culturally competent nursing care: A review of the literature. *Clinical Simulation in Nursing, 11*(4), 228–243. https://doi.org/10.1016/j.ecns.2015.01.004

Sanko, J., Schneidereith, T., Cowperthwait, A., & Onello, R. (2020). Findings from a human roles terminology survey: Consensus or chaos? *BMJ Simulation and Technology Enhanced Learning, 6*(3), 1–6. http://dx.doi.org/10.1136/bmjstel-2018-000378

Sanko, J., Shekhter, I., Rosen, L., Arheart, K., & Birnbach, D. (2012). Man versus machine: The preferred modality. *Clinical Teacher, 9*(6), 387–391. https://doi.org/10.1111/j.1743-498X.2012.00593.x

Sarmasoglu, S., Dinç, L., & Elçin, M. (2016). Using standardized patients in nursing education: Effects on students' psychomotor skill development. *Nurse Educator*, *41*(2), E1–E5. https://doi.org/10.1097/NNE.0000000000000188

Schlegel, C., Bonvin, R., Rethans, J. J., & Van der Vleuten, C. (2016). Standardized patients' perspectives on workplace satisfaction and work-related relationships: A multicenter study. *Simulation in Healthcare*, *11*(4), 278–285. https://doi.org/10.1097/SIH.0000000000000160

Shawler, C. (2008). Standardized patents: A creative teaching strategy for psychiatric-mental health nurse practitioner students. *Journal of Nursing Education*, *47*(11), 528–531. https://doi.org/10.3928/01484834-20081101-08

Shawler, C. (2011). Palliative and end of life care: Using a standardized patient family for Gerontological nurse practitioner students. *Nursing Education Perspectives*, *32*(3), 168–172.

Simmenroth-Nayda, A., Marx, G., Lorkowski, T., & Himmel, W. (2016). Working as simulated patient has effects on real patient life–preliminary insights from a qualitative study. *GMS Journal for Medical Education*, *33*(3). https://doi.org/10.3205/zma001041

Sittner, B. J., Aebersold, M. L., Paige, J. B., Graham, L. L., Schram, A. P., Decker, S. I., & Lioce, L. (2015). INACSL standards of best practice for simulation: Past, present, and future. *Nursing Education Perspectives*, *36*(5), 294–298. https://doi.org/10.5480/15-1670

Stillman, P. L., Brown, D. R., Redfield, D. L., & Sabers, D. L. (1997). Construct validation of the Arizona clinical interview rating scale. *Educational and Psychological Measurement*, *37*, 1031–1038.

Stillman, P. L., Gregorio, B. D., Michele, Y., Nicholson, G. I., Sabers, D. L., & Stillman, A. E. (1983). Six years of experience using patient instructors to teach interviewing skills. *Journal of Medical Education*. *58*(12), 941–946.

Stillman, P. L., Sabers, D. L., & Redfield, D. L. (1976). The use of paraprofessionals to teach interviewing skills. *Pediatrics*, *57*, 769–774.

Stillman, P. L., Sabers, D. L., & Redfield, D. L. (1977). Use of trained mothers to teach interviewing skills to first-year medical students: A follow-up study. *Pediatrics*, *60*(2), 165–169.

Swanson, D. B., & Stillman, P. L. (1990). Use of standardized patients for teaching and assessing clinical skills. *Evaluation & the Health Professions*, *13*(1), 79–103.

Swiggart, W. H., Ghulyan, M. V., & Dewey, C. M. (2012). Using standardized patient in continuing medical education courses on proper prescribing of controlled substances. *Journal of Substance Abuse*, *33*(2), 182–185. https://doi.org/10.1080/08897077.2011.640217

Talbot, T. B., Sagae, K., John, B., & Rizzo, A. (2012). Designing useful virtual standardized patient encounters. *Interservice Industry Training, Simulation, and Educational Conference proceeding*, *12354*, 1–11.

Tervalon, M., & Murray-Garcia, J. (1998). Cultural humility versus cultural competence: A critical distinction in defining physician training outcomes in multicultural education. *Journal of Health Care for the Poor and Underserved*, *9*(2), 117–125. https://doi.org/10.1353/hpu.2010.0233

Truglio, J., Lynch, G., Palermo, A. G., Hojsak, J., Sainte, M., & Karani, R. (2020). Deconstructing racism and bias in clinical medicine. In M. H. Swartz (Ed.), *Textbook of physical diagnosis* (8th ed., pp. 64–83). New York Elsevier.

Tuzer, H., Dinc, L., & Elcin, M. (2016). The effects of using high-fidelity simulators and standardized patients on the thorax, lung, and cardiac examination skills of undergraduate nursing students. *Nurse Education Today*, *45*, 120–125. https://doi.org/10.1016/j.nedt.2016.07.002

United States Medical Licensing Examination. (2019, September). *Step 2 clinical skills: Content description and general information*. https://www.usmle.org/pdfs/step-2-cs/cs-info-manual.pdf

van der Vleuten, C. P., & Swanson, D. B. (1990). Assessment of clinical skills with standardized patients: State of the art. *Teaching and Learning in Medicine: An International Journal*, *2*(2), 58–76. https://doi.org/10.1080/10401339009539432

Vessy, J. A., & Huss, K. (2002). Using standardized patients in advance practice nursing education. *Journal of Professional Nursing*, *18*(1), 29–35. https://doi.org/10.1053/jpnu.2002.30898

Wallace, P. (1997). Following the threads of an innovation: The history of standardized patients in medical education. *Caduceus (Springfield, Ill.)*, *13*(2), 5–28.

Wallerstein, N., Duran, B., Minkler, M., & Foley, K. (2005). Developing and maintaining partnerships with communities.In (Ed) Israel, BA, Eng, E, Schulz, AJ & Parker, EA *Methods in Community-Based Participatory Research for Health*, Second Ed. 31–51. San Francisco: Josey-Bass.

Weinick, R. M., Elliott, M. N., Volandes, A. E., Lopez, L., Burkhart, Q., & Schlesinger, M. (2011). Using standardized encounters to understand reported racial/ethnic disparities in patient experiences with care. *Health Services Research*, *46*(2), 491–509. https://doi.org/10.1111/j.1475-6773.2010.01214.x

Webster, D. (2013). Promoting therapeutic communication and patient-centered care using standardized patients. *Journal of Nursing Education*, 52(11), 645–648. https://doi.org/10.3928/01484834-20131014-06

Wilkerson, L., Fung, C. C., May, W., & Elliott, D. (2010). Assessing patient-centered care: one pproach to health disparities education. *Journal of General Internal Medicine*, *25*(2), 86–90. https://doi.org/10.1007/s11606-010-1273-5

Wisborg, T., Brattebø, G., Brinchmann-Hansen, A., & Hansen, K. S. (2009). Manikin or standardized patient: Participants' assessment of two training modalities in trauma team simulation. *Scandinavian Journal of Trauma, Resuscitation and Emergency Medicine*, 17, 59. https://doi.org/10.1186/1757-7241-17-59

Woolsey, C., & Narruhn, R. (2020). Structural competency: A pilot study. *Public Health Nursing*. https://doi.org/10.1111/phn.12756

Yoo, M. S., & Yoo, I. Y. (2003). The effectiveness of standardized patients as a teaching method for nursing fundamentals. *The Journal of Nursing Education,* 42(10), 444–448. https://doi.org/10.3928/0148-4834-20031001-06

Zhou, T., Huang, S., Cheng, J., & Xiao, Y. (2020). The distance teaching practice of combined mode of massive open online course micro-video for interns in emergency department during the COVID-19 epidemic period. *Telemedicine and e-Health,* 26(5), 584–588.

Zitzelsberger, H., Coffey, S., Graham, L., Papaconstantinou, E., & Anyinam, C. (2017). Exploring simulation utilization and simulation evaluation practices and approaches in undergraduate nursing education. *Journal of Education and Practice,* 8(3), 155–164.

Part II

Hospital-Based and Interprofessional Simulation

CHAPTER 4

Hospital-Based Simulation

J. Cedar Wang and Lori Podlinski

ABSTRACT

This chapter discusses the current state of hospital-based simulation, including the unprecedented events of 2020's global COVID-19 pandemic. Hospital-based simulation training requires a new approach. The realities of social distancing and the operational demands of hospital staffing ratios warrant creative adaptations of traditional simulation training methods. Hospitals used simulation to improve patient outcomes by training healthcare staff and students through telesimulation, and tested systems and equipment using in situ simulation (ISS). Latent safety threats (LSTs) were identified and corrected to improve patient outcomes. Hospital-based simulation has been incorporated into newly licensed registered nurses (NLRNs) residency programs to prepare them for competent practice. Simulations are also used for preparing staff for low-incidence, high-risk medical emergencies or disasters, such as active shooter events. Hospital-based simulation training adds value to healthcare systems, but requires more evidence of its quantitative and qualitative impacts.

http://dx.doi.org/10.1891/0739-6686.39.83

HOSPITAL-BASED SIMULATION

Hospitals compete for customers through "Five-Star Ratings," Leapfrog Safety Grades, and other reportable metrics by focusing on improving value and quality while attempting to spur innovation and differentiate themselves from competitors (Federal Trade Commission, 2020). Publicly reportable quality scores inform consumers about what goes on inside the doors of a hospital. These may even define the probability of making it out of the door alive (Agency for Healthcare Research and Quality [AHRQ], 2016). Currently, medical error is the third leading cause of death in the United States (Mackary & Daniel, 2016). The Joint Commission consistently identifies breakdowns in healthcare provider communication as the leading cause of sentinel events worldwide (Dingley et al., 2018). In response to market forces demanding excellence in healthcare delivery, alongside an ethical demand for improved patient safety, hospitals must equip a workforce that exceeds expectations. While skills and knowledge are acquired more readily through formal training, soft skills such as communication and emotionally intelligent behaviors are lacking (Jackson et al., 2016; Lavelle et al., 2019). How will hospitals manage to equip a workforce able to meet the high standards of quality and safety that is both morally above reproach and demanded by today's savvy consumers?

Becker's Hospital Review (2017) reported 58 hospitals with notable "innovation programs," but this list contains only a snapshot of programs existing across the United States. More than half of this list identified similar efforts to drive progress in patient care, enhance quality and safety, and promote a positive patient experience *through hospital-based simulation programs*. The controlled environment of simulation allows healthcare professionals the opportunity to practice technical and soft skills. More important than the acquisition of these skills, practicing in a simulated environment ensures maintenance of skills over time that can ensure consistent quality and safety outcomes (Bukhari et al., 2017; Lavelle et al., 2019).

In 2003, Dr. Amitai Ziv at Chaim Sheba Medical Center, Tel Aviv, Israel, and colleagues published a compelling article identifying simulation education as an "ethical imperative" for those training in hospitals (p. 786). The authors caution, "The application of modern medical technologies requires complex team interactions that mandate improved training techniques" (p.784). This message condemns the common practice of "see one, do one, teach one," in which patients are "commodities to be used as conveniences of training," and challenges the healthcare community to use simulation methods such as standardized patients (SPs) and human patient simulators to recreate real-life scenarios (Ziv et al., 2003, p. 784). The increase in simulation programs to train healthcare providers soon followed. However, the use of simulation in the hospital environment is not well represented in the literature (Harper et al., 2018).

Patient Safety

System or human error harms an estimated 1.5 million individuals in the United States. The Joint Commission requires that all healthcare institutions conduct root cause analysis (RCA) of adverse events and develop methods to prevent future incidents. RCA helps to identify underlying problems that might cause medical errors. Current literature on the use of simulation for investigating adverse events is lacking. Cooper (2020) discusses the use of a reenactment of an adverse event in the operating room in the mid-1980s. This reenactment would now be called simulation. A patient undergoing a CO_2 laser excision of a lesion suffered third-degree burns during an operating room fire initially thought to be spontaneously triggered by a malfunction of the laser. The use of high-fidelity simulation for RCA allowed the investigating team to recreate similar operating room conditions. The staff that was involved in the adverse event was also involved in the reenactment. The simulation determined that the most likely cause of the fire was an inadvertent step by the surgeon on the laser footswitch.

Using simulation for RCA allows the investigation team to view how individuals react in real time. Slakey et al. (2014) conducted a simulation of adverse outcomes (SOA) to investigate the RCA of three adverse surgical events: (a) patient death from failing to recognize a duodenal perforation after a laparoscopic cholecystectomy; (b) patient death from inability to recognize signs and symptoms of postoperative hemorrhage; (c) patient readied for cholecystectomy in operating room yet the patient had it removed in a previous surgery. This identified the failure to complete a thorough workup for right upper quadrant pain. The SOA revealed more potential causes of the adverse event than the traditional RCA format. The SOA identified the healthcare environment and organizational factors that affected medical decision-making.

In 2020, The Joint Commission released the National Patient Safety Goals, including one to improve communication effectiveness among caregivers (The Joint Commission, 2020). Groves et al. (2017) conducted a pilot study to evaluate patient safety behaviors. This group wanted to determine if identifying safety concerns during nursing handoff communication led to a change in nursing "safety-oriented" behaviors. The control group receive a brief handoff, "When he is awake, he's alert, and oriented X3, but restless" (Groves et al., 2017, p. 1401). The intervention group received the same handoff as the control group with the inclusion of embedded references to patient safety, "He's at risk for losing one of the peripheral IV lines because he moves around a lot" (Groves et al., 2017, p. 1401). The study showed a slight difference between the control group and the intervention group. Importantly, the intervention group recognized the specific safety concerns and was able to mitigate risk.

Credentialing/Performance Evaluation

There is limited literature that discusses simulation for Ongoing Professional Practice Evaluation (OPPE) and Focused Professional Practice Evaluation (FPPE) evaluation. OPPE and FPPE are competency assessments of healthcare professionals, required by The Joint Commission, who have been credentialed within the healthcare institution and earned practice privileges. OPPE is the process of evaluating a healthcare professional over time; it is needed to recommend credentialing and privileging. FPPE occurs with new privileges, which can occur at the time of appointment or when the healthcare professional requests new privileges, such as the administration of moderate sedation (Hunt, 2012).

According to The Joint Commission, simulation is a recommended method of data collection for OPPE and FPPE. Wang (2018) created a simulation for newly credentialed emergency medicine physicians seeking moderate sedation privileges. The Chair of Anesthesiology served as the content expert in the creation of the scenarios. To document compliance per The Joint Commission, the simulation staff created a checklist and the simulations were pilot-tested with an emergency room physician and an emergency room registered nurse (RN). After the pilot test, the emergency room staff made recommendations to edit the checklist items to reflect the correct sequence of actions (L. Podlinski, personal communication, March 13, 2017).

Another modality for addressing performance evaluation is web-based simulation that can use a computer, tablet, or mobile device to create a simulated environment (Anderson et al., 2020). Gorrindo et al. (2013) used a web-based simulation to assess physician competence to obtain informed consent before prescribing antipsychotic medications. This study concluded that web-based simulation can be used for competency assessments and is an efficient way to validate a large number of clinicians' competencies.

Nurse Residency Programs

The Institute of Medicine recommends that newly licensed registered nurses (NLRNs) participate in transition-to-practice programs to ease the shift from student to licensed professional (Gooch, 2015). The traditional, didactic form of teaching encourages passive learning. In addition, the clinical preparation students receive in nursing school is not sufficient enough to care for the increasing patient acuity. However, active learning and reflective practice inherent to simulation have proven to enhance critical thinking and teamwork. Rhodes et al. (2016)

evaluated the NLRN knowledge, confidence, and satisfaction following simulations with NLRN-only during the first month of hire and 9 to 12 months after hire with a multidisciplinary crisis scenario. The study found that the NLRN knowledge increased over time for both the NLRN-only and multidisciplinary scenario. The NLRN-only had a higher increase in confidence than those reported for the multidisciplinary scenario. The NLRN had higher satisfaction scores following the multidisciplinary scenario. The study concluded that repeated simulation might contribute to steady gains in knowledge, confidence, and satisfaction for up to 18 months. Rossler and Bennett (2017) conducted a pilot study to explore the NLRNs perceptions of manikin-based simulations incorporated into the medical-surgical residency program. Five simulation-based educational activities focused on patients with cardiac, neurological, gastrointestinal, and transfusion complications. The study found that incorporating simulation into a residency program provided a safe learning environment necessary to gain the knowledge needed to develop the professional role (Rossler & Bennett, 2017).

The American Nurses Credentialing Center (ANCC) offers a credentialing program for transition-to-practice. This program recognizes the increased use of advanced care practitioners (ACPs), such as nurse practitioners (NPs) and physician assistants, and requires nurse residents to practice as members of an interprofessional team (Cosme, 2015). Justus and Appel (2018) found that through simulation, NLRNs were more aware of the information that needed to be communicated to the ACPs during a critical patient incident so that the ACP could accurately diagnose the patient's problem.

As the demand for NPs in intensive care units increases, so does the need for a well-rounded orientation program. Simone et al. (2016) developed a comprehensive competency-based curriculum that included task training in skills labs and high-fidelity simulation exercises. The NPs stated that the skills labs and simulations were valuable to their learning and growth. Additionally, simulation-based education provides NPs with an opportunity to gain critical thinking skills and confidence through repetitive practice on task trainers. However, the creation of evaluation methods to establish competency before the simulation is crucial, and self-assessment and instructor evaluation at the beginning will provide a baseline of knowledge. A time frame should be created as well as a checklist to document competency. Incorporating these key elements can result in a successful transition to practice for the NP (Echenique & Wempe, 2018).

Drills

Drills and simulations provide a safe space for high-risk, low-volume medical emergencies in healthcare facilities (Sheen & Goffman, 2019), such as newborn resuscitation, where a delay of seconds can affect mortality and morbidity. The

Joint Commission Sentinel Event alert also recommends drills to improve team performance during obstetrical emergencies (Arafeh, 2017). Postpartum hemorrhage (PPH) is the most common obstetrical emergency in the United States and the most preventable cause of maternal mortality (Centers for Disease Control and Prevention, 2020; Watkins, 2020). Preparation is key to optimizing patient outcomes during PPH and in situ drills can enhance current clinical skills and improve upon communication and teamwork skills in an environment in which the clinicians will encounter a medical emergency (Inman, 2016; Spiegelman et al., 2018).

Active shooter incidents are rising in the United States and around the globe (Glasofer & Laskowski-Jones, 2019; U.S. Department of Justice et al., 2018). Since most active shooter events conclude prior to law enforcement's arrival, it is vital for hospital staff to be prepared to safely respond (Sanchez et al., 2018). Many healthcare institutions have online modules regarding how to respond to an active shooter event. However, simulation provides staff with an opportunity to be immersed in the event, providing a more realistic situation. There are multiple modalities to simulate an active shooter event: tabletop simulation, simulation with hospital staff only, and full-scale simulation drills with the involvement of local law enforcement. Tabletop simulation is a low-fidelity simulation where learners apply knowledge through a formal discussion and can be considered when hands-on cannot be achieved or before a higher fidelity simulation (Lehtola, 2007).

Mannenbach et al. (2018) conducted an ISS with hospital staff focused on an active shooter event's initial minutes. The simulation scenario lasted only 10 minutes, including the prebrief and debrief. The simulations were short so that they would minimize interference with patient care. It also heightened the participants' awareness of necessary split-second decision-making to run, hide, or fight. They found that some participants ran; however, many participants froze and did not know what to do in this situation. The debriefing following the drill allowed for teachable moments on how to respond to an active shooter event.

A full-scale active shooter drill involves hospital staff, as well as local law enforcement, to test and evaluate responses for all who would be involved in a real active shooter event. A full-scale simulation drill provides the most realistic experience, allowing the full immersion of participants (HNMC Media, 2012).

Being fully immersed can also affect the psychological safety of all participants. Some staff voiced that they found the simulation difficult because they were scared, and some froze and did not know how to respond (Sanchez et al., 2018). Wexler and Flamm (2017) conducted a full-scale simulation drill with the focus on evaluating (a) hospital staff communication, (b) staff communication with local law enforcement, (c) the ability of staff to recognize an armed intruder, (d) assess the emergency department (ED) staff's response to a mass casualty event, and (e) evaluate the ability to evacuate to an alternative care site. The evaluation of this drill assessed strengths and weaknesses. The ED's design was to minimize noise, which led to some staff not hearing the firearm discharge during the simulation.

Using SPs in simulation drills adds to the realism of the event. However, SPs in large-scale hospital drills provide a challenge because these simulations take place in an uncontrolled environment. It is crucial to prepare the SPs for their role thoroughly to help mitigate these challenges. This preparation includes planning a physical walk-through and developing a code word if the SP is uncomfortable at any point during the drill. An observer should be assigned to ensure that no provider performs any invasive procedure on an SP during the drill. This preparation aids in the physical and psychological safety of the SP (Holtscheider, 2017).

Finally, careful multidisciplinary planning of simulation drills is essential. Consider how the simulation drill will impact patient care and the effect of the drill on possible hospital visitors' psychological safety.

SYSTEMS DESIGN

Designing new clinical spaces provides an opportunity to rethink how the design impacts healthcare staff and patient safety. Petrosoniak et al. (2020) used a five-step process of design thinking during the construction of a new ED. This five-step process helped to mitigate patient safety threats and departmental issues.

- Step 1: Engage clinical staff feedback on the current workflow and challenges of the existing clinical space.
- Step 2: Hold interdisciplinary team meetings to define the current issues with workflow processes and systems.
- Step 3: Conduct brainstorming sessions to discuss how to alleviate the current problems in the new clinical space.
- Step 4: Conduct tabletop and mock-up simulations with staff working in the new area, at the same time, getting user feedback as well as observer feedback.
- Step 5: Test the new environment with ISSs before opening the new space with patients (Petrosoniak et al., 2020, p. 207).

ISSs take place in actual hospital rooms or units (Anderson et al., 2020). According to the Society for Simulation in Healthcare, ISS is defined as a simulation that occurs "in the actual patient care setting/environment in an effort to achieve a high level of fidelity and realism" (p. 17). ISS lends itself to timely education in a realistic environment and has been shown to improve teamwork and promote skill development (Petrosoniak et al., 2017; Walsh et al., 2019). This simulation method can help identify systems issues and LSTs that could only be determined if the simulation took place in the real-time work environment (Bapteste et al., 2020; Couto et al., 2018; Holtscheider, 2013; Knight et al., 2018). The definition of LST is "system-based threats to patient safety that can materialize at any time and are previously unrecognized by healthcare providers, unit directors, or hospital administration" (Kearney & Deutsch, 2017, p. 1017).

Francoeur et al. (2018) conducted a study using ISSs to prepare for a move to a new clinical setting. The design of the new facility was significantly different from the current model. This new design required nurses and respiratory therapists to adjust their patient care routines. The simulation found that when patient doors were closed, the hospital staff could not hear patients' call bells. The new system for storing and distributing medications added additional and time-consuming steps in medication acquisition. Power outlets caused a problem as the voltage-limited power outlets were not universal to all equipment and the healthcare provider was required to select the correct outlet for the equipment to function. The code blue button was also challenging to reach on the booms. Medical equipment booms centralize equipment in patient care areas such as the operating room, intensive care unit, and ED (STERIS Healthcare, 2018). The location of phones was outside patient rooms, which were not easily accessible during an emergency. Results from the simulations led to changes in the new clinical setting to promote patient safety. Doors are now left open for critical patients, the power outlets are now labeled, and phones are now located at the patient's bedside.

A similar simulation on relocating clinical operations to a new space was reported by Knippa and Senecal (2017). In this publication, staff nurses created a survey to evaluate confidence finding equipment and supplies, operating the new equipment, communicating with other healthcare professionals on the unit, and caring for patients in the newly designed space. The survey found that there was a decrease in the staff's perceived ability to know when other team members needed assistance or if an unsafe condition existed on the unit. Following the ISS, there was a statistically significant improvement in the confidence of staff who operated new equipment and their ability to safely care for patients (Knippa & Senecal, 2017). There were a few limitations in this study. Not all equipment was available at the time of this study, which may have impacted the staff's awareness of the new work environment. The wireless phones for communication were not fully functional, which may have contributed to the decrease in staff's knowledge of needed assistance or unsafe conditions. However, this study confirms the essential role that the nursing professional development practitioner plays in staff education and preparation for change.

Bender and Maryman (2018) used ISS to develop a new neonatal intensive care unit (NICU). The new space was two times the size of the previous, with a longer distance between areas, such as the operating room. Using simulation before opening the new unit to test systems and staff readiness identified LSS and resulted in their correction. One noted additional benefit, which was not an outcome measured in the study, was that staff felt positive about the anticipated move to a new unit.

Simulation can also be used to evaluate processes in existing patient care areas. Cardiac arrest is a rare complication, but cardiac arrest in an MRI scanner is loaded with additional challenges and complications related to the safety precautions required from the MRI's magnet. Czekajlo and Dabrowska (2017) conducted a pilot study to identify failure modes and causes in an adult cardiac arrest simulation scenario in an MRI scanner. Results of this pilot study validated the staff's awareness of the safety risks when healthcare providers respond to patient emergencies in an MRI scanner. The ISS also identified LST of a of a 45-second delay in activating the code team during the simulation. The MRI technician accurately called the operator to activate the code; however, the operator placed the call on hold for 45 seconds before confirming activation of the code team. This systems error delayed activation of appropriate personnel to respond to an emergency, which can lead to negative patient outcomes.

VALUE AND RETURN ON INVESTMENT

A hospital's decision to invest in operational and physical resources for simulation education requires a cost-benefit analysis that differs from that of an academic institution. Generally, hospitals calculate revenue by square footage based on the number of beds they house. Each bed is estimated to drive an average bottom line, allowing financial executives to build an operational budget (Kalman et al., 2015). Liu et al. (2012) describe how teaching and nonteaching hospitals generate income based on reimbursement from insurance companies including private and government plans (e.g., Medicare, Medicaid.) A hospital-based simulation center does not generate payer revenue. Simulation programs require considerable investment in physical and human capital; therefore, fees collected from individual clients or departments that use the center may be less than the center's costs for simulation planning and implementation. The onus of demonstrating value to the organization lies in the simulation center itself (Hippe et al., 2020).

Cost

Identifying the cost of simulation programs is an essential first step in establishing their value (Cook, 2013). Zendejas et al. (2013) identify a void of data related to the costs associated with creating and implementing simulation programs, making it difficult to determine the value of simulation or its effect on quality and safety outcome measures. Elements to consider include simulator and equipment prices and maintenance, development costs (including faculty time), facility overhead, and—most relevant in hospitals—replacement costs for simulation participants (Bukhari et al., 2017; Cook, 2013). For example, a nurse scheduled and paid to attend a day of simulation training requires the staffing of an additional nurse at the bedside to render patient care. This indirect cost of training staff who bill for services provided (e.g., physician, NP) can mount even faster than for an hourly employee (e.g., staff nurse). The first step in considering simulation's value requires careful consideration of both direct (e.g., invoices) and indirect (e.g., overhead) costs (Asche et al., 2020).

There is a void of data comparing the costs of creating and implementing simulation programs. Less than 1% of simulation research articles demonstrate sufficient cost data that can be used to compare simulation methods (e.g., manikin-based simulation, computer-based simulation; Asche et al., 2020; Zendejas et al., 2013). The lack of studies evaluating the impacts of simulation training on practicing nurses rather than student nurses further challenges the cost evaluation for hospital-based simulation programs (Elgin & Poston, 2019). The challenges of simulation costs in the hospital setting require careful analysis of costs versus benefits of various simulation modalities. Should nurses be required to physically attend manikin-based simulation training (more costly method), or would a cheaper, computer-based scenario reap the same educational benefits? Current studies focusing on cost and benefits do not include practicing nurses. However, one study compared learning outcomes and cost-effectiveness of manikin versus virtual simulation training on a cohort of nursing students. Haerling (2018) randomly assigned 84 nursing students to either a manikin-based simulation group or a virtual simulation group to complete the same scenario. The results yielded a favorable cost-utility ratio and no significant differences in learning outcomes or subsequent clinical performance. The manikin-based simulation scenario costs three times as much to implement as the virtual version, making the virtual simulation option a potential opportunity for training practicing nurses.

Value

The concept of simulation's value offsets the burden of cost and is an equally important consideration for hospital-based simulation programs. Bukhari et al. (2017) adapt the value measurement methodology (VMM) initially created by the United States government to identify five value categories applicable to a hospital-based simulation program's evaluation of simulation training. These include direct value, social value, operational value, strategic value, and financial value. The direct value represents the benefit of simulation to train someone to do their job function. The social value characterizes society's benefit, such as lower complication rates, infections, falls, and other quality indicators. The operational value constitutes the effect on productivity measures such as length of stay and throughput efficiencies. Consideration of the strategic value alludes to the impact on higher level concepts such as patient safety culture. Finally, the financial value assesses the simulation's economic impact on the organization through increased revenue and potential cost control. Utilizing VMM enables hospital-based simulation programs to identify the intangible and tangible benefits of simulation training, which serve as essential variables in calculating and communicating value to the organization.

Return on Investment

ROI and economic calculations yield an additional measure of simulation's value (Asche et al., 2020). Return on investment (ROI) is calculated as ROI% = (net profit/cost of investment) x 100, with a favorable ROI being greater than zero (Fiorillo, 2019). Net benefits, including profits and perceived improvements, are more difficult to define compared to cost of investments. Bukhari et al. suggest first differentiating between qualitative and quantitative benefits and then incorporating Phillip's ROI methodology (discussed below; Phillips et al., 2013). Qualitative benefits are more challenging to isolate but include perceived benefits in employee or patient satisfaction, public perception, and enhancements to patient safety culture. Quantitative benefits may include accomplishing an objective or procedure in less time, with greater accuracy, less error, and with measurable outcome improvements (Bukhari et al., 2017).

Phillips refers to Kirkpatrick's four levels of evaluation by adding a fifth element of "business value" to Dr. Kirkpatrick's standard four items: reaction, learning, behavior, and results (see Chapters 2 and 7). Phillip's fifth addition of business value requires an assessment of the impact of a training program on an organization. Trainees estimate the impact the training will have on their job performance or other outcomes in a quantifiable manner. Generally, a pre- and postevaluation tool measures perceived performance improvement in this manner. Subsequently, administrative stakeholders review the results and adjust the overall projected impact on the organization (Phillips et al., 2013). The Phillip's method incorporates both quantitative and qualitative benefits in calculating ROI.

Establishing the ROI of simulation education in the hospital setting requires identification of strategic initiatives that carry intrinsic value to an organization. Many hospitals have identified a preparation-practice gap in the new nursing workforce (Benner et al., 2010, as cited in Zimmerman & House, 2016). Nursing schools work on revising curricula to address this gap by promoting simulation training and opportunities to hone critical thinking skills. Hospitals will benefit from continuing these training efforts to mitigate the expensive errors resulting from knowledge gaps. Nursing students learn to safely administer medications in their schools of nursing. However, costly errors occur as novice nurses are more susceptible to commit medication errors due to lack of experience (Sanko & McKay, 2017). The cost burden of such errors thus lies with their employer, the hospital. Zimmerman and House (2016) propose simulation as a means to reduce the cost of medication errors. They estimate that adding an extra day of high-fidelity simulation-based medication administration training to nursing orientation can result in decreased medication errors and a cost savings of $461,200 per hospital within 7.5 months.

While this particular ROI example is only an estimate, simulation impacts other important nurse-driven safety initiatives. Elgin and Poston (2019) recognized a void of published simulation research assessing the impact of simulation training on practicing nurses' compliance with best-practice standards. The transfer of critical patient information is a noted safety hazard. Dingley et al. (2018) identified nurse-to-nurse bedside shift report as a potential training opportunity. After completing training based on best-practice standards and practicing these skills in two simulated scenarios, nurses were followed for 6 weeks in the clinical setting. The results yield a statistically significant ($p < .001$), sustained improvement in RN shift-to-shift report based on compliance with best practice (Elgin & Poston, 2019). Further application of these training methods and subsequent outcomes-based research will contribute to growing evidence of favorable ROI examples for hospital-based simulation programs.

HOSPITAL-BASED SIMULATION AND COVID-19

The novel COVID-19 virus has forced the reengineering of healthcare education. Social distancing requirements have left healthcare educators questioning how to train while protecting all learners and staff. Additionally, which technical, non-technical, and soft skills are viable options for distance learning? Telesimulation "a process by which telecommunication and simulation resources are utilized to provide education, training, and/or assessment to learners at an offsite location" (Papanagnou, 2017, p.137) is relatively new. The telesimulation platform offers access to simulation experiences in the social distancing era. Also, it provides a platform for learners who do not have access to a simulation center.

One of the major obstacles that resulted from the shutdown of nonessential medical interventions was the deployment of non-ICU healthcare providers needed to manage ICU-level patients. Telesimulation has allowed for remote training of staff to care for these individuals. Naik et al. (2020) report on the creation of a hybrid telesimulation that was used to educate nurses on COVID-19 ventilator strategies with just-in-time training. Prior to the telesimulation, the learners viewed an online video tutorial on the fundamentals of ventilator management. The learners then participated in a synchronous telesimulation of a virtual care team consisting of noncritical care providers to manage the ventilator of a COVID-19- positive patient experiencing respiratory distress. Simulation center staff operated the high-fidelity manikin via a wireless tablet computer. A monitor displayed the manikin's vital signs, and a band wrapped around the manikin's lungs created pulmonary resistance. A portable camera system provided real-time images of the ventilator and vital signs. The virtual meeting room provided images of the manikin, vital sign monitor, and ventilator throughout the simulation. The virtual care team was responsible for managing the ventilator in response to the patient's vital signs, lung compliance, ventilator pressures, and arterial blood gas values. Postsimulation evaluations showed that the participants felt that the telesimulation felt similar to how it would feel in an in-person simulation because they could remotely manipulate the ventilator settings using embedded (faculty) participants at the patient's bedside (Naik et al., 2020). An embedded participant is "an individual who is trained or scripted to play a role in a simulation encounter to guide the scenario, and may be known or unknown to the participants; guidance may be positive or negative, or a distractor based on the objectives, level of the participants, and the needs of the scenario" (Anderson et al., 2020 p. 16; Chapter 3).

Telesimulation can forge new relationships with other hospital systems and allied health schools. Based on the learning objectives, the instructional design of the telesimulation should account for the learner's knowledge level. Novice learners may not benefit from telesimulation, as they need more guidance at the beginning of their academic journey. Telesimulation provides the flexibility required for simulation education training to continue despite the social distancing restrictions. As telesimulation grows, there is a need to develop best practices and competencies to guide this integrative form of education (Papanagnou, 2017).

During the COVID-19 global pandemic, simulation also played a role in testing new equipment. An increase in the number of patients in a 361-bed, suburban, mid-Atlantic hospital created a shortage in isolation rooms. In collaboration with the hospital's simulation center, the engineering department designed and constructed isopods out of plexiglass and PVC piping. These isopods were connected to negative pressure ventilation, which allowed for more than one patient in a room, helped efficacy of care, and protected the staff. Moving patients throughout the hospital for diagnostic tests and surgeries also created a safety issue, and the creation of transport isopods helped alleviate this risk. The isopods had holes cut in the plexiglass so that staff could attend to the patient's respiratory needs or start an intravenous line if needed (Figure 4.1). While in the isopod, the healthcare provider had full access when necessary to provide emergency patient care (HNMC Media, 2020).

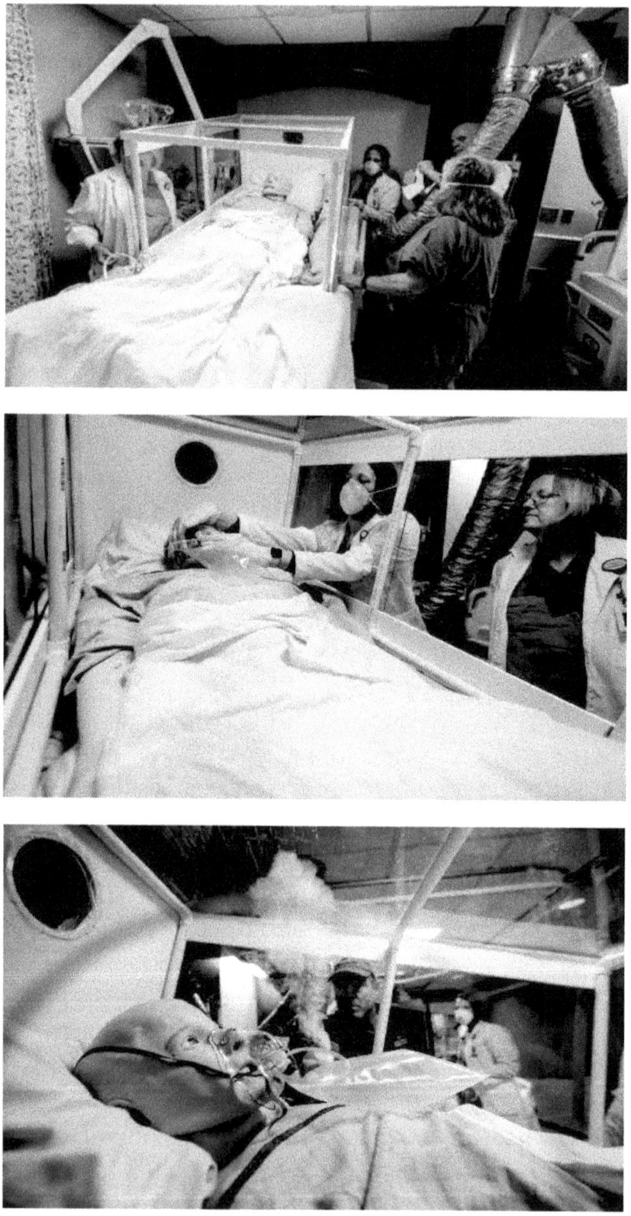

FIGURE 4.1 Photographs of Simulation of Isopod Effectiveness.
Note. Top: Picture of a manikin in an isopod. Middle: Picture of a manikin with a nurse applying 100% nonrebreather masks through hole cut-outs. Bottom: Picture of a manikin aerosolized in negative pressure. Source: Jeff Rhode/Holy Name Medical Center.

EVOLVING SIMULATION METHODS IN HOSPITALS

The new realities of social distancing, mandatory masking during classroom instruction, and the assumption that time spent educating staff is considered non-productive time require creativity and flexibility in designing simulation training. For many hospitals, dedicating otherwise revenue-generating square footage to expensive simulation programs presents challenges. Using existing clinical space for ISS allows for the added benefit of identifying environmental issues contributing to patient safety, operational efficiencies, and patient experience (Ventre et al., 2014).

As another alternative to live training in a simulation lab, virtual simulation provides additional opportunities for learners to engage in training activities without compromising personal or patient safety. Anderson et al. (2020, p. 54) define virtual simulation as "the recreation of reality on a computer screen." Virtual simulation includes augmented reality, virtual reality, and mixed reality applications discussed separately in another chapter.

More research is needed to compare the effectiveness of simulation training among diverse disciplines (Cook, 2013). The nature of hospital-based practice involves multiple disciplines working together. According to Weithholter et al. (2017), there is limited information on the impact of interprofessional collaborative practice (IPCP) of experienced, licensed providers practicing in hospitals today. In their study, 62 nurses, 10 pharmacists, and nine physicians participated in live simulation training, but only the impact of IPE on nurses was measured and found to enhance their perception of IPCP.

In the simulation center, what works for one discipline may not transfer to another. A randomized trial of medical residents training in mechanical ventilation skills showed that skill acquisition was significantly higher in the manikin-based than the computer-based training groups (Spadaro et al., 2017). A prospective, observational, ISS study comparing anesthesia, medical, and surgical critical care providers' procedural performance during central line insertion identified disparate practices. Simulation can uncover and address differences in multidisciplinary practice to ensure adherence to best-practice guidelines while still preserving the distinct realities of various practice environments (Golden et al., 2020).

CONCLUSION

Hospitals use simulation training modalities to equip a modern workforce. Training offerings exist for many clinical disciplines. However, there is an opportunity to include more support staff in this type of training. Societal and ethical demands require an attentive focus on quality and safety standards. Educators and administrators can work collaboratively to ensure accurate value and ROI measures in evaluating simulation methods and programs. These measures are particularly important when adapting to the "new normal" for education at all levels, both academic and practical. Simulation will continue to serve as an essential tool in evaluating participants and the environment of care. As technology advances and the body of simulation research expands, hospitals will leverage forms of immersive simulation training, including manikin-based and computer-based modalities, to promote sustainable performance and process improvements.

REFERENCES

Agency for Healthcare Research and Quality. (2016, March). *Examples of hospital quality measures for consumers*. https://www.ahrq.gov/talkingquality/measures/setting/hospitals/examples.html

Anderson, M., Chang, T., Diaz, D., Downing, D., Lioce, L., Robertson, J., & Spain, A. (2020). *Healthcare simulation dictionary* (2nd ed.). https://www.ssih.org/dictionary

Arafeh, J. M. R. (2017). Update: Simulation-based training. *The Journal of Perinatal & Neonatal Nursing, October/December*, *31*(4), 286–289. https://doi.org/10.1097/JPN.0000000000000288

Asche, C. V., Kim, M., Brown, A., Golden, A., Laack, T. A., Rosario, J., Strother, C., Totten, V. Y., & Okuda, Y. (2020). Communicating value in simulation: Cost benefit analysis and return on investment. *Academy of Emergency Medicine*. [Accepted Author Manuscript.] https://doi.org/10.1111/acem.13336

Bapteste, L., Bertucat, S., & Balanca, B. (2020). Unexpected detection of latent safety threats by in situ simulation: About two cases in an adult intensive care unit. *Clinical Simulation in Nursing*, *47*, 6–8. https://doi.org/10.1016/j.ecns.2020.07.001

Becker's Hospital Review. (2017, August 24). *58 hospitals with innovation programs*. https://www.beckershospitalreview.com/lists/58-hospitals-and-health-systems-with-innovation-programs.html

Bender, G. J., & Maryman, J. A. (2018). Clinical macrosystem simulation translates between organizations. *Simulation in Healthcare*, *13*(2), 96–106. https://doi.org/10.1097/SIH.0000000000000263

Benner, P., Sutphen, M., Leonard, V., & Day, L. (2010). *Educating nurses: A call for radical transformation*. Jossey-Bass.

Bukhari, H., Andreatta, P., Goldiez, B., & Rabelo, L. (2017). A framework for determining the return of investment of simulation-based training in health care. *The Journal of Health Care Organization, Provision, and Financing*, *54*, 1–7. https://doi.org/10.1177%2F0046958016687176

Centers for Disease Control and Prevention. (2020, February 4). *Pregnancy mortality surveillance system*. www.cdc.gov/reproductivehealth/maternalinfanthealth/pregnancy-mortality-surveillance-system.htm.

Cook, D. A. (2013). The literature on health care simulation education: What does it show? *Perspectives on Safety*. https://psnet.ahrq.gov/perspective/literature-health-care-simulation-education-what-does-it-show

Cooper, J. B. (2020). The case of the inadvertently triggered laser. *Simulation in Healthcare: The Journal of the Society for Simulation in Healthcare*. Advance online publication. https://doi.org/10.1097/SIH.0000000000000483

Cosme, S. (2015). Residency and fellowship programs for RNs and advanced practice RNs. *Journal of Nursing Administration*, *45*(9), 416–417. https://doi.org/10.1097/NNA.0000000000000224

Couto, T. B., Barreto, J. K., Marcon, F. C., Mafra, A. C. C. N., & Accorsi, T. A., D. (2018). Detecting latent safety threats in an interprofessional training that combines in situ simulation with task training in an emergency department. *Advances in Simulation*, *3*(23), 1–7. https://doi.org/10.1186/s41077-018-0083-4

Czekajlo, M., & Dabrowska, A. (2017). In situ simulation of cardiac arrest. *Disaster and Emergency Medicine Journal*, 2(3), 116–119. https://doi.org/10.5603/DEMJ.2017.0025

Dingley, C., Daugherty, K., Derieg, M. K., & Persing, R. (2018). Improving patient safety through provider communication strategy enhancements. In *Advances in patient safety: New directions and alternative approaches, Vol. 3: Performance and tools*. Agency for Healthcare Research and Quality. https://www.ncbi.nlm.nih.gov/books/NBK43663/

Echenique, A., & Wempe, E. P. (2018). Simulation-based training of the nurse practitioner in interventional radiology. *Techniques in Vascular and Interventional Radiology*, 22(1), 26–31. https://doi.org/10.1053/j.tvir.2018.10.006

Elgin, K. W., & Poston, R. D. (2019). Optimizing registered nurse bedside shift report. *Journal for Nurses in Professional Development*, *35*(2), E6–E14. https://doi.org/10.1097/NND.0000000000000526

Federal Trade Commission. (2020). *Competition in the healthcare marketplace*. https://www.ftc.gov/tips-advice/competition-guidance/industry-guidance/health-care

Fiorillo, S. (2019, February 13). *What is return on investment (ROI) and how is it calculated?* thestreet. https://www.thestreet.com/personal-finance/what-is-roi-14863482

Francoeur, C., Shea, S., Ruddy, M., Fontela, P., Bhanji, F., Razack, S., Gottesman, R., & Genova, T. (2018). It takes a village to move a hospital: Simulation improves intensive care team preparedness for a move to a new site. *Hospital Pediatrics*, *8*(3), 148–156. https://doi.org/10.1542/hpeds.2017-0112

Glasofer, A., & Laskowski-Jones, L. (2019). Active shooter incidents. *Nursing Management*, *50*(3), 18–25. https://journals.lww.com/nursingmanagement/Fulltext/2019/03000/Active_shooter_incidents__Awareness_and_action.4.aspx

Golden, A., Alaska, Y., Levinson, A. T., Davignon, K. R., Lueckel, S. N., Lynch, K. A., Jay, G., & Kobayashi, L. (2020). Simulation-based examination of arterial line insertion method reveals interdisciplinary practice differences. *Simulation in Healthcare: The Journal of the Society for Simulation in Healthcare*, *15*(2), 89–97. https://doi.org/10.1097/SIH.0000000000000428

Gooch, K. (2015, December 4). *IOM committee releases 10 recommendations for the future of nursing. Beckers Hospital Review*. https://www.beckershospitalreview.com/hr/iom-committee-releases-10-recommendations-for-the-future-of-nursing.html

Gorrindo, T., Goldfarb, E., Birnbaum, R. J., Chevalier, L., Meller, B., Alpert, J., Herman, J., & Weiss, A. (2013). Simulation-based ongoing professional practice evaluation in psychiatry: A novel tool for performance assessment. *The Joint Commission Journal on Quality and Patient Safety*, *39*(7), 319–323. https://doi.org/10.1016/s1553-7250(13)39045-x

Groves, P. S., Bunch, J. L., Cram, E., Farag, A., Manges, K., Perkhounkova, Y., & Scott-Cawiezell, J. (2017). Priming patient safety through nursing handoff communication: A simulation pilot study. *Western Journal of Nursing Research*, *39*(11), 1394–1411. https://doi.org/10.1177/0193945916673358

Haerling, K. A. (2018). Cost-utility analysis of virtual and mannequin-based simulation. *Simulation in Healthcare: The Journal of the Society for Simulation in Healthcare*, *13*(1), 33–40. https://doi.org/10.1097/SIH.0000000000000280

Harper, M. G., Gilbert, G. E., Gilbert, M., Markey, L., & Anderson, K. (2018). Simulation use in acute care hospitals in the United States. *Journal for Nursing in Professional Development*, *34*(5), 242–249. https://doi.org/10.1097/NND.0000000000000472

Hippe, D. S., Umoren, R. A., McGee, A., Bucher, S. L., & Bresnahan, B. W. (2020). A targeted systematic review of cost analyses for implementation of simulation-based education in healthcare. *SAGE Open Medical*, *8*, 1–9. https://doi.org/10.1177/2050312120913451

HNMC Media. (2012, June 27). *Live shooter drill at Holy name medical center*. [Video]. Youtube. https://www.youtube.com/watch?v=9xAgbYmQ7oY

HNMC Media. (2020, March 25). *DIY isopod with negative pressure and air scrubber*. https://www.youtube.com/watch?v=5FRBv3S252Q

Holtscheider, M. E. (2013). Simulation "programs" versus simulation "centers" in the hospital/workplace setting. *Journal for Nursing in Professional Development*, *29*(4), 213. https://doi.org/10.1097/NND.0b013e31829c521e

Holtscheider, M. E. (2017). Using standardized patients in large-scale hospital disaster drills. *Journal for Nursing in Professional Development*, *33*(2), 90–91. https://doi.org/10.1097/NND.0000000000000330

Hunt, J. L. (2012). Assessing physician competency: An update on the joint commission requirement for annoying and focused professional practice evaluation. *Advances in Anatomic Pathology*, *19*(6), 388–400. https://doi.org/10.1097/PAP.0b013e318273f97e

Inman, F. M. (2016). Using simulation drills to improve competency and team skill for rural perinatal nurses. *Journal of Obstetric, Gynecologic, and Neonatal Nursing*, *45*(3), S9–S10. https://doi.org/10.1016/j.jogn.2016.03.039

Jackson, K., Lower, C. L., & Rudman, W. J. (2016). The crossroads between workforce and education. *Perspectives in Health Information Management, 13, 1-11.*

The Joint Commission. (2020, July 1). *Hospital 2020: National patient safety goals*. https://www.jointcommission.org/standards/national-patient-safety-goals/hospital-2020-national-patient-safety-goals/

Justus, P. D., & Appel, S. A. (2018). Simulation with advanced care providers in a nurse residency program. *Journal for Nurses in Professional Development*, *34*(4), 180–184. https://doi.org/10.1097/NND.0000000000000453

Kalman, N. S., Bradley, G. H., Shulman, K. A., & Shah, B. R. (2015). Hospital overhead costs: The neglected driver of health care spending? *Journal of Healthcare Finance*, *41*(4), 1–15. https://healthfinancejournal.com/index.php/johcf/article/view/27

Kearney, J. A., & Deutsch, E. S. (2017). Using simulation to improve systems. *Otolaryngologic Clinics of North America*, *50*(5), 1015–1028. https://doi.org/10.1016/j.otc.2017.05.011

Knight, P., MacGloin, H., Lane, M., Lofton, L., Desai, A., Haxby, E., Macrae, D., Korb, C., Mortimer, P., & Burmester, M. (2018). Mitigating latent threats identified through an embedded in situ simulation program and their comparison to patient safety incidents: A retrospective study. *Frontiers in Pediatrics*, *5*(281), 1–8. https://doi.org/10.3389/fped.2017.00281

Knippa, S., & Senecal, P. (2017). Using simulation to prepare nursing stuff for the move to a new building. *Journal for Nurses in Professional Development*, *33*(2), E1–E5. https://doi.org/10.1097/NND.0000000000000329

Lavelle, M., Reedy, G. B., Attoe, C., Simpson, T., & Anderson, J. E. (2019). Beyond the clinical team: Evaluating the human factors-oriented training of non-clinical professionals working in healthcare contexts. *Advances in Simulation*, *4*(11), 1–11. https://doi.org/10.1186/s41077-019-0101-1

Lehtola, C. L. (2007). Developing and using table-top simulation as a teachingtool. *Journal of Extension*, *45*(4). https://www.joe.org/joe/2007august/tt4.php

Liu, L. L., Forgione, D. A., & Younis, M. Z. (2012). A comparative analysis of the CVP structure of nonprofit teaching and for-profit non-teaching hospitals. *Journal of Health Care Finance*, *39*(1), 12–38. https://pubmed.ncbi.nlm.nih.gov/23155742/

Mackary, M. A., & Daniel, M. (2016). Medical error - the third leading cause of death in the US. *British Medical Journal*, *359*, i2139. https://doi.org/10.1136/bmj.i2139

Mannenbach, M. S., Fahje, C. J., Sunga, K. L., & Sztajnkrycer, M. D. (2018). An *in situ* simulation-based training approach to active shooter response in the emergency department. *Disaster Medicine and Public Health Preparedness*, *13*(2), 345–352. https://doi.org/10.1017/dmp.2018.39

Naik, N., Finkelstein, R. A., Howell, J., Rajwani, K., & Ching, K. (2020). Telesimulation for COVID-19 ventilator management training with social-distancing restrictions during the coronavirus pandemic. *Simulation and Gaming*, *51*(4), 571–577. https://doi.org/10.1177/1046878120926561

Papanagnou, D. (2017). Telesimulation: A paradigm shift for simulation education. *AEM Education and Training: A Global Journal of Emergency Care*, *1*(2), 137–139. https://doi.org/10.1002/aet2.10032

Petrosoniak, A., Hicks, C., Barratt, L., Gascon, D., Kokoski, C., Campbell, D., White, K., Bandiera, G., Lum-Kwong, M. M., Nemoy, L., & Brydges, R. (2020). Design thinking -informed simulation: An innovative framework to test, evaluate, and modify new clinical infrastructure. *Simulation in Healthcare: The Journal of the Society for Simulation in Healthcare*, *15*(3), 205–211. https://doi.org/10.1097/SIH.0000000000000408

Petrosoniak, A., Ryzynski, A., Lebovic, G., & Woolfrey, K. (2017). Cricothyroidotomy *in situ* simulation curriculum (CRIC Study). *Simulation in Healthcare: The Journal of the Society for Simulation in Healthcare*, *12*(2), 76–82. https://doi.org/10.1097/SIH.0000000000000206

Phillips, J. J., Phillips, P. P., Phillips, Z. L., & Buzachero, V. V. (2013). *Measuring ROI in healthcare: Tools and techniques to measure the impact and ROI in healthcare improvement projects and programs*. McGraw Hill Education.

Rhodes, C. A., Grimm, D., Bradas, C., McClendon, S., & Noeller, T. P. (2016). Evaluation of nurse-specific and multidisciplinary simulation for nurse residency programs. *Clinical Simulation in Nursing*, *12*, 243–250. https://doi.org/10.1016/j.ecns.2016.02.010

Rossler, K. L., & Bennett, A. (2017). Restructuring a hospital nurse residency: Nursing and patient safety unite. *Clinical Simulation in Nursing*, *13*, 90–93. https://doi.org/10.1016/j.ecns.2017.01.001

Sanko, J. A., & McKay, M. (2017). Impact of simulation-enhanced pharmacology education in prelicensure nursing education. Nurse Educator, 42(5S), S32-S37. https://doi.org/10.1097/NNE.0000000000000409

Sanchez, L., Young, V. B., & Baker, M. (2018). Active shooter training in the emergency department: A safety initiative. *Journal of Emergency Nursing*, *44*(6), 598–604. https://doi.org/10.1016/j.jen.2018.07.002

Sheen, J., & Goffman, D. (2019). Emerging role of drills and simulations in patient safety. *Obstetrics and Gynecology Clinics of North America*, *46*(2), 305–315. https://doi.org/10.1016/j.ogc.2019.01.009

Simone, S., McComiskey, C. A., & Anderson, B. (2016). Integrating nurse practitioners into intensive care units. *Critical Care Nurse*, *36*(6), 59–69. https://doi.org/10.4037/ccn2016360

Slakey, D. P., Simms, E. R., Rennie, K. V., Garstka, M. E., & Korndorffer, J. R. (2014). Using simulation to improve root cause analysis of adverse surgical outcomes. *International Journal of Quality in Health Care*, *26*(2), 144–150. https://doi.org/10.1093/intqhc/mzu011

Spadaro, S., Karbing, D. S., Fogagnolo, A., Ragazzi, R., Mojoli, F., Astolfi, L., Gioia, A., Marangoni, E., Rees, S. E., & Volta, C. A. (2017). Simulation training for residents focused on mechanical ventilation. *Simulation in Healthcare: The Journal of the Society for Simulation in Healthcare*, *12*(6), 349–355. https://doi.org/10.1097/SIH.0000000000000249

Spiegelman, J., Sheen, J., & Goffman, D. (2018). Readiness: Utilizing bundles and simulation. *Seminars in Perinatology*, *43*, 5–10. https://doi.org/10.1053/j.semperi.2018.11.002

STERIS Healthcare. (2018, July 10). *What is a surgical boom?* https://www.steris.com/healthcare/knowledge-center/surgical-equipment/what-is-a-surgical-boom

United States Department of Justice, The Federal Bureau of Investigation, & The Advanced Law Enforcement Rapid Response Training (ALERRT) Center at Texas State University. (2018). *Active shooter incidents in the United States in 2018*. https://www.fbi.gov/file-repository/active-shooter-incidents-in-the-us-2018-041019.pdf/view

Ventre, K. M., Barry, J. S., Davis, D., Baiamonte, V. L., Wentworth, A. C., Pietras, M., Coughlin, & L., Barley, G. (2014). Using *in situ* simulation to evaluate operational readiness of a children's hospital-based obstetrics unit. *Simulation in Healthcare: The Journal of the Society for Simulation in Healthcare*, *9*(2), 102–111. https://doi.org/10.1097/SIH.0000000000000005

Walsh, B. M., Auerbach, M. A., Gawel, M. N., Brown, L. L., Byrne, B. J., & Calhoun, A. (2019). Community-based *in situ* simulation: Bringing simulation to the masses. *Advances in Simulation*, *4*(30), 1–12. https://doi.org/10.1186/s41077-019-0112-y

Wang, C. (2018, April 10). *How to: Using IPE simulation to satisfy regulatory requirements for practice assessment*. https://nlnteq.org/2018/04/10/how-to-using-ipe-simulation-to-satisfy-regulatory-requirements-for-practice-assessment/

Watkins, E., & Stem, K. (2020). Postpartum hemorrhage. *Journal of the American Academy of Physician Assistants*, *33*(4), 29–33. https://journals.lww.com/jaapa/Fulltext/2020/04000/Postpartum_hemorrhage.4.aspx

Weithholter, J. P., Grey, C., Howard, C., Johnson, B. N., Sween, R., & Rowlands, A. E. (2017). Interprofessional collaborative practice through an adult medicine based simulation. *Journal of Interprofessional Education & Practice*, *9*, 21–26. https://doi.org/10.1016/j.xjep.2017.07.011

Wexler, B., & Flamm, A. (2017). Lessons learned from an active shooter full-scale functional exercise in a newly constructed emergency department. *Disaster Medicine and Public Preparedness*, *11*(5), 522–525. https://doi.org/10.1017/dmp.2016.181

Zendejas, B., Wang, A. T., Brydges, R., Hamstra, S. J., & Cook, D. A. (2013). Cost: The missing outcome in simulation-based medical education research: A systematic review. *Surgery*, *153*(2), 160–176. https://doi.org/10.1016/j.surg.2012.06.025

Zimmerman, D. M., & House, P. (2016). Mediation safety: Simulation education for new RNs promises an excellent return on investment. *Nursing Economics*, *34*(1), 49–51.

Ziv, A., Wolpe, P. R., Small, S. D., & Glick, S. (2003). Simulation-based medical education: An ethical imperative. *Academic Medicine*, *78*(8), 783–788. https://doi.org/10.1097/00001888-200308000-00006

CHAPTER 5

Interprofessional Simulation: From the Classroom to Clinical Practice

Julie A. Poore and Dylan D. Cooper

ABSTRACT

Interprofessional simulation (IPS), frequently referred to in the literature as simulation-enhanced interprofessional education (IPE), has been widely studied in nursing and medical education. For decades, the literature has suggested IPE as a valuable strategy for enhancing communication and collaboration among health professionals. Interprofessional collaborative practice (IPCP) is foundational to developing high-functioning healthcare teams and can lead to reduced medical errors and increased patient safety. This chapter addresses IPS from both the academic and practice perspectives. The foundations of IPE and IPCP are reviewed, as well as the standards of best practice in simulation. Planning, development, and implementation will be discussed, including benefits, barriers, and possible solutions. Recommendations from relevant research on debriefing and evaluation of IPS are also reviewed. Outcomes from the growing body of research on IPS will be presented and include perceptions of interprofessional practice, better understanding of professional roles and responsibilities, development of communication and teamwork skills, and shared problem-solving and decision-making. Future implications and recommendations are provided based on the state of the science on IPS. Optimum design, implementation, and evaluation of IPS, along with a thorough understanding of the benefits, barriers, and opportunities, can

http://dx.doi.org/10.1891/0739-6686.39.105

help faculty and clinical educators prepare a collaborative healthcare workforce and reduce medical errors to ultimately improve patient outcomes.

INTRODUCTION

To better understand the significance of interprofessional simulation (IPS), one must recognize factors that led to the development of interprofessional education (IPE) alongside the associated terminology. Medical errors cost the United States approximately $20 billion annually and result in approximately 100,000 deaths (Rodziewicz & Hipskind, 2020). Ineffective and failed communication between health professionals was identified as a root cause of sentinel events in hospitals from 2004 to 2017 (The Joint Commission [TJC], 2012, 2017). For decades, the literature has suggested IPE as a valuable strategy for enhancing collaboration and communication among health professionals (Health Professions Accreditors Collaborative, 2019; Heuer et al., 2010; Institute of Medicine [IOM], 1972, 2001, 2003, 2011; National League for Nursing [NLN], 2012, 2015; Wilcock et al., 2009). Effective communication and collaboration among health professionals can reduce medical error and improve patient safety (Bhatt & Swick, 2017). Interprofessional collaborative practice (IPCP) is foundational to developing high functioning healthcare teams.

The most widely accepted definition of IPE, from the World Health Organization (2010), asserts that "IPE occurs when two or more professions learn about, from and with each other to enable effective collaboration and improve health outcomes" (p. 13). While the term interdisciplinary is sometimes used interchangeably with interprofessional, the strict definition of interdisciplinary involves multiple different disciplines within a profession, not different professions. Healthcare simulation is a pedagogy that has been widely used and studied in health profession education and has been suggested as a method for evaluating learner competency (King et al., 2016; Kostoff et al., 2016). Simulation replicates many aspects of the clinical setting in a safe learning environment where mistakes represent an opportunity for professional growth on the continuum from novice to expert (Lioce et al., 2020). The International Nursing Association for Clinical Simulation and Learning (INACSL) Standards of Best Practice: Simulation^{SM}: Simulation-Enhanced Interprofessional Education (2016b) declares that simulation-enhanced IPE "enables participants from different professions to engage in a simulation-based experience to achieve shared or linked objectives and outcomes" (p. S34). Simulation is currently the most common strategy for delivering IPE in nursing and medical programs (Rutherford-Hemming & Lioce, 2018).

BEST PRACTICES FOR IPS

Simulation and IPE are both costly and resource intensive. Expenses related to simulation include space, manikins, equipment, supplies, and personnel. Because most high-fidelity simulations include small numbers of learners, it is necessary to offer multiple sessions, which increases the workload for facilitators and requires additional supplies and equipment. Additional facilitators are needed for IPS encounters to ensure an adequate number of content experts from each participating profession. Facilitator training is essential for IPS and requires knowledge of IPE principles and competencies as well as simulation pedagogy. Facilitator training can be expensive and time-consuming. Therefore, commitment of financial and administrative support should be secured during the initial planning stages. Many universities with multiple health profession programs have created IPE centers to supervise and manage interprofessional initiatives, including IPS. In addition, IPE centers can provide direction while maintaining a neutral position that advocates for the needs of all professions.

Many IPS encounters occur in simulated hospital rooms using high-fidelity manikins. However, it is important to remember that IPS encompasses a wide range of approaches including tabletop exercises, counseling and discharge planning using standardized patients, and synchronous or asynchronous avatar-based virtual platforms (Wilhaus et al., 2013). IPS may also occur in situ, where manikins are taken into the hospital, clinic, operating room, or other healthcare site.

Like traditional simulation, IPS should be structured to include a prebriefing, simulation, and debriefing (Adamson, 2015; INACSL Standards Committee, 2016a). The prebrief (reviewed in Chapter 6) is an opportunity to set the stage for IPS. During the prebrief, facilitators share logistics, limitations, learning objectives, expectations, and evaluation methods; orient participants to space, manikins, and equipment; and discuss participant roles (INACSL Standards Committee, 2016b). The simulation encompasses the portion of the encounter where learners interact, through an authentic scenario, with the simulator or standardized patient. Debriefing is the portion of the simulation activity that allows learners an opportunity for collaborative reflection on the actions that occurred during the simulation (INACSL Standards Committee, 2016b).

CORE COMPETENCIES

Development, implementation, and evaluation of IPS should be guided by a theoretical framework (INACSL Standards Committee, 2016b). The primary definition of IPE activities comes from the World Health Organization (WHO) and identifies that “participants learn about, from, and with each other” (WHO, 2010,

p. 13). Following this consensus definition, there was a need for a common framework to guide multiple professions to work together. The Interprofessional Education Collaborative (IPEC), formed in 2009, includes the disciplines of dentistry, nursing, medicine, osteopathic medicine, pharmacy, and public health. The IPEC developed core competencies for IPCP that were released in 2011 and include four competencies: values/ethics for interprofessional practice, roles/responsibilities, interprofessional communication, and teams and teamwork (IPEC, 2011). Box 5.1 presents the 2016 IPEC core competencies, including a focus on disease prevention, improving individual care, and advancing population health (IPEC, 2016). Figure 5.1 depicts the interprofessional collaboration learning continuum from prelicensure through practice.

Another commonly used competency framework for IPS is TeamSTEPPS® (Bell & Fredland, 2020). Developed by the Department of Defense's Patient Safety Program, the TeamSTEPPS® curriculum is designed for team-based learning, with a focus on communication, teamwork skills, and patient safety. The course and all materials are available at no cost through the Agency for Healthcare Research and Quality (2020). Box 5.2 highlights the four teamwork training concepts covered in the TeamSTEPPS® curriculum.

Healthcare simulation provides an excellent opportunity to teach and assess both learners and teams in each of these competencies. While table-top and small group sessions supplement IPE endeavors, everything comes together when the team collaborates to manage a simulated patient (Reeves & van Schaik,

Box 5.1

Core Competencies for Interprofessional Collaborative Practice: 2016 Update

Work with individuals of other professions to maintain a climate of mutual respect and shared values. (**Values/Ethics for Interprofessional Practice**)

Use the knowledge of one's own role and those of other professions to appropriately assess and address the healthcare needs of patients and to promote and advance the health of populations. (**Roles/Responsibilities**)

Communicate with patients, families, communities, and professionals in health and other fields in a responsive and responsible manner that supports a team approach to the promotion and maintenance of health and the prevention and treatment of disease. (**Interprofessional Communication**)

Apply relationship-building values and the principles of team dynamics to perform effectively in different team roles to plan, deliver, and evaluate patient/population-centered care and population health programs and policies that are safe, timely, efficient, effective, and equitable. (**Teams and Teamwork**)

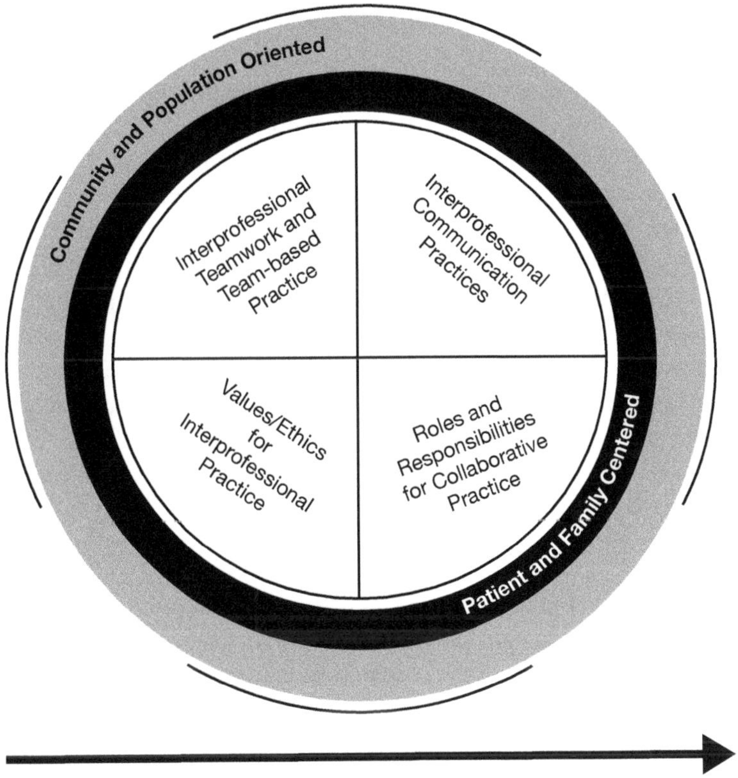

FIGURE 5.1 The learning continuum prelicensure through practice trajectory.

Box 5.2
TeamSTEPPS® 2.0

- Leadership
- Communication
- Situational Monitoring
- Mutual Support

2012). In addition, patient-centered simulation creates a more realistic and stressful environment for all professions (van Soeren et al., 2009). Therefore, either the IPEC or TeamSTEPPS® competencies can be used by educators to identify appropriate IPS opportunities within the curriculum and develop new IPS opportunities to meet curricular needs.

DEVELOPMENT

Goals and Objectives

Performing a needs assessment is the first step in designing effective IPS (INACSL Standards Committee (2016a). Curricular mapping is crucial as it aligns IPS to program outcomes and reveals opportunities for integration and scaffolding of simulation throughout each program. Sequencing IPS throughout the curricula allows learners to reflect on their simulation experiences and apply the newly gained skills to future clinical or simulation experiences (Astbury et al., 2020).

Each discipline must actively participate in designing and implementing IPE activities beginning with the creation of goals and objectives. Measurable learning objectives should have relevance and significance for each participating discipline. The IPS modality as well as goals and objectives should match the level of the learners (Health Professions Accreditors Collaborative, 2019). Objectives should also determine the appropriate disciplines and participant numbers to be included in each scenario.

Planning

Once the goals and objectives have been identified, educators must begin planning the simulation event. Success of the final product is highly dependent on the amount of work that goes into the preparation. Educators from all professions as well as simulation support staff should be involved in this phase of the process. Scheduling should be done well in advance to identify the most appropriate timing to meet availability and curricular appropriateness. Both learners and educators should be available for the event. While some professions may not have enough facilitators to support IPS, highly effective IPE includes the presence of faculty from all professions (Paige et al., 2015). Creativity in scheduling must be considered; for example, evening events may increase participation (Poore et al., 2017). Next, faculty should ensure that learners are at similar levels of training. For example, nursing students often gain clinical training earlier than medical students, so running a simulation for all second-year nursing and second-year medical students may not have prepared them with equivalent experiences. It is important that educators work together to identify times in training when clinical experiences align.

Once the date(s) of the IPS events have been finalized, the team can begin to retrograde plan for the IPS event(s). First, dates must be blocked off in all curricular and simulation calendars to include setup time. Next, the team identifies space, equipment, manikins, and personnel needs. Goals and objectives will drive every step in the process.

Space

The optimal space for IPS is a clinical setting where all professions will interact, whether it be in the simulation lab, emergency department, intensive care unit

(ICU), or outpatient clinic. Allow enough room for all participants to be around the simulated patient, avoiding smaller spaces where learners feel isolated from the rest of the team. In addition, ensure there is enough space for faculty and staff to observe the event. Finally, if available, a separate debriefing room allows for a neutral, safe location for all participants.

Equipment

All professions should ensure that equipment normally used in the clinical setting is available for the simulation scenario. Learner engagement and participation will be maximized if the simulation environment and equipment replicate what is used in clinical practice (Cook et al., 2012). In addition, it can heighten realism while reducing learner stress. For example, in a resuscitation scenario, ensure that there are stocked medications for the pharmacist, defibrillator pads for nursing, airway supplies for respiratory therapy, and imaging/labs for the provider.

Manikins

There exist a multitude of different manikins for simulation education. While the highest fidelity manikins can provide more realism, they are expensive and may not achieve improved learning outcomes when compared to low-fidelity manikins (Cheng, Lockey et al., 2015). Therefore, educators should choose the manikin fidelity that will best meet the goals and objectives. As with the equipment, it is paramount to select a manikin with functionality appropriate for all professions. For example, if the simulation involves cardiac arrest with defibrillation, the manikin will need cardiopulmonary resuscitation (CPR) and defibrillation capabilities.

Personnel

If possible, IPS should include a simulation operations technician or specialist to run the manikin while educators concentrate on the interactions of learners as they meet the goals and objectives of the session (Bailey et al., 2015). Identifying faculty with simulation expertise and/or IPE expertise is essential to the success of IPS. With IPS, a heightened level of skill is required, therefore more novice faculty may struggle to successfully facilitate both IPE and simulation. Figure 5.2 provides an example of an IPS design template.

Scenario Development

Development of IPS should follow the best practices for simulation and IPE (INACSL Standards Committee, 2016a). When developing scenarios, it is essential to begin with the goals and objectives. Key faculty representatives from all specialties involved in the event should be engaged in selecting the appropriate goals and objectives for their learners. In addition to profession-specific goals and

<table>
<tr><td colspan="2">Interprofessional Simulation Design Template

IPE Simulation Opportunities:
1. Curriculum
2. Learners
3. Faculty</td></tr>
<tr><td>Goals and Objectives
•
•
•</td><td>IPEC Core Competencies
• Values & Ethics
• Roles & Responsibilities
• Communication
• Team & Teamwork</td></tr>
<tr><td colspan="2">Case(s)
•
•
•</td></tr>
<tr><td colspan="2">Debriefing Focus</td></tr>
<tr><td colspan="2">Assessment</td></tr>
<tr><td colspan="2">Sustainability
1. Scholarship
2. Grants</td></tr>
</table>

FIGURE 5.2 Example of an interprofessional simulation design template.

objectives, the case should also have overall goals and objectives for the team (Astbury et al., 2020).

Several key factors in determining the simulation case include complexity, timeline, roles, and debriefing format. Complexity of the case is dependent upon the learner level of training. Faculty must ensure learners have the appropriate knowledge and skills to be successful in the simulation. Usually, the more straightforward and simpler the case, the less likely learners will lose focus on goals and objectives. Case timeline involves location of the scenario and progression of events, which should reflect clinical practice as closely as possible. Learners should portray appropriate professional roles in the simulation: nurses in nursing roles, pharmacy in pharmacy roles, and so on. Faculty must use extreme caution when participants role play other professions in IPS. There are significant healthcare stereotypes that could inhibit learning from, about, and with other professions if not addressed before the simulation (Cook & Stoecker, 2014; Price et al., 2019). Finally, given the multiple approaches and strong opinions toward different debriefing formats, the IPS faculty team should discuss and agree upon a debriefing framework early during case development.

Once the simulation curriculum is developed, the next steps include manikin selection and programming, room and equipment identification, use of audio-video recording, and piloting. The most appropriate manikin to meet goals and objectives should be selected; again, the most technically advanced manikin may not be needed for the simulation. In terms of programming the scenario flow, allow for significant flexibility as teams may not follow the anticipated course of action. Next, simulation staff and educators should work together to identify the location (e.g., inpatient, outpatient, home setting) and equipment (e.g., monitor, medications, ventilator) needed for the case. In addition, a decision should be made about use of audio-video recording and determination of necessary consents from learners and faculty. The final, and perhaps most important step in developing the simulation, is the pilot session. Given the complexity of IPS, a pilot session within the same space, and with the same manikin, equipment, and faculty, should be run well in advance of the actual session to allow time for modifications. Learners from all professions should be at the pilot and should be about the same level of training to ensure they have similar knowledge and skills as the intended participants.

IPS is expanding in both academic and practice settings. Educator training is critical to the development and implementation of IPS across professions. In order to maximize learner outcomes, IPS facilitators should be trained in simulation and IPE (Alexander et al., 2015; INACSL Standards Committee, 2016a; Lemoine et al., 2015). IPS knowledge and skills can be gained through literature review, formal workshops, and working with and observing experienced simulation educators (Anderson et al., 2012). Therefore, IPS planning and preparation should include faculty and educator development through formal training or homegrown solutions (Stephenson et al., 2019).

IMPLEMENTATION

On the day of the simulation event, faculty from all professions should be present. If this is not possible, additional time should be spent with members of each profession individually to ensure specific needs of each group are addressed. Technicians and support staff should ensure each room is set up appropriately and that manikins are up and running. In addition, faculty should work with simulation staff to review the room setup and examine all equipment, including ensuring sufficient battery charge, to limit technological failures during the simulation.

The IPS prebriefing or orientation is conducted to (a) establish ground rules, (b) share logistics for the day, (c) provide an icebreaker, and (d) orient participants to the simulation space and equipment. A successful simulation can be derailed within the first few minutes if a prebriefing is not conducted appropriately (Boet et al., 2014; Rutherford-Hemming et al., 2019; Stephenson & Poore, 2016). The initial phase of the IPS prebriefing is establishing ground rules, specifically to build a foundation of trust and safety. Specific statements can include "simulation is safe for both patients and participants," "you and/or your colleagues will likely make mistakes today," "what happens in simulation stays in simulation," and so on. Next, instructors explain the participant responsibilities in simulation. Participants must act professionally and treat manikins as they would an actual patient. Other rules include verbalizing orders, communicating with the manikin, and working together as a team (Rutherford-Hemming et al., 2019). Finally, a discussion of the importance of debriefing and expectations of participants during debriefing is essential.

Second, a presentation of logistics should follow the ground rules, including goals and objectives for the simulation. Participants will be better engaged when they are aware of overall goals and objectives and do not feel they are being tricked in a simulation (Calhoun et al., 2020). The role of the embedded participant, an actor in the case who can provide additional information to the learner, should be explained to all professions (Lioce et al., 2020). Logistics may also include an opportunity for the learners from different professions to participate in a group session or icebreaker to learn from, about, and with one another. A schedule of events is shared with participants to include number of cases or scenarios, debriefings, breaks, and overall session length.

Third, allowing learners from different professions the opportunity to interact with one another through an icebreaker activity prior to IPS can help with the initial stage of team development (Wen et al., 2019). IPS scenarios should be based on realistic situations and replicate the practice environment. Professions should not be added to an IPS session unless they would work together in the actual clinical environment.

Finally, all IPS participants should be oriented to the simulation space, manikins, and equipment. To establish a level field for all professions, orientation should occur in the space with a description of the available supplies and equipment. Specific equipment that may be new, different, or potentially dangerous should be demonstrated. For example, if live defibrillators will be used during simulation cases, participants should be shown how the defibrillator functions and connects to the manikin during the orientation. Also, manikin functionality can be demonstrated through direct interaction. Allowing participants the opportunity to auscultate heart and lung sounds or palpate pulses on the manikin will improve their experience with the technology. During the orientation, the instructor may converse with the manikin to demonstrate both realism and professionalism.

Interprofessional competencies cannot be achieved through a single experience, rather they take multiple encounters to accomplish expected outcomes (INACSL Standards Committee, 2016a). Sigalet et al. (2015) found an improvement in team performance as nursing, medical, and respiratory therapy students progressed from one simulation to the next. In addition, each discipline must feel the IPE experience is contributing to the development of their individual professional identities. Poore et al. (2017) noted decreased participation in IPS when faculty did not feel there was a substantial role in the patient case for students from their discipline.

DEBRIEFING

During debriefing, participants reflect on the IPS performance and recognize educational gaps in order to improve future performance (Boet et al., 2014; INACSL Standards Committee, 2016b; Salik & Paige, 2020). Interprofessional debriefing should be conducted by content experts from all participating disciplines. Additionally, educators facilitating the debriefing should be trained in debriefing techniques.

Cheng, Palaganas et al. (2015) define codebriefing as “more than one facilitator conducting a debriefing session” (p. 69). In this case, codebriefing may include multiple discipline-specific content experts alongside expert simulation facilitators. Benefits of codebriefing include a wider breadth of knowledge, experience, and viewpoints. While codebriefing can enhance the simulation experience for learners, it can also be challenging for facilitators. Common challenges include lack of knowledge of learning objectives, differing personal agendas, facilitator dominance, facilitator disagreement, and inequitable engagement of learners. In order to ameliorate challenges, facilitators should meet in advance to discuss individual strengths and areas of expertise, ground rules, and strategies for facilitation. Issues among facilitators can still arise even with thorough advanced preparation. Cheng, Palaganas et al. (2015) offer suggestions for managing challenges that arise during the debriefing, including open negotiation and a pulse check. They describe open negotiation as a sharing of concerns through cordial dialogue. A pulse check is a technique a facilitator uses to help clarify something a cofacilitator said that may have been confusing to learners. A postdebriefing huddle serves the dual purpose of allowing for discussion of any issues that arose and setting ground rules for future codebriefing sessions.

All learners should be actively engaged during the debriefing which is often difficult when learners have varying learning styles. Trained debriefers can better manage learners who may dominate or withdraw from the conversation, but this can be particularly difficult for novice educators. Poore et al. (2019) developed a tool to aid in debriefing interprofessional competencies that includes questions for each phase of debriefing and probing questions to gain more insight into critical thinking and clinical judgment. The debriefing tool also provides facilitators an opportunity to address interprofessional competencies in both uniprofessional and interprofessional groups.

BARRIERS AND BENEFITS

Barriers to IPS cited in the literature include scheduling, money, distance, lack of common curriculum across disciplines, disproportionate numbers of learners per program, and culture (Leclair et al., 2018; Palaganas et al., 2014; Poore et al., 2017; Umoren et al., 2017). Conducting a needs assessment to determine organizational readiness can ameliorate some barriers to IPS. Table 5.1 identifies common barriers and possible solutions to IPS in both the educational and practice environments.

The literature supports the use of IPS among both health profession students and practicing professionals (Alanazi et al., 2017; Cantrell et al., 2017; IOM, 2001, 2003, 2011, 2015; Labrague et al., 2018; NLN, 2012, 2015; Poore et al., 2017). Effective implementation of IPS can offer significant benefits to the patient by developing a healthcare team that functions in a unified, cooperative manner utilizing best practices to promote improved patient outcomes and patient-centered care (Poore et al., 2019). In addition, health professionals must understand that interdependence is crucial to providing quality care because performance levels of even the most skilled health professionals will be limited if collaborative processes are flawed (Wilcock et al., 2009). Riggall and Smith (2015) facilitated 17 IPSs focused on team training with internal-medicine residents, registered nurses, respiratory therapists, and patient care technicians. Participants felt that IPS was effective in reinforcing teamwork and communication skills (Riggall & Smith, 2015). Oncology nurses and fellows also rated IPS as an effective method for developing teamwork and communication skills (James et al., 2016). The benefits of IPS based upon literature review and author experience are listed in Box 5.3.

TABLE 5.1
Common Barriers and Possible Solutions

Buy-in	**Academic and practice** • Identify faculty/educator champions from each profession. • Effective leadership can add sustainability to IPS. Leaders must have a vested interest in IPS and be willing to support the IPS efforts by providing adequate financial support, training, and resources. • Highlight ROI for each environment (e.g., patient safety, improved teamwork, decreased turnover).
Scheduling	Coordinating IPS is complex and requires cooperation and flexibility from each health profession. **Academic** • Designate specific dates on the academic calendar as protected IPS dates for all health profession programs. **Practice** • IPS is often difficult to schedule due to the uncertainty of patient census and daily staffing needs. Schedule IPS to overlap with shift change to allow health professionals to attend IPS without having patient care responsibilities.
Disproportionate numbers of learners	As the largest health profession, nursing has significantly more learners than most other professions. **Academic** • Partner with other local health profession programs to increase diversity and engagement. **Practice** • Balance the mix of professions. • Schedule only those who accurately represent the clinical environment.
Geographic location of learners	**Academic** • Consider virtual IPS. • Consider a geographic location that is equidistant to all learners. • Consider a rotating travel schedule so no one program has the burden of traveling every semester.

TABLE 5.1
Common Barriers and Possible Solutions (Continued)

Workload	**Academic** • Distribute workload between faculty of different professions. • Consider stipend or protected time for IPS faculty. • Recognize benefits of IPS for promotion and tenure. Practice • Protect educator time for IPS. • Utilize IPS to help achieve Magnet Hospital designation. Academic and practice • Ensure facilitators receive education and training related to the foundations of interprofessional education and simulation.
Learner engagement	**Academic and practice** • Develop common goals, objectives, and learning outcomes collaboratively and relate to learners from each profession.
Social hierarchy	**Academic and practice** • Consider meeting in advance to discuss roles and responsibilities of facilitation to prevent one facilitator from dominating one or all parts of the simulation. • Role model collaborative behavior to provide an example for learners.
Cost	**Academic and practice** • While the expense associated with implementing and sustaining IPE initiatives is often a challenge, financial opportunities may be available to support and sustain IPE. Support for IPE from national health organizations and accrediting bodies has generated increased funding opportunities for IPE research. • Several grants specific to IPE are available and may improve the prospects of acquiring external funding. • Share resources and costs among the participating departments. • Provide ROI data to executive management.

Notes. IPE = interprofessional education; IPS = interprofessional simulation; ROI = return on investment.

EVALUATION AND SUSTAINABILITY

IPS is an excellent opportunity to evaluate individual and/or team performance. While many evaluations can be completed live during an event, some are better done afterward through video review. The most appropriate evaluators are those trained and experienced with the evaluation tool. Both qualitative and quantitative data can provide a more robust assessment of team performance

Box 5.3

Benefits of IPS

- Realistic patient-centered clinical environment, practices, and processes
- Safe learning environment
- Improved teamwork and communication
- Ability to practice and evaluate clinical competencies
- Opportunity for repeated practice
- Opportunity for feedback and reflection
- Increase understanding of professional roles and responsibilities
- Dedicated simulation roles
- Organizational support for simulation
- Potential for reduced provider turnover
- Opportunity to improve patient care

Note. IPS = interprofessional simulation.

(Boet et al., 2014). Multiple tools for IPS evaluation can be found online (National Center for Interprofessional Practice and Education, 2020) and in the Wooding et al. (2020) systematic review.

Given the effort that goes into developing and delivering IPS, sustainability should also be a focus of the faculty involved. Grant funding can facilitate ongoing IPS curricula and can be found through the Association for Healthcare Research and Quality (AHRQ), Josiah Macy Jr. Foundation, Robert Wood Johnson Foundation, Gordon and Betty Moore Foundation, John A. Hartford Foundation, and other organizations.

Scholarship is another way to build sustainability. Through working together, the faculty can study, measure, and publish IPS findings in journals of multiple professions. Finally, perhaps the most reliable form of sustainability is support from leadership. If schools can agree to write IPS into curricula, IPS will continue year after year (Kumar et al., 2018). Therefore, facilitators should consider inviting high-level leadership to IPS events to highlight the importance of working together.

CONCLUSION

Socioeconomic demands, an aging population, and workforce shortages have necessitated changes in healthcare delivery systems that includes coordinated efforts among all professions to efficiently and effectively manage patient populations. IPS can play an integral role in shaping the future of health professions through opportunities to learn about, from, and with one another in a realistic, safe learning environment (Box 5.4).

Box 5.4

Resources for Interprofessional Education and Simulation

- AHRQ TeamStepps® (https://www.ahrq.gov/teamstepps/index.html)
- AMA ©—Code of Medical Ethics: Interprofessional Relationships (https://www.ama-assn.org/delivering-care/ethics/code-medical-ethics-inter-professional-relationships)
- Canadian Interprofessional Health Collaborative (http://www.cihc-cpis.com/)
- Healthcare Simulation Dictionary (https://www.ssih.org/dictionary)
- IPEC © (https://www.ipecollaborative.org/)
- International Nursing Association for Clinical Simulation and Learning (https://www.inacsl.org/inacsl-standards-of-best-practice-simulation/)
- National Center for Ethics in Healthcare (https://www.ethics.va.gov/index.asp)
- NEXUSIPE (https://nexusipe.org/)
- NLN © Interprofessional Education Resources (http://www.nln.org/professional-development-programs/teaching-resources/interprofessional-education-(ipe))
- QSEN © (https://qsen.org/faculty-resources/interprofessional-resources/)
- Society for Simulation in Healthcare (C:.S.org)
- University of Washington ©—CHSIE (https://collaborate.uw.edu/resources-and-training/online-training-and-toolkits/interprofessional-preceptor-toolkit/)

Notes. AHRQ = Agency for Healthcare Research and Quality; AMA = American Medical Association; CHSIE = Center for Health Sciences Interprofessional Education, Research, and Practice; IPEC = Interprofessional Education Collaborative; NEXUSIPE = National Center for Interprofessional Practice and Education; NLN = National League for Nurses; QSEN = Quality and Safety Education for Nurses.

REFERENCES

Adamson, K. (2015). A systematic review of the literature related to the NLN/Jeffries simulation framework. *Nursing Education Perspectives*, 36(5), 281–291. https://doi.org/10.5480/15-1655

Agency for Healthcare Research and Quality. (2020, August 8). *TeamSTEPPS®*. https://www.ahrq.gov/teamstepps/index.html

Alanazi, A. A., Nicholson, N., & Thomas, S. (2017). The use of simulation training to improve knowledge, skills, and confidence among healthcare students: A systematic review. *Internet Journal of Allied Health Sciences and Practice*, 15(3), 2.

Alexander, M., Durham, C. F., Hooper, J. I., Jeffries, P. R., Goldman, N., Kesten, K. S., & Tillman, C. (2015). NCSBN simulation guidelines for prelicensure nursing programs. *Journal of Nursing Regulation*, 6(3), 39–42. https://doi.org/10.1016/S2155-8256(15)30783-3

Anderson, M., Bond, M. L., Holmes, T. L., & Cason, C. L. (2012). Acquisition of simulation skills: Survey of users. *Clinical Simulation in Nursing*, 8(2), e59–e65. https://doi.org/10.1016/j.ecns.2010.07.002

Astbury, J., Ferguson, J., Silverthorne, J., Willis, S., & Schafheutle, E. (2020). High-fidelity simulation-based education in pre-registration healthcare programmes: A systematic review of reviews to inform collaborative and interprofessional best practice. *Journal of Interprofessional Care*. 1–11. https://doi.org/10.1080/13561820.2020.1762551

Bailey, R., Taylor, R. G., FitzGerald, M. R., Kerrey, B. T., LeMaster, T., & Geis, G. L. (2015). Defining the simulation technician role: Results of a survey-based study. *Simulation in Healthcare*, *10*(5), 283–287. https://doi.org/10.1097/SIH.0000000000000103

Bell, R., & Fredland, N. (2020). The use of theoretical frameworks guiding interprofessional simulation: An integrative review. *Nursing Education Perspectives*, *41*(3), 141–145. https://doi.org/10.1097/01.NEP.0000000000000615

Bhatt, J., & Swick, M. (2017). *Focusing on teamwork and communication to improve patient safety*. *American Hospital Association*. https://www.aha.org/news/blog/2017-03-15-focusing-teamwork-and-communication-improve-patient-safety

Boet, S., Bould, M. D., Burn, Layat., C, & Reeves, S. (2014). Twelve tips for a successful interprofessional team-based high-fidelity simulation education session. *Medical Teacher*, *36*(10), 853–857. https://doi.org/10.3109/0142159X.2014.923558

Calhoun, A., Pian-Smith, M., Shah, A., Levine, A., Gaba, D., DeMaria, S., Goldberg, A., & Meyer, E. C. (2020). Exploring the boundaries of deception in simulation: A mixed-methods study. *Clinical Simulation in Nursing*, *40*, 7–16. https://doi.org/10.1016/j.ecns.2019.12.004

Cantrell, M. A., Franklin, A., Leighton, K., & Carlson, A. (2017). The evidence in simulation-based learning experiences in nursing education and practice: An umbrella review. *Clinical Simulation in Nursing*, *13*(12), 634–667. https://doi.org/10.1016/j.ecns.2017.08.004

Cheng, A., Lockey, A., Bhanji, F., Lin, Y., Hunt, E. A., & Lang, E. (2015). The use of high-fidelity manikins for advanced life support training—A systematic review and meta-analysis. *Resuscitation*, *93*, 142–149. https://doi.org/10.1016/j.resuscitation.2015.04.004

Cheng, A., Palaganas, J., Eppich, W., Rudolph, J., Robinson, T., & Grant, V. (2015). Co-debriefing for simulation-based education. A primer for facilitators. *Simulation in Healthcare*, *10*(2), 69–75. https://doi.org/10.1097/SIH.0000000000000077

Cook, D. A., Brydges, R., Hamstra, S. J., Zendejas, B., Szostek, J. H., Wang, A. T., Erwin, P. J., & Hatala, R. (2012). Comparative effectiveness of technology-enhanced simulation versus other instructional methods: A systematic review and meta-analysis. *Simulation in Healthcare*, *7*(2), 308–320. https://doi.org/10.1097/SIH.0b013e3182614f95

Cook, K., & Stoecker, J. (2014). Healthcare student stereotypes: A systematic review with implications for interprofessional collaboration. *Journal of Research in Interprofessional Practice and Education*, *4*(2), 1–13. https://doi.org/10.22230/jripe.2014v4n2a151

Health Professions Accreditors Collaborative. (2019). *Guidance on developing quality interprofessional education for the health professions*. https://healthprofessionsaccreditors.org/wp-content/uploads/2019/02/HPACGuidance02-01-19.pdf

Heuer, A. J., Geisler, S. L., Kamienski, M., Langevin, D., & O'Sullivan-Maillet, J. ((2010). Summer). Introducing medical students to the interdisciplinary health care team: Piloting a case-based approach. *Journal of Allied Health*, *39*(2), 76–80. https://doi.org/10.1136/bmjopen-2011-000417. https://pubmed.ncbi.nlm.nih.gov/20539929

INACSL Standards Committee. (2016a). INACSL standards of best practice:. Simulation[SM] Simulation-Enhanced Interprofessional Education (sim-IPE). *Clinical Simulation in Nursing*, *12*, S34–S38. https://doi.org/10.1016/j.ecns.2016.09.011

INACSL Standards Committee. (2016b). INACSL standards of best practice: Simulation[SM]: Simulation. *Clinical Simulation in Nursing*, *12*, S5–S50. https://doi.org/10.1016/j.ecns.2016.09.009

Institute of Medicine. (1972). *Educating for the health team. The National Academies Press.*

Institute of Medicine. (2001). *Crossing the quality chasm: A new health system for the 21st century*. http://www.nap.edu/catalog.php?record_id=10027

Institute of Medicine. (2003). *Health professions education: A bridge to quality*. National. Academies Press.

Institute of Medicine. (2011). *The future of nursing: Leading change, advancing health*. National Academies Press.

Institute of Medicine. (2015). *Measuring the impact of interprofessional education on collaborative practice and patient outcomes*. The National Academies Press. https://doi.org/10.17226/21726

Interprofessional Education Collaborative. (2011). *Core competencies for interprofessional collaborative practice: Report of an expert panel*. Author. https://nebula.wsimg.com/3ee8a4b5b5f7ab794c742b14601d5f23?AccessKeyId=DC06780E69ED19E2B3A5&disposition=0&alloworigin=1

Interprofessional Education Collaborative. (2016). *Core competencies for interprofessional collaborative practice: 2016 update*. Author. https://nebula.wsimg.com/2f68a39520b03336b41038c370497473?AccessKeyId=DC06780E69ED19E2B3A5&disposition=0&alloworigin=1

James, T. A., Page, J. S., & Sprague, J. (2016). Promoting interprofessional collaboration in oncology through a teamwork skills simulation programme. *Journal of Interprofessional Care*, *30*(4), 539–541. https://doi.org/10.3109/13561820.2016.1169261

Joint Commission. (2012). *Sentinel event data*. http://www.jointcommission.org/assets/1/18/Root_Causes_by_Event_Type_2004-1Q2012.pdf

Joint Commission. (2017). Inadequate hand-off communication. *Sentinel Event Alert*, *58*, 1–6. https://www.jointcommission.org/resources/patient-safety-topics/sentinel-event/sentinel-event-alert-newsletters/sentinel-event-alert-58-inadequate-hand-off-communication/

King, J., Beanlands, S., Fiset, V., Chartrand, L., Clarke, S., Findlay, T., Morley, M., & Summers, I. (2016). Using interprofessional simulation to improve collaborative competences for nursing, physiotherapy, and respiratory therapy students. *Journal of Interprofessional Care*, *30*(5), 599–605. https://doi.org/10.1080/13561820.2016.1189887

Kostoff, M., Burkhardt, C., Winter, A., & Shrader, S. (2016). An interprofessional simulation using the SBAR communication tool. *American Journal of Pharmaceutical Education*, *80*(9), 157. 1–8. https://doi.org/10.5688/ajpe809157

Kumar, A., Kent, F., Wallace, E. M., McLelland, G., Bentley, D., Koutsoukos, A., & Nestel, D. (2018). Interprofessional education and practice guide No. 9: Sustaining interprofessional simulation using change management principles. *Journal of Interprofessional Care*, *32*(6), 771–778. https://doi.org/10.1080/13561820.2018.1511525

Labrague, L. J., M, McEnroe–Petitte, D., Foronda, D. C., & Obeidat, A. A. (2018). Interprofessional simulation in undergraduate nursing program: An integrative review. *Nurse Education Today*, *67*, 46–55. https://doi.org/10.1016/j.nedt.2018.05.001

Leclair, L. W., Dawson, M., Howe, A., Hale, S., Zelman, E., Clouser, R., Garrison, G., & Allen, G. (2018). A longitudinal interprofessional simulation curriculum for critical care teams: Exploring successes and challenges. *Journal of Interprofessional Care*, *32*(3), 386–390. https://doi.org/10.1080/13561820.2017.1405920

Lemoine, J. B., Chauvin, S. W., Broussard, L., & Oberleitner, M. G. (2015). Statewide interprofessional faculty development in simulation-based education for health professions. *Clinical Simulation in Nursing*, *11*(3), 153–162. https://doi.org/10.1016/j.ecns.2014.12.002

Lioce, L., Lopreiato, J., Downing, D., Chang, T. P., Robertson, J. M., Anderson, M., Diaz, D. A., Spain, A. E., & and the Terminology and Concepts Working Group. (2020, January). *Healthcare simulation dictionary* (2nd ed.). Agency for Healthcare Research and Quality. AHRQ Publication No. 20-0019. https://doi.org/10.23970/simulationv2

National Center for Interprofessional Practice and Education. (2020). *Assessment and evaluation*. https://nexusipe.org/advancing/assessment-evaluation-start

National League for Nursing. (2012). *A nursing perspective on simulation and Interprofessional Education (IPE): A report from the national league for nursing's think tank on using simulation as an enabling strategy for IPE*. http://www.nln.org/

National League for Nursing. (2015). *Interprofessional collaboration in education and practice: A living document from the National League for Nursing*. http://www.nln.org/docs/default-source/default-document-library/ipe-ipp-vision.pdf?sfvrsn=14

Paige, J. T., Garbee, D. D., Brown, K. M., & Rojas, J. D. (2015). Using Simulation in interprofessional education. *Surgical Clinics of North America*, *95*(4), 751–766. https://doi.org/10.1016/j.suc.2015.04.004

Palaganas, J. C., Epps, C., & Raemer, D. B. (2014). A history of simulation-enhanced interprofessional education. *Journal of Interprofessional Care*, *28*(2), 110–115. https://doi.org/10.3109/13561820.2013.869198

Poore, J. A., Dawson, J. C., Dunbar, D. M., & Parrish, K. (2019). Debriefing interprofessionally: A tool for recognition and reflection. *Nurse Educator*, *44*(1), 25–28. https://doi.org/10.1097/NNE.0000000000000518

Poore, J. A., Stephenson, E., Jerolimov, D., & Scott, P. J. (2017). Development of an interprofessional teaching grand rounds. *Nurse Educator*, *42*(4), 164–167. https://doi.org/10.1097/NNE.0000000000000351

Price, S. L., Sim, M., Little, V., Almost, J., Andrews, C., Davies, H., Harman, K., Khalili, H., Reeves, S., Sutton, E., & LeBrun, J. (2019). Pre-entry perceptions of students entering five health professions: Implications for interprofessional education and collaboration. *Journal of Interprofessional Care*, 1–9. https://doi.org/10.1080/13561820.2019.1702514

Reeves, S., & van Schaik, S. (2012). Simulation: A panacea for interprofessional learning? *Journal of Interprofessional Care*, *26*(3), 167–169. https://doi.org/10.3109/13561820.2012.678183

Riggall, V. K., & Smith, C. M. (2015). Creating a sustainable, interprofessional-team training program: initial results. *Clinical Nurse Specialist*, *29*(3), 147–155. https://doi.org/10.1097/NUR.0000000000000121

Rodziewicz, T. L., & Hipskind, J. E. (2020). Medical error prevention. In *StatPearls [Internet]*. StatPearls Publishing.

Rutherford-Hemming, T., & Lioce, L. (2018). State of interprofessional education in nursing: A systematic review. *Nurse Educator*, *43*(1), 9–13. https://doi.org/10.1097/NNE.0000000000000405

Rutherford-Hemming, T., Lioce, L., & Breymier, T. (2019). Guidelines and essential elements for prebriefing. *Simulation in Healthcare*, *14*(6), 409–414. https://doi.org/10.1097/SIH.0000000000000403

Salik, I., & Paige, J. T. (2020). Debriefing the interprofessional team in medical simulation. In *StatPearls [Internet]*. StatPearls Publishing.

Sigalet, E. L., Donnon, T. L., & Grant, V. (2015). Insight into team competence in medical, nursing and respiratory therapy students. *Journal of Interprofessional Care*, *29*(1), 62–67. https://doi.org/10.3109/13561820.2014.940416

Stephenson, E., & Poore, J. (2016). Tips for conducting the pre-brief for a simulation. *The Journal of Continuing Education in Nursing*, *47*(8), 353–355. https://doi.org/10.3928/00220124-20160715-05

Stephenson, E., Poore, J., Byrne, B. J., Dwyer, J., Ebert, D., Hasty, G., Schroedle, K., Turner, J., & Cooper, D. (2019). Interprofessional educator development course for simulation. *Journal of Continuing Education in Nursing*, *50*(10), 463–468. https://doi.org/10.3928/00220124-20190917-08

Umoren, R. A., Poore, J. A., Sweigart, L., Rybas, N., Gossett, E., Johnson, M., Allen, M., Scott, P., Truman, B., & Das, R. (2017). TeamSTEPPS virtual teams: Interactive virtual team training and practice for health professional learners. *Creative Nursing*, *23*(3), 184–191. https://doi.org/10.1891/1078-4535.23.3.184

van Soeren, M., Macmillan, K., Cop, S., Kenaszchuk, C., & Reeves, S. (2009). Development and evaluation of interprofessional care practices through clinical simulation. *Journal of Interprofessional Care*, *23*(3), 304–306. https://doi.org/10.1080/13561820802432463

Wen, A., Wong, L., Ma, C., Arndt, R., Katz, A. R., Richardson, K., Deutsch, M., & Masaki, K. (2019). An interprofessional team simulation exercise about a complex geriatric patient. *Gerontology & Geriatrics Education*, *40*(1), 16–29. https://doi.org/10.1080/02701960.2018.1554568

Wilcock, P. M., Janes, G., & Chambers, A. (2009). Health care improvement and continuing interprofessional education: Continuing interprofessional development to improve patient outcomes. *Journal of Continuing Education in the Health Professions*, 29, 84–90. https://doi.org/10.1002/chp.20016

Wilhaus, J., Palaganas, J., Manos, J., Anderson, J., Cooper, A., Jeffries, P., & Mancini, M. E. (2013). *Interprofessional education and healthcare simulation symposium [White paper]*. http://www.nln.org/docs/default-source/professional-development-programs/white-paper-symposium-ipe-in-healthcare-simulation-2013-(pdf).pdf?sfvrsn=0

Wooding, E. L., Gale, T. C., & Maynard, V. (2020). Evaluation of teamwork assessment tools for interprofessional simulation: A systematic literature review. *Journal of Interprofessional Care*, 34(2), 162–172. https://doi.org/10.1080/13561820.2019.1650730

World Health Organization. (2010). *Framework for action on interprofessional education and collaborative practice*. http://apps.who.int/iris/bitstream/10665/70185/1/WHO_HRH_HPN_10.3_eng.pdf

Part III

Simulation Practices, Operations, and Professional Development

CHAPTER 6

Evidence-Based Debriefing

Kate J. Morse, Mary K. Fey, and Susan Gross Forneris

ABSTRACT

Ongoing shifts in the healthcare system require practitioners who possess metacognitive skills to evaluate their decisions and the thinking and rationale guiding those decisions. In an effort to design learning activities that support metacognition in nursing education, undergraduate and graduate faculty, are embracing simulation-based education (SBE) as an effective teaching and learning strategy. SBE includes prebriefing, the simulation scenario, and debriefing, all of which are supported by psychological safety. Prebriefing precedes the entire learning process and is integral to engagement in the simulation and to the effectiveness of the debriefing. Debriefing provides educators with the opportunity to explore and develop those metacognitive skills with learners. In this chapter on evidence-based debriefing, the authors will explore the evidence and theories surrounding best practices in SBE, specifically the prebriefing and debriefing components of the learning experience. The chapter explores the theoretical foundation of SBE and theory-based debriefing; educational best practices of prebriefing as an integral part of an effective debriefing; theory-based debriefing models; research evidence of debriefing outcomes; evaluation of the prebriefing and debriefing process; and finally, provides recommendations on the priorities for further research in debriefing. Within this chapter, the term educator is inclusive of undergraduate, graduate, and professional development nurse educators and reflects the educator role in SBE.

http://dx.doi.org/10.1891/0739-6686.39.129

THEORY

This section will present foundational theories and highlight the importance of understanding the influence and usefulness of theory in simulation-based education (SBE) and more broadly in nursing education. Theory is a driver of innovation and change in contemporary teaching and learning as evidenced in the recent Horizon reports (Educause, 2019, 2020). The Horizon reports come from an initiative to chart emerging technologies for teaching and learning and serves as a reference planning guide for higher education. The most current Horizon reports underscore the importance of the changes in teaching and learning in higher education that are being shaped by larger macrotrends. A significant challenge cited in these reports is rethinking the practice of teaching. This challenge is defined as moving educators from transmitters of knowledge to facilitators of knowledge. SBE has also pushed the boundaries of the widely held belief of educators as the holders of all knowledge and instead views the role of the educator as a collaborator with learners. This is especially true during the debriefing process.

Two influential theories that SBE is predicated on include Kolb's experiential learning theory (ELT; Kolb, 1984) and Mezirow's transformational learning theory (TLT; Mezirow, 2003). Kolb's ELT provides a means to describe the cycle of experiential learning that takes place in SBE (Kolb, 1984). It was built primarily upon the work of Kurt Lewin, John Dewey, and Jean Piaget and describes the process by which learners perceive and then transform their experiences in order to create knowledge. The elements of *concrete experience, reflective observation, abstract conceptualization,* and *active experimentation* are among the main constructs in Kolb's ELT and represent the recursive cycle of experiential learning (see Chapter 1). *Concrete experience* is described as the perception, through the senses, of the learning experience; it is dependent on the ability of learners to involve themselves fully and without bias in new experiences. This precedes the reflective period and influences it to the extent that the learners were adequately prepared for the experience and that the experience was meaningful to them. *Reflective observation,* the next step in the cycle, is the ability to reflect on the experience from many perspectives. *Abstract conceptualization* is the ability to create concepts that integrate current observations into logically sound theories. *Active experimentation* is the ability to use these theories to make decisions and solve problems in similar future situations (Kolb & Kolb, 2009).

The *reflective observation, abstract conceptualization,* and *active experimentation* elements in Kolb's experiential learning model are most directly connected to debriefing as the time to reflect on events and examine their meaning through the participant's mental models. Following reflection, new understandings are applied to future situations. The opportunity to engage in the critical self-reflection described in *reflective observation* and *abstract conceptualization* creates the opportunity for the learner to engage in transformative learning.

Transformative learning is learning that transforms problematic frames of reference to make them more inclusive, discriminating, open, reflective, and emotionally able to change. These frames of reference include habits of mind, cultural biases, ideologies, schemata, stereotyped attitudes and practices, religious doctrine, moral–ethical norms, psychological preferences and schema, paradigms in science and mathematics, frames in linguistics and social sciences, and aesthetic values and standards (Mezirow, 2003). TLT offers an explanation for change in these frames of reference or meaning structures. Behavior change is a consequence of a transformation in these frames of reference. The transformation occurs through self-reflection by identifying and judging premises, presuppositions, and taken-for-granted assumptions. This change often starts with a disorienting dilemma, that is, an experience in which our "usual" interpretations and actions do not result in success. A transformed perspective is one that is more: (a) inclusive, (b) differentiating, (c) permeable, (d) critically reflective, and (e) integrative of experience.

Rational discourse is the essential medium through which transformation is promoted and developed (Mezirow, 1991). Discourse in transformative learning rests on the following assumptions:

- It is rational only as long it meets the conditions necessary to create understanding with another.
- It is driven by objectivity.
- All actions and statements are open to question and discussion.
- Understanding is created through the weighing of evidence and by measuring the insight and strength of supporting arguments.
- The primary goal is to promote mutual understanding among others.

Mezirow posits 10 phases of transformation and describes transformation as more commonly a process, not always linear, rather than a sudden blinding moment in time:

- Experiencing a disorienting dilemma
- Self-examination with discontent
- Critically assessing assumptions
- Recognizing the connection between discontent and the process of transformation
- Exploring options for new roles, relationships, and actions

- Planning/revising a course of action
- Acquiring knowledge and skills for implementing one's plan
- Trying new roles on a provisional basis
- Building competence and self-confidence in new roles and relationships (Mezirow, 1991)

When the debriefing process is a structured, facilitated process that supports transformative learning, it provides the opportunity for the learner to engage in critical self-reflection and possibly perspective transformation. For some learners, self-reflection may continue after debriefing and perspective change may occur postdebriefing. (Morse, 2015). The theories of Kolb (1984) and Mezirow (2003) provide the theoretical support for the subsequent SBE models. Because SBE aims to improve decision-making and resultant performance, theories of behavior change are relevant.

Undergraduate nursing education began exploring the use of simulation as early as 2003 through the work of the National League for Nursing (NLN) under the direction of Dr. Pamela Jeffries and Dr. Mary Anne Rizzolo (Jeffries & Rizzolo, 2006). This seminal work resulted in the NLN Jeffries Simulation Framework (Jeffries, 2005, 2007, 2012) that evolved into the first nursing midrange theory focused on simulation: The NLN Jeffries Simulation Theory (Jeffries, 2015; Jeffries et al., 2015).

In particular, the role of the educator in facilitating debriefing is supported by the work of the NLN Jeffries Simulation Theory and educational practices. Educational practices as a theoretical component are derived from the seminal work of Chickering and Gamson's seven principles of good practice in undergraduate education (1987). Techniques such as active learning, communicating high expectations, and direct interactions between learner and educator lay the strong foundation for the teaching and learning benefits derived from debriefing. The main objectives of debriefing provide opportunities for learners to critically reflect on their experience and react to the simulation learning encounter. Guided by the educator, debriefing engages reflective thinking, a metacognitive activity for the learner to reflect on their thinking and uncover or make explicit the decision-making process behind their actions during the learning encounter. Debriefing provides a deep dive into examining real-life experiences, engaging in critical self-reflection, *normalizing* behaviors, and acknowledging emotions.

Moving the "transforming nursing education dialogue" further, the NLN published a vision statement entitled *Debriefing Across the Curriculum* (2015). The vision statement was developed and written based on the strong theoretical underpinnings of debriefing and the reflective and critical nature of conversations. The NLN advocates for these conversations to be used in teaching and learning across the curriculum—not just in simulation. Among factors affecting the expanded use of debriefing as a critical conversation are the elements of context and active learning. The call to *teach with and about context* is imperative to transform nursing education. Contextualizing learning in the moment shifts the focus from learners as doers of actions to learners as *meaning makers*. As discussed briefly earlier, active learning is a key principle in effective teaching and embraces the meaning-making conversation rather than the traditional *depositing* of content. The intent of the NLN *Debriefing Across the Curriculum* vision statement was the call to action for nurse educators to integrate theory-based debriefing principles into everyday teaching and learning. The NLN has since then published a number of resources to develop faculty expertise in this area. *Critical Conversations: The NLN Guide for Teaching Thinking* (Forneris & Fey, 2016, 2017) was published as a beginning foundation to provide a structure for educators that guides students to discern what is meaningful and relevant and to use their knowledge to work through the problems of nursing practice. It is a learner-centered approach involving a three-part conversation structure: *context*, *content*, and *course*. *The NLN Guide for Teaching Thinking* lays a foundation for reflective learning conversations. The philosophical and theoretical underpinnings used in this guide are derived from those that underpin theory-based debriefing. This coupled with experiential learning and TLT lay a strong foundation for reflective learning in SBE.

PREBRIEFING

Prebriefing is intended to create psychological safety that promotes learner engagement in the simulation scenario and debriefing. The two components, prebriefing and debriefing, are intertwined to create and maintain psychological safety for the learners. To discuss one without the other does a grave disservice to the reader; therefore, the discussion of the learning process in debriefing starts with prebriefing.

Prebriefing and debriefing as components of simulation are essential components of simulation design. These educational practices are used by the educator to create a dynamic interaction between the educator and the learner. Key to this dynamic interaction is the creation of a psychologically safe learning environment. Psychological safety can be defined as a perception, on the part of the learners, that they are comfortable taking interpersonal risks such as admitting error, discussing mistakes, receiving feedback, sharing their thinking, and valuing diverse points of view (Edmonson et al., 2016; Rudolph et al., 2014). The idea of creating a safe and trusted learning space—psychological safety in learning—has been described in a concept analysis (Turner & Harder, 2018). The authors describe the three defining attributes of psychological safety as: (a) the ability of the learners to make mistakes without consequences, (b) the qualities of the educator influencing the creation and maintenance of psychological safety, and (c) the inclusion of activities such as orientation, preparation, objectives, and expectations. The educator who is facilitating the learning process is pivotal to creating and maintaining psychological safety throughout the learning process.

Transformation requires critical self-reflection in the setting of psychological safety. This leverages the learning experience and supports the process of shifting learners' internal frames or mental models, which has been described as perspective transformation or transformative learning (Mezirow, 2003).

During prebriefing, the educator has the responsibility to begin or continue the teaching–learning relationship, orient the learners, and provide an adequate context to allow the learners to proceed. The International Nursing Association for Clinical Simulation and Learning (INACSL) Standards of Best Practice: Simulation^{SM}: Simulation Design describes the essential elements of simulation (INACSL Standards Committee, 2016). Within this standard, Criterion 7 describes beginning every simulation experience with a prebriefing. The standard goes on to describe required elements, including a structured approach that occurs immediately prior to the experience and: (a) explores learners' expectations, (b) establishes ground rules, (c) provides an orientation, (d) acknowledges the limitations of simulation, and (e) promotes learner engagement through the discussion of a fiction contract.

These essential elements have also been described in concept analyses (Chamberlain, 2015; Page-Cutrara, 2015). Chamberlain (2015) identified the consequences of prebriefing as enhanced satisfaction, increased participation, and learning effectiveness of the simulation experience. Page-Cutrara (2015) similarly recognized that prebriefing identified learner engagement, enhanced a readiness to receive cues during the simulated case, and reinforced or revised ways of thinking. Both authors described the key elements of prebriefing: supporting learning prior to engagement in the simulated case; time to consider the upcoming situation; perceiving meaning and anticipating a plan (Page-Cutrara, 2015); and the role of the educator in creating a safe and trusted learning space (Chamberlain, 2015).

The attributes described in the concept analyses (Chamberlain, 2015; Page-Cutrara, 2015) are consistent with Element 1 of the Debriefing Assessment for Simulation in Healthcare© (DASH). The DASH is a behaviorally anchored rating scale that was designed to develop and evaluate debriefing skills. Element 1 speaks to the facilitator's skill in establishing an engaging learning environment (Brett-Fleegler et al., 2012; Simon et al., 2010). Element 1 further describes the key dimensions as "clarifies course objectives, environment, roles and expectations; establishes a 'fiction contract'; attends to logistical details; and conveys a commitment to respecting learners and understanding their perspective" (Simon et al., 2010, pp. 5–6). The "fiction contract" refers to the process of partnering with the learner to create a shared agreement in which both have obligations to each other, primarily related to recognizing that the simulated learning environment has limitations. Included in this agreement is recognition that the educator has done as much as they can to make the experience as real as possible; the clinical problems and conversations are real despite the patient being a manikin; and a request for the learner to enter into the contract by engaging in the case's clinical problems.

Prebriefing prior to engaging in simulation has been shown to contribute to the learning experience. Dileone et al. (2020) conducted an integrative review of simulation prebriefing in nursing education. The review spanned from 2012 to 2019 and included six articles in the final analysis. The authors concluded that, while there are robust descriptions of prebriefing activities, there is a lack of consistency and consensus on how prebriefing should be conducted, resulting in an inability to compare studies and draw meaningful conclusions (Dileone et al., 2020). McDermott (2020) reviewed the history of prebriefing and proposed a Know:Do:Teach model that is based on adult learning principles and Benner's novice to expert framework. This model is intended to be a guide for facilitators in prebriefing.

A number of studies have examined the impact of prebriefing on nursing students' clinical competency and judgment (Kim et al., 2017; Page-Cutrara & Turk, 2017; Sharoff, 2015). Page-Cutrara and Turk (2017) conducted an experimental study examining the impact of a structured prebriefing compared to the standard prebriefing. Both included orientation to the equipment, simulation space, patient (manikin), learning objectives, and the clinical situation, but the structured prebriefing also included an author-designed, structured prebriefing model with reflection-before-action (anticipating a clinical plan), concept mapping, and activating prior learning and bringing it into the current learning context. There was a significant difference between standard and structured prebriefing in competency performance ($p < .001$), clinical judgment ($p < .001$), and prebriefing experience ($p < .001$).

Sharoff (2015) demonstrated the positive impact of prebriefing materials on students' perceptions of the effectiveness of the written prebriefing materials, and subsequent planning, implementation of effective nursing actions, and reflections on the experience. This study was limited due to the lack of a control group and the self-report tools used for outcome measures; however, it did present an innovative approach to prebriefing with written materials and videos.

Kim et al. (2017) explored the impact of a step-based prebriefing approach on the students' flow (defined as the fluidity of the performance of the student and level of engagement) and clinical competency through a quasiexperimental study. The step-based approach to prebriefing included: Step 1—a verbal presentation of learning objectives, students roles, and introduction to the simulation process; Step 2—experiencing the simulation environment (vital signs, assessment of the manikin location of equipment); and Step 3—practice in a similar learning environment with guidance from a trained nurse. Three groups of learners participated in the study with Group 1 receiving only Step 1, Group 2 receiving Steps 1 and 2, and Group 3 receiving all three steps. Group 2 demonstrated the highest levels of satisfaction, flow, and self-confidence. Clinical competency was significantly higher in Group 2 but not when compared to Group 3 (control group) ($F = 5.19$, $p = .006$).

The studies reviewed demonstrate the importance of prebriefing to overall learning outcomes. An evidence-based prebriefing supports an evidence-based debriefing.

THEORY-BASED MODELS OF DEBRIEFING

Debriefing is a purposeful, structured, reflective learning conversation. In a now-classic work, Fanning and Gaba (2007) describe the structure of a debriefing as having an initial phase during which the emotional impact of the simulation is acknowledged; a phase of systematic reflection and analysis; and a conclusion with application to the future behaviors. Most methods of debriefing in wide use in prelicensure and graduate nursing education today follow this general structure, including Debriefing With Good Judgment© (Rudolph et al., 2006), Debriefing for Meaningful Learning© (DML; Dreifuerst, 2012), and Promoting Excellence and Reflective Learning in Simulation (PEARLS; Eppich & Cheng, 2015). This section will briefly review these methods of debriefing.

These collective works illustrate the value of the conversation in the teaching and learning process. The theoretical underpinnings of these debriefing methods have at their core an emphasis on being critical, that is, the ability to examine and share perspectives (Freire, 1970). This requires reflection, perspective taking, examining one's biases and beliefs to understand the whole of the situation—to be truly *critical*. Critical pedagogy, while not new, is the philosophical foundation that underpins and guides many contemporary teaching strategies, like debriefing, that use reflection as a core attribute. The learning process is one of assessing what is relevant and determining the reasons for our actions. As a process of assessing relevancy, the educator facilitates learners' reflection to help them to examine the thought processes guiding the actions taken during the learning encounter. It is a conversation that moves from *let me show you how do this* to *tell me how you understand this*. This pivot to dialogue from monologue has been part of the disruption in nursing education (Waxman et al., 2019). That is, nurse educators pivot from teaching moments to *creating learning moments*.

Many of the theories guiding today's debriefing methods were contemporary ideas in the 1980s (Schön, 1987), so, not really new today. The difference between teaching moments and learning moments is the shift from a focus on content to teaching students how to directly apply content knowledge. In this approach, students are presented with structured learning situations and asked to apply their knowledge in a logical, coherent way to achieve an end point. Schön (1983 and 1987) would suggest that our real-world situations do not come to us as shaped case studies, but rather in scattered pieces, that we find, make sense of, and then fit together. In this approach, learners create meaning as they encounter and work through the bits and pieces. The learning moment is enhanced by the conversations the educator has to uncover learner rationale; the thoughts guiding decision and action. The ability to connect to thinking *in the moment* to actions taken is so important for successful work in today's complex healthcare environments.

Debriefing With Good Judgment

Debriefing With Good Judgment is in widespread use throughout the world (Rudolph et al., 2006). Based on theories from diverse fields (adult learning, behavior change, cognitive psychology) and research from organizational behavior, this method of debriefing aims to discover the thought processes driving observable actions. During a multiphase debriefing discussion, the facilitator uses the "advocacy/inquiry" conversational strategy as a reflective learning technique to uncover the thought processes, or cognitive frames, behind the actions observed in simulation. Through discussion and teaching, the facilitator reinforces positive cognitive frames, or helps to facilitate the creation of new cognitive frames that will support improved practice moving forward.

Debriefing for Meaningful Learning

DML (Dreifuerst, 2012) is a method that is used in hundreds of prelicensure nursing programs throughout the world. It uses reflective discourse to uncover relationships between thought processes and nursing actions. This method is based on six elements that facilitate thinking processes: engage, explore, explain, elaborate, evaluate, and extend. These elements serve to guide learners through a reflective learning conversation to facilitate sensemaking of the learning experience and apply current learning to potential future experiences (Bradley & Dreifuerst, 2016). DML promotes clinical reasoning by actively teaching prelicensure students to use reflection-in-action, reflection-on-action, and reflection-beyond-action (Dreifuerst, 2015).

Promoting Excellence and Reflective Learning in Simulation

PEARLS is a method of debriefing described by Eppich and Cheng (2015). It is a blended approach to debriefing that includes three educational strategies: learner self-assessment, focused facilitation for reflective learning, and providing directive feedback and/or teaching. These educational strategies are combined with scripting for the debriefer. The PEARLS framework and script provide scaffolding for developing debriefers, as it helps guide the facilitator in making choices about the use of the educational strategies.

The three widely used theory-based debriefing methods discussed earlier all have critical reflection as the method for examining thought processes. There is no definitive research demonstrating the superiority of any one of these methods over the other. Rather, the research cited supports use of structured, theory-based debriefing versus debriefing that is unstructured and does not follow a specific method. A review of literature on debriefing from aviation, psychology, education, medicine, and nursing identified several factors important to the practice of debriefing (Lusk & Fater, 2013). These include:

- The debriefer as a facilitator provides a safe learning environment
- Active listening techniques
- Facilitating reflective discussion by all participants as a role of the debriefer
- Debriefing should be planned and satisfy learning objectives
- Generalizability of lessons learned to broader contexts should be included in debriefing
- The time frame for debriefing should be at least as much time as is spent in the simulation but is often longer
- A structured framework is important to the process (Lusk & Fater, 2013)

OUTCOMES OF DEBRIEFING RESEARCH IN NURSING EDUCATION

The National Council of State Boards of Nursing (NCSBN; Hayden et al., 2014) led the effort to transform undergraduate nursing education (Benner et al., 2010). Since this landmark study, simulation and debriefing have continued to push the boundaries of traditional teaching and learning in nursing education (Waxman et al., 2019). Debriefing is a vital step in the process of the simulation learning experience and is one of the key design features to consider when operationalizing a simulation learning encounter (Jeffries, 2005). Recent nursing education research across the discipline of nursing (i.e., undergraduate, graduate, and professional development) with specific emphasis on the impact of theory-based debriefing is limited to date (Allen et al., 2020; Cant & Cooper, 2011; Mariani et al., 2019; Morse, 2015; Shinners et al., 2016; Vanderzwan et al., 2020).

Research was reviewed that focused on debriefing as a primary intervention. Theory-based debriefing has been supported empirically to enhance learning (Dreifuerst, 2012; Eppich & Cheng, 2015; O'Donnell et al., 2009; Morse et al., 2015; Shinnick & Woo, 2010) and advances in these methods continue to illustrate the value of conversation on the teaching–learning process.

Theory-based debriefing as an evidence-based contextual teaching–learning strategy facilitates experiential learning and fosters critical thinking and clinical reasoning (Dreifuerst, 2012; Forneris et al, 2015; Minehart et al., 2014). Several empirical studies underscore that, in the absence of debriefing in a simulation learning encounter, learning does not occur (Mahmood & Darzi, 2004; Savoldelli et al., 2006; Shinnick & Woo, 2010). Jeffries (2012) found that poorly conducted debriefing can result in poor clinical judgment. While these studies' findings were based on simulation learning encounters, the importance of their outcomes has significance for other learning encounters. Debriefing as an education best practice has relevance according to findings in a meta-analysis (Tannenbaum & Cerasoli, 2012) that reported a positive correlation between debriefing and improved individual and team performance. Similarly, a recent systematic review and meta-analysis of debriefing methods and learning outcomes found that simulation plus structured debriefing improves learning outcomes, such as clinical performance, problem-solving ability, confidence to perform, critical thinking, and clinical reasoning (Lee et al., 2020).

EVALUATION OF PREBRIEFING/DEBRIEFING PROCESS

Prebriefing

There are no known instruments that specifically evaluate prebriefing alone. Rather, prebriefing is often included as a component of debriefing evaluation instruments or as part of overall simulation evaluation tools. Element 1 of the DASH specifically evaluates facilitator behaviors that contribute to creating an engaging environment for learning and can provide feedback from three perspectives: rater version, instructor (self-evaluation), and student (Simon et al., 2010). While this provides guidance and evaluation data for faculty development, it does not examine the impact of prebriefing on learner outcomes.

The Simulation Effectiveness Tool, Modified (SET-M), is a self-report instrument completed by learners in simulation-based learning experiences (Leighton et al., 2015). The instrument has four identified subscales, one of which is prebriefing. Self-report is an effective way to measure phycological safety, as psychological safety is a perception, on the part of the learner, that they can trust the educator to help them manage the stresses of challenging experiential learning, and that they will be viewed positively even if they make a mistake (Rudolph et al., 2014).

Debriefing Evaluation

In the literature, several instruments that evaluate the skill of the debriefer are intended for use with specific debriefing approaches, while others can be used regardless of debriefing method.

Instruments that are used by more experienced debriefers to assess developing debriefers include:

- The DASH Rater Version© (Simon et al., 2011)
- The Objective Structured Assessment of Debriefing (OSAD; Arora, 2012)
- DML Evaluation Scale (Bradley & Dreifuerst, 2016)

Two instruments used for self-assessment:

- The DASH Instructor Version© (Simon et al., 2012)
- The DML Inventory (Bradley, 2018)

Two instruments that allow learners to assess the debriefing:

- The DASH Student Version© (Simon et al., 2010)
- Debriefing Experience Scale (DES; Reed, 2012)

The Debriefing Assessment for Simulation in Healthcare

The DASH (Simon et al., 2010) is a six-element, unweighted, criterion-referenced, behaviorally anchored rating scale that evaluates instructor behaviors that are believed to represent optimal behaviors (Brett-Fleegler et al., 2012). There are six elements of the instrument: establishes an engaging learning environment; maintains an engaging learning environment; structures the debriefing in an organized way; provokes engaging discussions; identifies and explores performance gaps; and helps trainees achieve or sustain good future performance. Each of the elements is rated from 1 (extremely ineffective) to 7 (extremely effective). Each element is further described through the use of behavioral descriptors that should be demonstrated by the facilitator, such as "described the simulation environment"; "described what would be expected during the activity"; "introduced the learning objectives"; and "clarified issues of confidentiality." The DASH is the most frequently used facilitator assessment in prelicensure nursing education programs in the United States (Fey, 2014) and was used to assess debriefers during the NCSBN simulation study (Hayden et al, 2014).

The Objective Structured Assessment of Debriefing

The OSAD instrument was developed for use in surgical simulation experiences (Arora, 2012). A rigorous development process included extensive literature review, interviews with 360 end users, and review by experts. Interviews included practicing surgeons who conduct debriefing, surgical residents who receive debriefing, operating room nurses, and anesthesiologists from the United States, the United Kingdom, and Australia. Eight key features pertaining to an effective debriefing were identified as:

- Approach
- Learning environment
- Learner engagement
- Reaction
- Reflection
- Analysis
- Diagnosis
- Application

Each of the categories is rated on a scale of 1 (minimum) to 3 (maximum) regarding how well the facilitator conducts the debriefing element. Descriptive anchors at the low, mid, and highpoint guide the rater.

The Debriefing Experience Scale

The DES (Reed, 2012) was developed from a comprehensive literature review by three nursing simulation experts. Using factor analysis, the 20 items were identified that represent four subscales. Each of the items is rated on two Likert-type scales. One scale represents learners' perception of the quality of the experience; the other represents learners' perception of the importance of the items to the overall debriefing experience. Experience is rated from 1 (strongly disagree) to 5 (strongly agree) and importance is rated from 1 (not important) to 5 (very important). The subscales are:

- Analyzing thoughts and feelings
- Learning and making connections
- Facilitator skill in conducting the debriefing
- Appropriate facilitator guidance

The DML Evaluation Scale

The DML Evaluation Scale (Bradley & Dreifuerst, 2016) is a behaviorally anchored rating scale that was developed specifically for DML debriefers. It is used by proficient DML facilitators to evaluate others through the six elements of DML: engage, explore, explain, elaborate, evaluate, and extend.

The DML Inventory

The DML Inventory was developed based on the DML Evaluation Scale. The DML Inventory is a self-report measure of understanding and application of DML in debriefing. In contrast to the DML Evaluation Scale, which measures observable behaviors, the DML Inventory is a self-report of the debriefer's understanding and application process, and provides a window into the thinking of the debriefer. The DML Evaluation Scale and DML Inventory can be used together for formative assessment of debriefers.

Debriefer Development

The NCSBN national simulation study (Hayden et al., 2014) and subsequent guidelines (Alexander et al., 2015) recommend that educators debriefing in simulation-based learning have training in a theory-based debriefing method. As a critical component of learning in SBE and other learning contexts, debriefing should follow an evidence-based approach. This evidence base includes theories of learning and behavior change. The elements of these theories have been used to develop assessment tools with objective criteria against which debriefer skills can be assessed. Training debriefers and assessing their competence increases the likelihood that debriefers will conduct theory-based debriefing (Fey & Jenkins, 2015).

The metacognitive strategy of critical reflection that is used to debrief learners can also be used for formative assessment in the development of debriefing skills. Those who are responsible for faculty development of simulation educators can "debrief the debriefing" and explore the actions taken and thought processes used by the debriefing facilitator. This is generally done soon after the conclusion of the debriefing. There is no universal approach to this developmental strategy.

A flexible assessment model that is often used in health professions education is Miller's pyramid (1990). This assessment framework can be used to guide both the cognitive and behavioral aspects of debriefer skill development. The hierarchy embedded in this framework begins with learning basics facts and builds through knowing how to apply that factual knowledge to achieve competent performance (Miller, 1990). Within this assessment framework, however, the specific knowledge and behaviors of an effective debriefing facilitator are not described. Combining Miller's framework with debriefing-specific evaluation instruments can guide the ongoing professional development of educators.

CONCLUSION

This chapter reviewed the current state of nursing research on the prebriefing and debriefing aspects of SBE. The literature discussed in this chapter supports that prebriefing and debriefing are essential elements of SBE and that a structured theory-based approach is associated with better outcomes. While the nature of debriefing and critical self-reflection is an individual journey and primarily an internal process requiring self-report tools, learner satisfaction is no longer an important contribution to the field. As early as 2011 the paucity of research primarily focused on debriefing was discussed in the simulation literature (Raemer et al., 2011). While there have been a number of studies published since then, there are still areas that require further exploration:

- Prebriefing (alternative methods—written, e-mail, prerecorded), and the influence of different learning environments such as in situ.
- Debriefing the debriefer models and evaluating different feedback models.
- Replicating debriefing studies focused on enhancing learners' critical thinking and moving toward behavior change in practice.
- Leveraging collaborative research that brings together schools of nursing, graduate, and undergraduate, to diversify the sample population and increase the power of the findings.
- Connecting SBE in training to future patient safety events in clinical practice.
- A deeper exploration of the impact of psychological safety on learner outcomes and the key educator behaviors is an area of future research.

SBE, in particular prebriefing and debriefing, will always have variations in practice with consistent theoretical threads. While there are many paths to reflective practice, examining our educational process with a critical eye and continuing to deepen our evidence-based teaching and learning practices is an ongoing journey.

REFERENCES

Alexander, M., Durham, C. F., Hooper, J. I., Jeffries, J. R., Goldman, N., Kesten, Kardong-Edgren., A, K., Spector, N., Tagliareni, E., Radtke, B., & Tillman, C. (2015). NCSBN simulation guidelines for prelicensure nursing programs. *Journal of Nursing Regulation*, 6(3), 39–42. https://doi.org/10.1016/S2155-8256(15)30783-3

Allen, L., Bulat, T., Uphold, C. R., Johnson, T., & Winkler, S.L. (2020). Using a post fall assessment simulation to examine nurse thought processes. *Journal for Nurses in Professional Development*, 36, 266–270. 35(6) https://doi.org/10.1097/NND.0000000000000662

Arora, S. (2012). Objective structured assessment of debriefing bringing science to the art of debriefing in surgery. *Annals of Surgery*, *256*(6), 982. https://doi.org/10.1097/SLA.0b013e3182610c91

Benner, P., Sutphen, M., Leonard, V., & Day, L. (2010). *Educating nurses: A call for radical transformation*. Jossey-Bass.

Bradley, C. S. (2018). Confirmatory factor analysis of the debriefing for meaningful learning inventory©. *Clinical Simulation in Nursing*, *14*, 15–20. http://doi.org/10.1016/j.ecns.2017.09.004

Bradley, C. S., & Dreifuerst, K. T. (2016). Pilot testing the debriefing for meaningful learning evaluation scale. *Clinical Simulation in Nursing*, *12*(7), 277–280. https://doi.org/10.1016/j.ecns.2016.01.008

Brett-Fleegler, M., Rudolph, J., Eppich, W., Monuteaux, M., Fleegler, E., Cheng, A., & Simon, R. (2012). Debriefing assessment for simulation in healthcare: Development and psychometric properties. *Simulation in Healthcare*, *7*(5), 288–294. https://doi.org/10.1097/SIH.0b013e3182620228

Cant, R. P., & Cooper, S. J. (2011). The benefits of debriefing as formative feedback in nurse education. *Australian Journal of Advanced Nursing*, *29*(1), 37–47. https://www.ajan.com.au/archive/Vol29/29-1_Cant.pdf

Chamberlain, J. (2015, July). Prebriefing in nursing simulation: A concept analysis using Roger's methodology. *Clinical Simulation in Nursing*, *11*(7), 318–322. http://doi.org/10.1016/j.ecns.2015.05.003

Chickering, A. W., & Gamson, Z. F. (1987). Seven principles of good practice in undergraduate education. *AAHE Bulletin*, *40*(7), 1–6.

Dileone, C., Chyun, D., Diaz, D., & Maruca, A. (2020). An examination of simulation prebriefing in nursing education: An integrative review. *Nursing Education Perspectives*. *41*(6), 345–348. Advanced Online Publication. https://doi.org/1097/01.NEP.0000000000000689

Dreifuerst, K. T. (2012). Using debriefing for meaningful learning to foster development of clinical reasoning in simulation. *Journal of Nursing Education*, *51*(6), 321–333. https://doi.org/10.3928/01484834-20120409-02

Dreifuerst, K. T. (2015). Getting started with debriefing for meaningful learning. *Clinical Simulation in Nursing*, *11*(5), 268–275. https://doi.org/10.1016/j.ecns.2015.01.005

Edmonson, A. C., Higgins, M., Singer, S., & Weiner, J. (2016). Understanding psychological safety in health care and educational organizations: A comparative perspective. *Research in Human Development*, *13*(1), 65–83. https://doi.org/10.1080/15427609.2016.1141280

Educause. (2019). *Educause horizon report: 2019 Higher education edition*. Author. https://library.educause.edu/-/media/files/library/2019/4/2019horizonreport.pdf?la=en&hash=C8E8D444AF372E705FA1BF9D4FF0DD4CC6F0FDD1

Educause. (2020). *Educause horizon report: 2020 Teaching and learning edition*. Author. https://library.educause.edu/-/media/files/library/2020/3/2020_horizon_report_pdf.pdf?la=en&hash=08A92C17998E8113BCB15DCA7BA1F467F303BA80

Eppich, W., & Cheng, A. (2015). Promoting Excellence and Reflective Learning in Simulation (PEARLS): Development and rationale for a blended approach to health care simulation debriefing. *Simulation in Healthcare*, *10*(2), 106–115. https://doi.org/10.1097/SIH.0000000000000072

Fanning, R. M., & Gaba, D. M. (2007). Summer). The role of debriefing in simulation-based learning. *Simulation in Healthcare*, 2(2), 115–125. https://doi.org/10.1097/SIH.0b013e3180315539

Fey, M. K. (2014). *Debriefing practices in nursing education programs in the United States*. University of Maryland, Baltimore Maryland. Doctoral dissertation. https://search-proquest-com.ezproxy2.library.drexel.edu/pqdtglobal/docview/1545890423/2194BA9FA58442C6PQ/1?accountid=10559

Fey, M. K., & Jenkins, L. S. (2015). Debriefing practices in nursing education programs: Results from a national study. *Nursing Education Perspectives*, *36*(6), 361–366. https://doi.org/10.5480/14-1520

Forneris, S. G., & Fey, M. (2016). Critical conversations: The NLN guide for teaching thinking. *Nursing Education Perspectives*, 37(5), 248–249. https://doi.org/10.5480/15-1672

Forneris, S. G., & Fey, M. (Eds.). (2017). *Critical conversations: The NLN guide for teaching thinking*. National League for Nursing.

Forneris, S. G., Neal, D. O., Tiffany, J., Kuehn, M. B., Meyer, H. M., Blazovich, L. M., Holland, A. E., & Smerillo, M. (2015). Enhancing clinical reasoning through simulation debriefing: A multi-site study. *Nursing Education Perspectives*, *36*(5), 304–310. https://doi.org/10.5480/15-1672

Freire, P. (1970). *Pedagogy of the oppressed* (30th anniversary ed.). Continuum International Publishing Group.

Hayden, J. K., Smiley, R. A., Alexander, M., Kardong-Edgren, S., & Jeffries, P. R. (2014). Supplement: The NCSBN National Simulation Study: A longitudinal, randomized, controlled study replacing clinical hours with simulation in prelicensure nursing education. *Journal of Nursing Regulation*, 5(2), C1–S64. https://doi.org/10.1016/S2155-8256(15)30062-4

INACSL Standards Committee. (2016, December). INACSL standards of best practice: SimulationSM: Simulation design. *Clinical Simulation in Nursing*, *12*(5), S5 S12. https://doi.org/10.10.1016/j.ecns.2016.09.05

Jeffries, P. R. (2005). A framework for designing, implementing, and evaluating simulations used as teaching strategies in nursing. *Nursing Education Perspectives*, *26*(2), 96–103.

Jeffries, P. R. (Ed.). (2007). *Simulation in nursing education: From conceptualization to evaluation*. National League for Nursing.

Jeffries, P. R. (Ed.). (2012). *Simulation in nursing education: From conceptualization to evaluation* (2nd ed.). National League for Nursing.

Jeffries, P. R. (Ed.). (2015). *The NLN Jeffries simulation theory*. Wolters Kluwer.

Jeffries, P. R., & Rizzolo, M. A. (2006). *Designing and implementing models for the innovative use of simulation to teach nursing care of ill adults and children: A national, multi-site, multi-method study*. http://www.nln.org/docs/default-source/professional-development-programs/read-the-nln-laerdal-project-summary-report-pdf.pdf?sfvrsn=0

Jeffries, P. R., & Rogers, K. J. (2012). Theoretical framework for simulation design. In P. R. Jeffries (Ed.), *Simulation in nursing education: From conceptualization to evaluation* (2nd ed., pp. 25–42). National League for Nursing.

Jeffries, P. R., Rodgers, B., & Adamson, K. (2015). NLN Jeffries simulation theory: A brief narrative description. *Nursing Education Perspectives*, *36*(5), 292–293. https://doi.org/10.5480/1536-5026-36.5.292

Kim, Y. J., Noh, G. O., & Im, Y. S. (2017). Effect of step-based prebriefing activities on flow and clinical competency of nursing students in simulation-based education. *Clinical Simulation in Nursing*, *13*(11), 544–551. http://doi.org/10.1016/j.ecns.2017.06.005

Kolb, A. Y., & Kolb, D. A. (2009). The learning way: Meta-cognitive aspects of experiential learning. *Simulation & Gaming*, *40*(3), 297–327. https://doi.org/10.1177/1046878108325713

Kolb, D. A. (1984). *Experience as the source of learning and development*. NV Basic Books.

Lee, J., Lee, H., Kim, S., Choi, M., Ko, I. S., Bae, J., & Kim, S. H. (2020). Debriefing methods and learning outcomes in simulation nursing education: A systematic review and meta-analysis. *Nurse Education Today*, *87*, 104345. https://doi.org/10.1016/j.nedt.2020.104345

Leighton, K., Ravert, P., Mudra, V., & Macintosh, C. (2015). Updating the simulation effectiveness tool: Item modifications and reevaluation of psychometric properties. *Nursing Education Perspectives*, *36*(5), 317–323. https://doi.org/10.5480/15-1671

Lusk, J. M., & Fater, K. (2013). Postsimulation debriefing to maximize clinical judgment development. *Nurse Educator*, *38*(1), 16–19. https://doi.org/10.1097/NNE.0b013e318276df8b

Mahmood, T., & Darzi, A. (2004). The learning curve for a colonoscopy simulator in the absence of any feedback: No feedback, no learning. *Surgical Endoscopy*, *18*(8), 1224–1230. https://doi.org/10.1007/s00464-003-9143-4

Mariani, B., Zazyczny, K. A., & Decina, P. (2019). Preparation for clinical preparedness in pediatric emergencies: A pilot study. *Journal for Nurses in Professional Development*, *35*(1), 6–11. https://doi.org/10.1097/NND.0000000000000500

McDermott, D. S. (2020). Prebriefing: A historical perspective and evolution of a model and strategy (Know:Do:Teach. *Clinical Simulation in Nursing*, *X*, 1–10. https://doi.org/10.1016/j.ecns.2020.05.005

Mezirow, J. (1991). *Transformative dimensions of adult learning*. Jossey-Bass.

Mezirow, J. (1997). Transformative learning: Theory to practice. *New Directions for Adult and Continuing Education*, *74*, 5–12. http://dx.doi.org/10.1002/ace.7401

Mezirow, J. (2003). Transformative learning as discourse. *Journal of Transformative Education*, *1*(1), 58–63. https://doi.org/10.1177/1541344603252172

Miller, G. E. (1990). The assessment of clinical skills/competence/performance. *Academic medicine*, *65*(9), S63–S67. https://doi.org/10.1097/00001888-199009000-00045

Minehart, R. D., Rudolph, J., Pian-Smith, M. C., & Raemer, D. B. (2014). Improving faculty feedback to resident trainees during a simulated case: A randomized, controlled trial of an educational intervention. *Anesthesiology*, *120*(1), 160–171. https://doi.org/10.1097/ALN.0000000000000058

Morse, K. J. (2015). Structured model of debriefing on perspective transformation for NP students. *Clinical Simulation in Nursing*, *11*(3), 172–179. https://doi.org/10.1016/j.ecns.2015.01.001

National League for Nursing. (2015). *Debriefing across the curriculum*. http://www.nln.org/docs/default-source/about/nln-vision-series-(position-statements)/nln-vision-debriefing-across-the-curriculum.pdf?sfvrsn=0

O'Donnell, J., Rodgers, D., Lee, W., Edelson, D., Haag, J., Hamilton, M., & Meeks, R. (2009). *Structured and supported debriefing*. American Heart Association.

Page-Cutrara, K. (2015). Prebriefing in nursing simulation: A concept analysis. *Clinical Simulation in Nursing*, *11*(7), 335–340. http://doi.org/10.1016/j.ecns.2015.05.001

Page-Cutrara, K., & Turk, M. (2017). Impact of prebriefing on competency performance, clinical judgment and experience in simulation: An experimental study. *Nurse Education Today*, *48*, 78–83. https://doi.org/10.1016/j.nedt.2016.09.012

Savoldelli, G. L., Naik, V. N., Park, J., Joo, H. S., Chow, R., & Hamstra, S. J. (2006). Value of debriefing during simulated crisis management: Oral versus video-assisted oral feedback. *Anesthesiology*, *105*(2), 279–285. https://doi.org/10.1097/00000542-200608000-00010

Sharoff, L. (2015). Simulation: Pre-briefing, clinical judgement and reflection. What is the connection? *Journal of Contemporary Medicine*, *5*(2), 88–101. https://doi.org/10.16899/ctd.49922

Raemer, D., Anderson, M., Cheng, A., Fanning, R., Nadkarni, V., & Savoldelli, G. (2011, August). Research regarding debriefing as part of the learning process. *Simulation in Healthcare*, *6*, S52–S57. https://doi.org/10.1097/SIH.0b013e31822724d0

Reed, S. (2012). Debriefing experience scale: Development of a tool to evaluate the student learning experience in debriefing. *Clinical Simulation in Nursing*, *8*(6), e211–e217. https://doi.org/10.1016/j.ecns.2011.11.002

Rudolph, J. W., Raemer, D. B., & Simon, R. (2014). Establishing a safe container for learning in simulation: The role of the presimulation briefing. *Simulation in Healthcare*, *9*, 339–349. https://doi.org/10.1097/sih.0000000000000047

Rudolph, J. W., Simon, R., Dufresne, R. L., & Raemer, D. B. (2006). There's no such thing as "nonjudgmental" debriefing: A theory and method for debriefing with good judgment. *Simulation in Healthcare*, *1*(1), 49–55. https://doi.org/10.1097/01266021-200600110-00006

Schön, D. (1983). *The reflective practitioner*. Basic Books.

Schön, D. (1987). *Educating the reflective practitioner*. Jossey-Bass.

Shinner, J., Africa, L., & Hawkes, B. (2016). Debriefing as a supportive component for registered nurses in transition. *Journal for Nurses in Professional Development*, *32*(4), 212–218. https://doi.org/10.1097/NND.0000000000000273

Shinnick, M. A., Woo, M., Horwich, T. B., & Steadman, R. (2011). Debriefing the most important component in simulation? *Clinical Simulation in Nursing*, *7*(3), e105–e111. https://doi.org/10.1016/j.ecns2010.11.005

Simon, R., Raemer, D. B., & Rudolph, J. W. (2010). *Debriefing assessment for simulation in healthcare (DASH)© rater's handbook*. Center for Medical Simulation. https://harvardmedsim.org/wp-content/uploads/2017/01/DASH.handbook.2010.Final.Rev.2.pdf

Simon R, Raemer DB, Rudolph JW. 2011. Debriefing Assessment for Simulation in Healthcare (DASH)© – Rater Version, Short Form. Center for Medical Simulation, Boston, Massachusetts. https://harvardmedsim.org/wp-content/uploads/2017/01/DASH.RV.ShortScoresheet.2011.pdf. English, French, German, Japanese, Spanish.

Simon R, Raemer DB, Rudolph JW. 2012. Debriefing Assessment for Simulation in Healthcare (DASH)© – Instructor Version, Long Form. Center for Medical Simulation, Boston, Massachusetts. https://harvardmedsim.org/wp-content/uploads/2017/01/DASH.IV.LongForm.2012.05.pdf. English, French, Japanese, Spanish.

Tannenbaum, S. I., & Cerasoli, P. (2012). Do team and individual debriefs enhance performance? A meta-analysis. *Human Factors: The Journal of the Human Factors and Ergonomics Society*, *55*(1), 231–245. https://doi.org/10.1177/0018720812448394

Turner, S., & Harder, N. (2018). Psychological safe environment: A concept analysis. *Clinical Simulation in Nursing*, *18*, 47–55. https://doi.org/10.1016/j.ecns.2018.02.004

Waxman, K. T., Bowler, F., Forneris, S. G., Kardong-Edgren, S., & Rizzolo, M. A. (2019). Simulation as a nursing education disrupter. *Nursing Administration Quarterly*, *43*(4), 300–305. https://doi.org/10.1097/naq.0000000000000369

CHAPTER 7

Evaluation of Simulation Outcomes

Susan Prion and Katie Anne Haerling

ABSTRACT

Simulation has been used in nursing education and training since Florence Nightingale's era. Over the past 20 years, simulation learning experiences (SLEs) have been used with increasing frequently to educate healthcare professionals, develop and increase the expertise of practicing professionals, and gain competency in key interprofessional skills. This chapter provides a brief overview of simulation evaluation history, beginning in the late 1990s, and the initial focus on learner self-report data. Using Kirkpatrick's Levels of Evaluation as an organizing model, four types of SLE evaluation are reviewed as well as suggestions for future research.

INTRODUCTION

Simulation has a long history as a teaching strategy in nursing. Florence Nightingale used a "jointed skeleton" and anatomical models in her nurse training in the 1850s (Sanko, 2017). In 1910, full-body manikins were available and have become increasingly popular since the 1950s (Moule, 2011; Sanko, 2017). In the 1930s, nursing schools began to create skills laboratories and began to use various manikins and partial anatomic models to teach skills to students (Sanko, 2017). The military and aviation industry have long been and continue to be leaders in the use of simulation to not only train, but evaluate performance (McNeal, 2010; Palaganas et al., 2014).

http://dx.doi.org/10.1891/0739-6686.39.149

During the 1980s, the healthcare industry recognized the advantages of simulation for training and evaluation, and simulation began to be used in the education, training, and certification of physicians. Because the gear, including manikins, training models, specialized equipment, and computers, was expensive, many nursing and ancillary healthcare professionals did not adopt high-fidelity, mannequin-based simulation as an instructional approach until the early 1990s (Sanko, 2017). At that point, the decreased availability of traditional clinical learning opportunities and increasingly complex patient care needs necessitated the adoption of clinical simulation as a routine part of nursing education (Sanko, 2017).

Simulation is an instructional strategy that "uses a situation or environment created to allow persons to experience a representation of a real healthcare event for the purpose of practice, learning, evaluation, testing or to gain understanding of systems or human actions" (Council for the Accreditation of Healthcare Simulations Programs [CAHSP], 2013, p. 46). Current nursing simulation practice involves a variety of modalities including task trainers, standardized patients, interactive mannequins, role-play, virtual simulation, and gaming (Sanko, 2017). A study in 2013–2014 by the National Council of State Boards of Nursing (NCSBN) suggests that up to 50% of healthcare institution-based clinical hours for prelicensure nursing students can be replaced safely by clinical simulation if there are clearly defined learning outcomes, administrative support, adequate resources, and sufficient faculty preparation (Alexander et al., 2015; Greenawalt, 2014).

Nursing is a practice-oriented profession involving theoretical knowledge, psychomotor skills, and important affective attributes such as ethics and compassion. The simulation learning experience (SLE) reflects the real-life situations that a nurse will encounter in clinical practice, and allows the student to apply and integrate knowledge, skills, and affective attributes in a safe environment without risk of harm to the patient. In addition, the SLE encourages deliberate practice (McGaghie et al., 2009), self-paced learning, real-time analysis and evaluation, interactive learning, timely feedback from the instructor and peers, and the opportunity to learn from mistakes with the option of a do-over. Simulation-based research has offered many insights into the usefulness of SLE as demonstrated by self-reports of perceived changes in satisfaction, confidence, and competence toward interventional studies that explore skill development, and subsequent skill transfer into patient care settings for improved patient care outcomes (Franklin et al., 2015).

Kirkpatrick's levels of evaluation (2019) provide a useful conceptual model for summarizing and analyzing efforts to measure the impact of SLEs. The model describes four sequential stages of assessment and evaluation efforts (Figure 7.1).

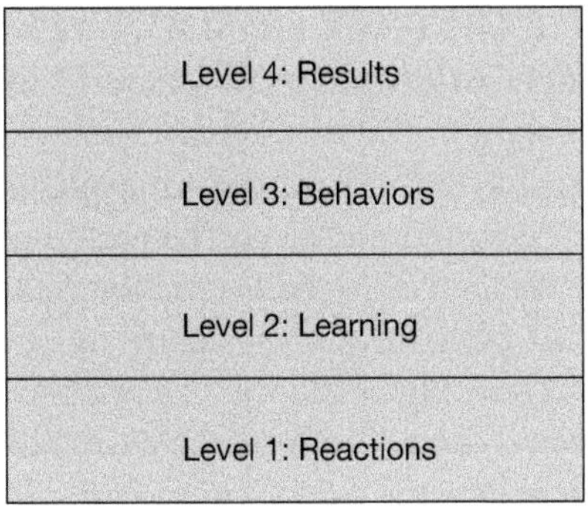

FIGURE 7.1 Kirkpatrick's Four Levels of Evaluation.

Each level corresponds to a different type of assessment and evaluation. Level 1: Reaction focuses on the learner's feelings and reactions to the learning experience. This type of evaluation asks the learner if the instructional experience was favorable, engaging, and relevant. The most common instrument used for this level of evaluation is a posttraining instrument with items related to the participants' satisfaction with the training activities, prebriefing, and debriefing. Level 2: Learning focuses on whether the learner acquired the expected or intended knowledge, skills, attitudes, confidence, and commitment planned for the instructional experience. Commons methods for this level of evaluation include pre- and posttests, questions about change in confidence and commitment, and analyzing learners' responses to case studies. Level 3: Behavior evaluates whether the learner can apply what they have learned in the instructional experience to a real world. Methods used at Level 3 include skills checkoffs and repeat demonstrations. Level 4: Results examines whether the expected or desired outcomes result from the learning experience. At this level of evaluation, demonstrable changes in behaviors should occur, such as decreased medication errors and patient falls.

The following narrative used Kirkpatrick's model as an organizing framework. The three sections (Overview of the History of Simulation Evaluation, Evaluation Strategies and Resources used for Simulation Practice, and Current Research Exploring the Relationship between Simulation and Outcomes) use the four levels to describe and analyze research efforts directed at (a) reactions including learner self-report of satisfaction, change in confidence, and change in competence; (b) learning including research designs to measure pre- to posttest changes in knowledge and self-report changes in learning; (c) behaviors including demonstrated improvement in selected skill performance; and (d) results that are focused on linking simulation to patient and system outcomes including costs.

OVERVIEW OF THE HISTORY OF SIMULATION EVALUATION

Level 1 Reactions: Early Attempts to Evaluate SLEs

Early nursing research about SLEs focused on Kirkpatrick's Evaluation Level 1: Reactions (Kirkpatrick, 2019). These studies explored learner and instructor satisfaction with the SLE, and perceived changes in confidence and competence (knowledge) that resulted from the instructional experience. The research used indirect methods of assessment and evaluation, usually self-reporting by study participants, and often employed locally developed instruments (Baillie & Curzio, 2009; Bambini et al., 2009; Bearnson & Wiker, 2005; Cioffi, 2001; Feingold et al., 2004; Goldenberg et al., 2005; Gore et al., 2011; Kaddoura, 2010; Kenny, 2002; Madorin & Iwasiw, 1999; Rhodes & Curran, 2005; Ross & Tuovinen, 2001; Schoening et al., 2006).

As an example, Heinrich et al. (2002) explored the perceptions of nurse anesthetist students about an anesthesia patient simulator. This qualitative study was designed to collect learners' reactions to the simulation experience and describe "the perceptions" (p. 219) of the learners related to the SLE. The authors asked four additional reaction questions:

- What are the behavioral responses and reported anxiety level of the students?
- How is the SLE perceived by the students as a part of their anesthesia education?
- What are the most favorite and least favorite aspects of the simulator?
- Should the simulator be used for certification and recertification? (p. 219)

Twelve learners participated in the qualitative study. The learners reported (in rank order):

- Improved critical thinking and decision-making skills
- Opportunities to practice crisis management skills
- Valuable practice in administering anesthesia without harm to the patient
- Enhanced confidence
- Permission for harm-free evaluation of cognitive and psychomotor skills
- The opportunity to learn about rare events or unusual complications
- The chance to critique self and peers via videotape
- A motivation to learn more about a specific topics
- Improved leadership skills

Reported disadvantages included the learner's lack of knowledge of the appropriate action to take in the situation, fixation errors (defined as "getting stuck on a specific issue" and not being able to move on), anxiety, and the lack of reality of the manikin. Learners also felt like "sitting ducks" during parts of the simulation and complained about malfunctioning equipment that decreased the reality (p. 223). The authors summarized their results by noting "the value of the anesthesia patient simulation is just beginning to be appreciated and realized" (p. 225).

In 2004, Feingold, Calaluce, and Kallen published a study investigating learner satisfaction and performance. Nursing students in an Advanced Acute Care of the Adult course completed two SLEs and were evaluated by faculty members for skill performance and clinical decision-making using a checklist of critical behaviors. At the end of the semester, students completed a survey with 20 items asking for their perceptions of the value of the experience, their ability to transfer skills from simulation to clinical practice, the realism of the SLE, and the value of the overall learning experience. Study results indicated that even though most reported that the simulation was realistic, valuable, that they received good feedback about their performance from the faculty member, only about half of the participants thought the experience increased confidence, improved competence, or prepared them to function effectively in a real clinical environment.

Level 2 Learning: Subsequent Attempts to Evaluate SLEs

Kirkpatrick's second level is the evaluation of learning. Based on the initial attempts of the National League for Nursing (NLN) and the International Nursing Association for Clinical Simulation and Learning (INACSL) to describe best practices for SLEs, researchers next attempted to describe and define the types and amount of learning that resulted from a single or multiple SLEs (Ballard et al., 2012; Buckley & Gordon, 2010; Lapkin et al., 2010; Radhakrishnan et al., 2007; Rauen, 2004; Schubert, 2012; Wolf, 2008).

An excellent example of this approach is the Alinier et al. (2006) research study investigating "the effect of scenario-based simulation training on nursing students' clinical skills and competence" (p. 359). This was a pretest/posttest design using 99 volunteer undergraduate nursing students and a 15-station objective structured clinical exam (OSCE). The learners in the experimental group were exposed to simulation training in addition to their normal learning activities. In this study, both the control and experimental groups showed improved performance on the second OSCE, but the simulation group demonstrated a statistically significant improvement that was double that of the control group (14% vs. 7%). Both groups self-reported stress and confidence levels very similar to the first and second OSCE. The authors conclude that simulation is an important instructional addition to nursing education, but issue the warning that it "can only be beneficial to students if it is used appropriately and in a way that improves the quality of teaching and learning" (Alinier et al., 2006, p. 368). They also conclude that greater standardization of the simulation experience, including diminishing the role of the instructor and placing the students as the major players, will help to establish this approach as a valuable and necessary healthcare education and training tool.

Level 3 Behavior: Direct Measures of the Effect of Simulation on the Learner's Performance

The third level of Kirkpatrick's evaluation model is behavior. Evidence at this level demonstrates that the learner can apply and transfer skills and knowledge from the simulation performance to real clinical situations. The problem for simulation researchers is the difficulty collecting data in a real clinical situation, so many studies of behavior use simulation for both the instructional intervention and the evaluation approach (e.g., see Bergen & Barber, 2019; Colman et al., 2019; Kirkpatrick et al., 2019; Persaud & Thornton, 2018; Pollard & Wild, 2014; Schneidereith, 2014).

An early example is DeBourgh and Prion's (2011) study examining the impact of a simulation-enhanced patient fall instruction module with beginning nursing students. The researchers conducted a quasiexperimental, pretest/posttest design study using standardized patients to teach 285 students about patient falls. Using three different scenarios, students interacted with the standardized patient (an acting student at the same university) to conduct a basic physical assessment. The standardized patient was instructed either to get out of bed while remaining in character as (a) a confused elderly man, (b) a young man with hepatitis, or (c) an obese woman after knee replacement surgery. The simulation provided each student with the opportunity to interact with a live patient, to conduct a safety and physical assessment, and to problem-solve managing a patient fall. The postsimulation debriefing questions helped the students to reflect on the simulation and identify content and skills topics for additional practice and study. The groups demonstrated an effect size improvement of 1.32 between pretest and posttest knowledge scores. The authors note in their conclusions that studying patient falls is important, but "it is essential to provide learning experiences that engage students in opportunities to develop and apply advanced reasoning, decision making, and rapid recognition and response to unfolding clinical situations that place patients at risk" (p. e55).

Level 4 Results and Outcomes: Kirkpatrick's Ultimate Level of Evaluation

Demonstrating the effect of simulation-based learning experiences on patient outcomes is challenging. The gap between the simulation-based learning experience

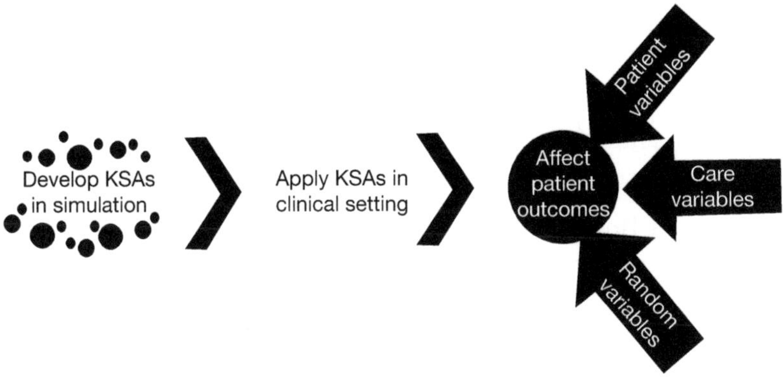

FIGURE 7.2 The ultimate goal of a simulation learning experience.

and the patient care outcome allows ample room for confounding variables. Referencing Kirkpatrick's levels of evaluation (Kirkpatrick & Kirkpatrick, 2016), the simulation-based learning experience must result in improved patient outcomes in the patient care setting (Figure 7.2).

It is much simpler to demonstrate the effect of simulation-based learning experiences on reactions, learning, and even behavior. A systematic review of the literature and meta-analysis by Brydges et al. (2015) included 33 articles representing 1,203 participants, and concluded that simulation-based assessments, while not without their limitations, were positively correlated with patient care outcomes. However, "just one study in the review (Yudkowsky et al., 2013) reported evidence indicating how changes in the simulation-based outcome corresponded with changes in the patient-related outcome" (p. 251). The article demonstrated that simulation-based learning activities improved medical residents' performance in both live and simulated ventriculostomy procedures (Yudkowsky et al., 2013).

A logical argument is often used where simulation participants' reactions to simulation-based learning experiences affect their learning, their learning affects their behavior, and their behavior affects patient outcomes. The following examples suggest it is difficult, but not impossible, to demonstrate more direct relationships between simulation-based learning experiences and patient outcomes.

Several recent reviews have confirmed this unsurprising gap in the literature (Kaplonyi et al., 2017; Lewis et al., 2019; Seaton et al., 2019). Theory and less direct evidence support the connection between simulation-based learning experiences and improved patient care; however, within nursing research, there is limited evidence directly linking simulation-based learning experiences with improved patient outcomes. For example, Kaplonyi et al. (2017) completed a review of the literature summarizing the impact of simulation-based learning experiences on participants' communication skills. Of the 60 studies included in the review, only two demonstrated patient outcomes. Both studies (Curtis et al., 2013; Jay et al., 2010) were published in medical journals, although notably Curtis et al. (2013) included nurse practitioners and used survey-based measures to assess quality of communication, quality of end-of-life care, depression, and functional status. However, they found the simulation-based learning experience (a) did not improve the clinicians' quality of communication or end-of-life care, (b) was associated with an increase in patient depression, and (c) was not associated with improvements in patients' functional status.

Barleycorn and Lee (2018) completed a systematic review of the literature on simulation-based learning experiences to improve trauma patient outcomes. In their review, only seven studies met the criteria for the synthesis, and "... no studies found any specific correlation of simulation-based learning in trauma to wider effects such as patient outcomes, length of stay or morbidity" (p. 37). Seaton et al. (2019) conducted a scoping review of the literature examining evidence supporting the relationship between simulation-based learning experiences and patient safety. While they identified an emerging body of work demonstrating the link between simulation-based learning experiences and improved patient outcomes, they lamented the large proportion of the literature reflecting, "lower level measures of simulation effectiveness such as satisfaction, and/or skills and knowledge acquisition" (Seaton et al., 2019, p. 202). Goldshtein et al. (2020) completed a systematic review of the literature examining the effects of in situ simulation on patient outcomes and identified seven studies that demonstrated a relationship between simulation-based learning experiences and improved patient morbidity and/or mortality outcomes. All studies, however, had a moderate or serious risk of bias and multiple limitations or methodological "issues."

EVALUATION RESOURCES USED FOR SIMULATION PRACTICE

Evaluation Used in Development of the NLN Jeffries Simulation Theory

From 2003 to 2006, the NLN and Laerdal Medical sponsored two projects on simulation. The first phase resulted in the development of the initial NLN simulation model and included educational practices, learner outcomes, and design characteristics of the intervention (simulation). This was the first attempt to collate research and anecdotal results of simulation practice into a working model and provided simulationists with evidence-based guidelines for simulation design and implementation.

The second phase of the project resulted in nine online faculty development modules including "Evaluating Simulations" (Prion, 2008a). Using the NLN simulation model, this module described techniques and approaches to measure multiple aspects of the simulation experience, including the effectiveness of various education practices, a variety of learner outcomes, and specific, embedded design characteristics (such as fidelity, complexity, cueing, debriefing, and objectives/information). Prion (2008b) elaborated on the evaluation strategies by reconceptualizing the NLN model as an input-environment-output/outcomes design.

The NLN revised and validated the NLN/Jeffries Simulation Framework and published the NLN Jeffries Simulation Theory in 2015 (Jeffries et al., 2015). The new model attends to the simulation context (including place and purpose of the SLE), background (goals of the sim, curricular fit, and resources), design (learning objectives, fidelity, facilitator responses, participant and observer roles, activity progression, prebriefing, and debriefing), simulation experience (experiential, interactive, collaborative, and learner centered), facilitator and educational strategies, participant attributes, and outcomes (reaction, learning, and behavior).

The International Nursing Association for Clinical Simulation and Learning Standards of Best Practices[SM]

In 2002, the INACSL was established. The organization grew out of the need for "a professional organization to meet the growing needs of nursing educators using simulation" (INACSL, n.d.-a). In 2010, the INACSL Board of Directors commissioned a process to develop standards for best practice in simulation, and the first edition of *Standards of Best Practice: Simulation* was published in 2011 (INACSL Board of Directors, 2011). Originally, there were seven standards, and in 2015, Standard VIII: Simulation-Enhanced Interprofessional Education (Decker et al., 2015) and Standard IX: Simulation Design (Lioce et al., 2015) were added.

In 2016, the standards were revised following internal and external constituent feedback and a standardized format of components was established (standard, background, criteria, and required elements; INACSL Standards Committee, 2016). The revisions also included two new areas of expertise: simulation-enhanced interprofessional education and simulation design. In 2017, an additional standard for operations (INACSL Standards Committee, 2017) was added and others were condensed to form a total of eight standards, as shown in Box 7.1.

These standards support evaluation of simulation in many ways. The INACSL Standards of Best Practice describe the behaviors and outcomes expected of simulation practitioners and learners, thus offering multiple evidence-based

Box 7.1
The 2016 INACSL Standards of Best Practice: Simulation

Standard
Professional integrity
Outcomes and objectives
Facilitation
Debriefing
Participant evaluation
Simulation-enhanced IPE
Simulation design
Operations

options for evaluation. Taken as a whole, the INACSL Standards of Best Practice can serve as a blueprint for competency assessment, evaluation and feedback for instructors, focused assessment and evaluation information for learners, and provide helpful ideas for possible research topics.

Instruments Used in Simulation Research

A wide variety of instruments have been used to evaluate the effect of SLEs (Table 7.1). Two important reviews (Adamson et al., 2013; Kardong-Edgren et al., 2010) analyzed published simulation evaluation instruments. The authors of both reviews found that many instruments were widely used but had not been fully validated and that many researchers were still reliant on locally developed instruments without adequate psychometric testing for validity and reliability.

TABLE 7.1
Evaluation Instruments

Instrument Name	Primary Focus of Tool	Primary Reference
Sweeny-Clark Simulation Evaluation Rubric	Evaluation of observed learner performance using a blended model of Benner's novice to expert framework and Bloom's taxonomy	Sweeney et al. (2020)

TABLE 7.1
Evaluation Instruments (Continued)

Instrument Name	Primary Focus of Tool	Primary Reference
Lasater Clinical Judgment Rubric	Evaluation of observed learner performance using Benner's novice to expert framework and Tanner's clinical judgment model	Lasater (2007)
CSET	Evaluation of basic clinical practice skills such as assessment skills, safety, prioritization, problem-focused assessment, interventions, delegation, and communication in a two-patient simulated assignment	Radhakrishnan et al. (2007)
C-CEI	Evaluation of 22 general nursing behaviors divided into the broad categories of assessment, communication, clinical judgment, and patient safety	Todd et al. (2008)
National League for Nursing's Simulation Design	Evaluation of the five design features of successful simulations including objectives/information, support, problem-solving, feedback, and fidelity	Jeffries and Rizzolo (2006) National League for Nursing
NLN Educational Practices in Simulation Questionnaire	Evaluation of four key educational practices are present in the simulation: active learning, collaboration, diverse ways of learning, and high expectations	Jeffries and Rizzolo (2006) National League for Nursing
NLN Student Satisfaction and Self-Confidence in Learning Scales	Evaluation of student satisfaction with the simulation and self-confidence in learning	Jeffries and Rizzolo (2006)

(Continued)

TABLE 7.1
Evaluation Instruments (Continued)

Instrument Name	Primary Focus of Tool	Primary Reference
SET	Evaluation of student perceptions of learning, confidence, and satisfaction with the simulation learning experience	Cordi et al. (2012)
SET-M	Evaluation of the simulated clinical experience	Leighton et al. (2015)
Center for Medical Simulation's DASH	Evaluation of debriefing skills	Brett-Fleegler et al. (2012)
GITCS	Evaluation of culturally appropriate provider–patient communication	Campbell and Aredes (2019)
Quint Leveled Clinical Competency Tool	Evaluation of observed learner performance for ten competencies derived from Tanner's model	Prion et al. (2017)
TBAT-ELN	Evaluation of individual teamwork skills by an entry-level nurse	Gilbert et al. (2018)
FCR	Evaluation of simulation facilitators based on a novice-to-expert competency scale	Leighton et al. (2018)
SCORS	Evaluation of leadership and organizational readiness to integrate simulation into the curriculum	Leighton et al. (2018)
Clinical Learning Environment Comparison Survey 2.0	Evaluation of how well learning needs are met in the traditional and simulated undergraduate clinical environments	Leighton et al. (2015)

TABLE 7.1
Evaluation Instruments (Continued)

Instrument Name	Primary Focus of Tool	Primary Reference
IICR	Evaluation of students' communications	Foronda et al. (2019)
Actions, Communication and Teaching in Simulation Tool	Evaluation of performance of confederates participating in a simulation	Sanko et al. (2016)

Notes. C-CEI = Creighton Competency Evaluation Instrument; CSET = Clinical Simulation Evaluation Tool; DASH = Debriefing Assessment for Simulation in Healthcare; FCR = Facilitator Competency Rubric; GITCS = Global Interprofessional Therapeutic Communication Scale©; IICR = ISBAR Interprofessional Communication Rubric; NLN = National League for Nursing; SCORS = Simulation Culture Organizational Readiness Survey; SET = Simulation Effectiveness Tool; SET-M = Simulation Effectiveness Tool-Modified; TBAT-ELN = Team Behavior Assessment Tool for Entry Level Nurses.

Four instruments with established psychometrics have been used extensively for simulation evaluation, including the Sweeny-Clark Simulation Performance Evaluation Tool now called the Sweeney-Clark Simulation Evaluation Rubric (Sweeney et al., 2020); the Lasater Clinical Judgment Rubric (Lasater, 2007); the Clinical Simulation Evaluation Tool (CSET; Radhakrishnan et al., 2007); and the Creighton Competency Evaluation Instrument (a derivation of the original Creighton Simulation Evaluation Instrument; Todd et al., 2008). The NLN's simulation design, educational practices in simulation, and student satisfaction and self-confidence in learning scales (Jeffries & Rizzolo, 2006) continue to be used extensively. The Simulation Effectiveness Tool (SET; Cordi et al., 2012) has undergone several revisions and has been renamed the SET-M. The new instrument has added prebriefing and debriefing subscales to the original confidence and perceived learning subscales (Leighton et al., 2015). Hemman et al. (2007) note that it is very difficult to validate a performance-based evaluation instrument because the process is highly dependent on the experience, training, perspective, knowledge, and skill of the evaluator. As Adamson et al. (2013) lament, "Reaction and learning are often the low-hanging fruit of simulation evaluation" (p. 397).

Newer and promising instruments to evaluate SLEs from the perspective of both learner and instructor include the Center for Medical Simulation's Debriefing Assessment for Simulation in Healthcare (DASH; Brett-Fleegler et al., 2012), the Global Interprofessional Therapeutic Communication Scale© (GITCS) by Campbell & Aredes (2019), the Quint Leveled Clinical Competency Tool (Prion et al., 2017), and the Team Behavior Assessment Tool for Entry Level Nurses

(TBAT-ELN) by Gilbert et al. (2018). Additional tools for free download and use through Evaluating Healthcare Simulation (Evaluating Healthcare Simulations, 2020) include the Facilitator Competency Rubric (FCR), the Simulation Culture Organizational Readiness Survey (SCORS), the Clinical Learning Environment Comparison Survey 2.0, the ISBAR Interprofessional Communication Rubric (IICR), and the Actions, Communication and Teaching in Simulation Tool.

The International Nursing Association of Clinical Simulation and Learning (INACSL) offers the Instrument Repository of Instruments used in Healthcare Simulation (INACSL, n.d.-b). This categorized citation list is organized using the domains described in the NLN Jeffries Simulation Theory, including skill performance, learner satisfaction, knowledge and learning, critical thinking and clinical judgment, and self-confidence and self-efficacy (Jeffries, 2015). Additional categories for debriefing, facilitatory competencies, and organizational evaluation are also searchable. The resources, which may or may not contain the full research instrument, can also be used to gain additional background information and for potential research collaborations.

CURRENT RESEARCH EXPLORING THE RELATIONSHIP BETWEEN SIMULATION AND OUTCOMES

With almost 20 years of use as an instructional strategy, simulation is an important approach for most nursing education and training. Lab-based, in situ, and community-based simulations are common, as are interprofessional simulations involving a variety of healthcare professionals (Chapter 5). Unfortunately, much of the published simulation research continues to rely on indirect measures of low-level phenomena such as reactions and learning (Kirkpatrick's Levels 1 and 2). The difficulties in conducting meaningful research about the impact of simulation on behaviors and outcomes (Kirkpatrick's Levels 3 and 4) continue to confront researchers, and the reliance on locally developed, untested instruments continues to hamper advances in simulation practice (Prion & Adamson, 2012).

Level 1: Reactions

An interesting example of the scope and breadth of SLEs is described in a Korean study by Hwang and Kim (2020). They developed and evaluated a simulation scenario for senior community health nursing students that was based in a home visit with an elderly person with diabetes mellitus who lived alone. A standardized patient was used and the students observed their peers interact with the patient. The researchers used questionnaires and the SET to collect self-report data from 87 nursing students about self-efficacy, learning effectiveness, and critical thinking. After the SLE, the participants reported slightly increased critical thinking, self-efficacy, self-confidence, and learning effectiveness. There were no statistically significant correlations among these variables.

Nunes and Harder (2019) offer a innovative example of current research at the Kirkpatrick's Level 1 of evaluation. The researchers conducted a mixed-methods concurrent triangulation study to explore the perceived value and usefulness of debriefing in palliative simulation process feelings and emotions. A nursing student's first experience with a patient death has been shown to profoundly influence their subsequent practice (Kirkpatrick et al., 2017), so the potential of guiding the experience through simulation debriefing has great merit. Ninety-eight third-year nursing students participated in a dying patient simulation, then completed both the DASH evaluation and an adapted version of the Debriefing Experience Scale (DES). Based on the learner's self-report data, the results indicated that the debriefer for a palliative care simulation needed an additional skill set. Not only did the debriefer need to be highly skilled with the debriefing process, but also needed to be comfortable and competent with emotionally stressful situations and encouraging students to talk about their feelings in response to the simulation outcome. Learners reported that hearing other students express their emotions during the debrief helped to normalize their own feelings and view the simulation as a positive learning experience.

Level 2: Learning

Kirkpatrick's second level, focused on learning, is often measured in simulation with a pre- and posttest design. Graham (2020) conducted a study on learning gains of safe patient handling made by 34 associate degree nursing students after a low-fidelity SLE. Learners completed a pre-and posttest assessing safe patient handling knowledge and also a competency exam using the same equipment from the simulation. Learners demonstrated significant increases in knowledge scores on the posttest when compared to the pretest,and also enhanced competency properly using equipment.

In response to pandemic-necessitated changes in healthcare, another innovative research study used a pretest–posttest design to measure the learning gains of nurse practitioner students engaged with a pediatric virtual visit simulation using text messaging (Merritt, 2020). Learning was measured using a diagnostic accuracy rubric developed by pediatric nurse experts and scored as a percentage of a perfect total score. Learners were also asked to self-report their confidence and competence in dealing with common pediatric assessment and diagnosis skills. The results returned a statistically significant ($p < .05$) difference between the self-rating before and after the virtual visit simulation.

Karnish et al. (2019) conducted a study to examine the effects of an interprofessional simulation on the socialization and knowledge of medical imaging, nursing, and physical therapy students. Learners participated in one acute care interprofessional simulation and then completed three postactivity open-ended descriptive questions and the Interprofessional Socialization and Valuing Scale (ISVS-21). Forty-two nursing students, 47 physical therapy students, and 20 medical imaging students demonstrated a significant positive change in knowledge about the other professions and reported the development of a culture of communication and teamwork and enhanced professional role discernment. The researchers did not measure behavior but conducted statistical analysis on the pre- and postexperience ISVS-21 responses. The postsimulation score was 24 points higher than the presimulation score ($p < .001$). This innovative simulation study demonstrated that even a single SLE can be successful in exposing different types of healthcare students to interprofessional practice and to improve attitudes toward collaboration. Further research to measure actual changes in collaboration behaviors is needed.

Level 3: Behaviors

A 2019 study by Bergen and Barber examined identification and demonstration of caring behaviors during SLEs. The Caring Behaviors Checklist for Scenario-Based High-Fidelity Simulation (CBC-HFS) was used as both a self-assessment and observer-generated data tool (Dunnington & Farmer, 2015) with 78 senior-level prelicensure students from two nursing programs in the southeastern United States. Three scenarios were used: a patient with pneumonia who experienced an anaphylactic reaction to a medication, a patient with a myocardial infarction experiencing chest pain and clinical deterioration, and a postoperative patient who exhibited signs and symptoms of a pulmonary embolism. Two observers watched the students in the scenario and completed the CBC-HFS, and the students completed a student version of the CBC-HFS to indicate which of the caring behaviors listed they demonstrated during the simulation. Results showed that "actively listens to the patient," "verbally responded to an expressed concern," and "treats patient with gentleness, sensitivity, kindness, reverence or respect" were most often self-reported and observed (Bergen & Barber, 2019, p. 226). The researchers conclude that there are opportunities for students to demonstrate caring behaviors in a simulated patient care experience and that students are mostly aware of these opportunities. Historically, high-fidelity simulation has been identified primarily with cognitive and psychomotor skill development and evaluation. This study opens the opportunity for students to develop and practice affective skills during the SLE. The authors note that additional research in caring behaviors is essential to collect evidence to "target opportunity for demonstration of caring behaviors known to be essential to positive patient outcomes in the clinical setting" (Bergen & Barber, 2019, p. 231).

Level 4: Outcomes

Lewis et al. (2019) completed a review of the literature on the role of simulation-based learning experiences for nurses on patient safety outcomes. Of the 12 articles included in the review, nine used measures of direct observation (Ballangrud et al., 2013; Gerolemou et al., 2014; Klipfel et al., 2011; Liaw et al., 2016; Nevo et al., 2010; Pati et al., 2012; Raurell-Torreada et al., 2015; Trbovich et al., 2010; Wilson et al., 2010) and four (discussed later) documented improved patient outcomes (Braddock et al., 2014; Gerolemou et al., 2014; Kim et al., 2014; Liaw et al., 2016). Additionally, Cant et al. (2020) conducted a scoping review that examined the impact of simulation-based education for hospital-based nurses on patient outcomes. While only two of the 20 articles included changes in nurses' behavior or actual impacts on patient outcomes, these articles highlighted nursing research (Harvey et al., 2019; Mariani & Doolen, 2016) as discussed later in this chapter.

SIMULATION-BASED LEARNING EXPERIENCES AND PATIENT OUTCOMES

The following sections describe specific examples of research linking simulation-based learning experiences to patient outcomes. The studies use a wide variety of data sources and cover a range of patient-related outcomes. The first and second sections include *structured observation of performance in the simulation setting* representing Kirkpatrick's Level 3: Behavior and *structured observation of performance in the patient care setting* representing Kirkpatrick's Level 4: Results. The next sections review "big" outcomes such as survival and code or trauma registry data, and nurse-sensitive outcomes—both in terms of care quality and care outcomes.

Structured Observations Within the Simulation Setting

Authors consistently highlight the logical link between the effect simulation-based learning experiences have on performance in the simulation lab and patient care/patient outcomes. Prakash et al. (2014) used structured observations to examine the effect of simulation-based training on rates of medication errors among nurses in an outpatient chemotherapy setting. The specific aim of the simulation-based training was to reduce medication errors associated with interruptions during medication "verification and administration" (Prakash et al., 2014, p. 884). In this study, however, the structured observations took place in simulation and not during actual patient care. The list and description of tasks and performance metrics used to assess the nurses' performance is included in the article.

Colman et al. (2019) implemented simulation-based training with rapid cycle deliberate practice to improve communication/teamwork of rapid response teams. Their work demonstrated improved team performance within the simulated setting (as measured by the Clinical Training Scale [Guise et al., 2008]). However, they did not include measures to assess translation of improved practice to the bedside. Abram et al. (2020) looked at the use of simulation to improve advanced practice registered nurses' safe implementation of medication-assisted treatment for opioid use disorder. Outcomes used participant feedback and observation-based assessment with a checklist to "ensure competency in each of the core domains of patient safety and mastery of the prescriber's role" (Abram et al., 2020, pp. 39–40).

A recent special issue of *Clinical Simulation in Nursing* highlighted the use of simulation to improve patient safety. In the issue, Dick-Smith et al. (2020) compared the effects of three different feedback options during simulation-based learning experiences aimed at teaching Basic Life Support (visual, visual-embodied metaphoric, and audio-visual). The outcome variable was technical accuracy in cardiopulmonary resuscitation (CPR) performance in the simulation environment. Hazwani et al. (2020) used retrospective data about simulation performance to assess "the impact of simulation-based training on resuscitation skills" (p. 43). The outcome variables were time to initiation of CPR, time to first epinephrine dose, and nontechnical team performance assessment using assessments based on the Ottawa Global Rating Scale (Nunnink et al., 2014) and Team Emergency Assessment Measure (Cooper et al., 2010).

Harvey et al. (2014) compared the effects of simulation-based learning and a case study review on a variety of outcomes, including nurses' performance in a failure to rescue simulation. The investigators used the TeamSTEPPS Team Performance Observation Tool to assess teamwork performance in the simulation setting (Agency for Healthcare Research and Quality, n.d.).

Structured Observations of Performance in Patient Care Setting

While it may be reasonable to assume behaviors demonstrated in the simulation setting should translate to the patient care setting, it is important to test this assumption. Ford et al. (2010) examined rates of medication errors among coronary care unit (CCU) and intensive care unit (ICU) nurses before and after an educational intervention involving either didactic lecture or simulation. In addition to knowledge exams administered before and after the educational interventions, the investigators employed structured observations of medication administration in the patient care setting to assess and compare the outcomes of the interventions. They discovered a significant and sustained reduction in medication error rates after the simulation-based intervention, but not after the didactic lecture intervention. This use of structured observation is a resource-intensive but validated method for detecting medication error and demonstrating the relationship between simulation-based training and patient care (Barker et al., 2002).

In addition to direct observation of individuals, direct observation of teams has been used to demonstrate the effect of simulation-based learning experiences on patient care. Berkenstadt et al. (2008) implemented and assessed the effects of specific training on patient handoffs in a simulation-based teamwork and communication workshop. To assess the effect of the training, the investigators observed actual patient handoffs in a critical care setting before and after the intervention and noted the inclusion or exclusion of specific content including patient demographic data, medical history, physiologic parameters, medical orders, and fluid balance. The "Handoff Protocol/Checklist" revealed a significant increase in nurses' inclusion of many but not all the items on the checklist during patient handoffs after the intervention as compared with before the intervention (Berkenstadt et al., 2008, p.162).

Two studies that examined performance of resuscitations in the patient care setting include Haug et al. (2020) and Patterson et al. (2013). Haug et al. (2020) used video recordings of newborn resuscitations and found that most resuscitations deviated from the Helping Babies Breath training. Patterson et al. (2013) used a variety of assessment measures including a modification of the Behavioral Markers for Neonatal Resuscitation Scale (Thomas et al., 2004) to assess the effect of an interdisciplinary simulation-based learning experience. These assessments were completed in both the patient care and simulation settings and findings showed that the simulation-based training was associated with a decrease in patient safety events.

Patient Survival to Discharge

In addition to evaluating the effect of simulation-based learning experiences on patient care performance, it is most useful to demonstrate the effect on patient outcomes. Survival to discharge is frequently used to examine the effect that simulation-based learning experiences have on patient outcomes. A benefit of this metric is the ability to analyze data without needing to complete additional assessments on patients. Much of the data used to demonstrate the efficacy of simulation-based learning experiences on survival to discharge comes from the medical literature. Dillon et al. (2018) used simulation-based training with an interprofessional group of learners to improve rapid response/code team performance. They studied a "national registry of CPR data used to compare the proportion of Codes/Rapid Response Teams over time and by shift and the change in the proportion of patients who survived to discharge for those patients who received codes" (Dillon et al., 2018, p. 69). Andreatta et al. (2011) provides another example of research using survival to discharge as an outcome variable. This group examined survival rates before and after the implementation of a simulation-based mock code program. Examples also exist from institutional (Sodhi et al., 2015) and interdisciplinary (Knight et al., 2014) studies.

To examine the efficacy of simulation-based learning experiences on nurses' ability to identify deteriorating patients, Mariani and Doolen (2016) used a range of data including patient transfer rates and patient survival to discharge. Crowe et al. (2018) used simulation as part of a training specifically focused on deteriorating patients. These researchers used unit-level data that demonstrated improved performance as evidenced by an "increase in the percentage of recognized patient deteriorations, a decrease in the number of code blue arrest calls, a decrease in the number of pulseless cardiac arrests and an increase in pre-arrests called, as well as an improved success rate in the return of spontaneous cardiac circulation" (Crowe et al., 2018, p.73).

Trauma Registry and Other Data Sources

The trauma registry is another common source of data used to demonstrate the efficacy of simulation-based learning experiences. A benefit of this data is, like the survival to discharge data, it does not require additional patient assessments. However, it does require the investigator to access and analyze the data. Murphy et al. (2018) used trauma registry data to assess the effect of team training on time to critical treatment in trauma. The implementation of the simulation-based training was associated with a decreased time to treatment and an increased average length of stay in emergency department (ED). In addition to observation-based assessments of trauma team performance, Harvey et al. (2019) used trauma registry data to examine whether their simulation-based, advanced nurse TeamSTEPPS training affected patient care and patient outcomes. They noted a decrease in the time to ultrasonography after the training as compared to before the training.

In addition to the trauma registry, there are novel sources of patient outcome data that can be used to examine the effect of simulation-based learning experiences without the need to complete further assessments on patients. An example can be found in the study by Kim et al. (2014) that used data from the Collaborative Alliance for Nursing Outcomes (CALNOC) nursing sensitive quality indicators database to demonstrate the effect of an interprofessional communication and teamwork simulation-based learning experience on patient fall and hospital-acquired pressure ulcer rates. This study found "notable improvements in falls and pressure ulcer rates," but noted a lack of conclusive evidence that the simulation-based training was responsible for these improved patient outcomes (Kim et al., 2014, p. 96).

Healthcare Records

The healthcare record holds many opportunities for assessing the efficacy of simulation-based learning experiences. Kinsman et al. (2012) sought to examine the effect of simulation-based education intervention aimed at improving nurses' responses to deteriorating patients in a rural hospital. The investigators used data from patients' medical records reflecting quality of nursing care, including frequency of observation, assessment of pain, SPO2, vital signs, and neurologic status and application of O2 therapy. Results indicated improvements in some, but not all quality-of-care indicators after the intervention. While the instrument used for extracting data from patients' charts is not included in the article, the concept is readily applicable to future research examining not only the effect of simulation on nursing practice, but on patient outcomes.

Using an interdisciplinary approach, Theilen et al. (2013) examined how ongoing simulation-based team training affected the care and outcomes of deteriorating pediatric patients. The investigators used prospective audits of unplanned admissions to the pediatric intensive care unit (PICU), reflecting length of time from deterioration to first response and the length of time from first response to admission to the PICU. They also examined indicators of care quality, including frequency of nursing observations and level of care. Finally, the investigators were able to assess the effect of the simulation-based team training on patient outcomes by examining morbidity, mortality, and length of stay. Findings indicate that deteriorating patients were recognized sooner and received higher levels of care after the training. The training also corresponded with a significant reduction in patient mortality.

Siassakos et al. (2009) assessed the effect of a multidisciplinary simulation-based training program on patient outcomes. Patient and hospital records were used to compare performance and outcomes before and after the training. Performance measures included recognition and management of cord prolapse and reduction in time from diagnosis to delivery. Patient outcomes included APGAR scores and rates of neonatal intensive care unit (NICU) admissions. Braddock et al. (2015) used a wide range of patient-safety-focused activities, including in situ simulation, and observed for changes in "Hospital-acquired severe sepsis/septic, shock and acute respiratory failure; unplanned transfers, to higher level of care (HLOC); weighted risk-adjusted Mortality" (p. 425). Gibbs et al. (2018) demonstrate a decrease in the number of methicillin-resistant *Staphylococcus aureus* (MRSA) infections after in situ simulation training in NICU.

Several nurse-focused studies used patient care data to demonstrate the efficacy of simulation-based learning experiences (Gerolemou et al., 2014; Justus et al., 2016; Liaw et al., 2016; Stephens & Mosser, 2013). Gerolemou et al. (2014) revealed an 85% reduction in catheter-related bloodstream infections after critical care nurses completed a simulation-based training about sterile technique. Liaw et al. (2016) demonstrated efficacy of a web-based SLE by comparing the number of deteriorating patients identified by nurses before and after the implementation of the program. Justus et al. (2016) used a blended model, including simulation-based learning experiences, to improve catheter insertion and care practices. Their research demonstrated not only a reduction in catheter-associated urinary tract infections, but a cost savings for the institution. Finally, Stephens and Mosser (2013) implemented a simulation-based learning experience for nurses on peripheral IV insertion and demonstrated a decrease in the number of peripheral IV insertion attempts.

FUTURE DIRECTIONS

Nursing research about the effects of SLEs has been rich and plentiful, exploring the use of simulation in a wide variety of settings and for a diverse set of purposes and goals. Until now, the research has mostly been conducted at the lower levels of Kirkpatrick's evaluation framework, focusing on participant reactions and learning. As understanding of the complexities of SLE becomes more sophisticated, studies examining changes in actual behaviors (Level 3) and outcomes (Level 4) are becoming more common. The NLN Jeffries Simulation Theory and the INACSL Standards of Best Practice provide a conceptual framework from which to pose perceptive and meaningful research questions.

An umbrella review by Cantrell et al. (2017) offers hope that there is more sophistication in the design of nursing research in simulation and "increasing number of studies focused on skill transfer to the practice setting, patient safety, and outcomes" (p. 635). These authors also advocate for more emphasis on translational research, research into measurement of higher order thinking skills, and increased methodological rigor in simulation research designs.

During the recent pandemic, many educators turned to virtual simulation to provide clinically focused, no-touch educational experiences for healthcare students. The efficacy of this approach is emerging in the literature, but much of the work is focused in Kirkpatrick's Levels 1 and 2 evaluation strategies. Hopefully, virtual simulation research will move quickly to evaluating behaviors (Kirkpatrick's Level 3: Behaviors) and positive changes in patient outcomes (Kirkpatrick's Level 4: Results).

Nurse scientist should strive to document the effects of simulation on nurse-sensitive indicators. The National Database of Nursing Quality Indicators® is an excellent place to find examples of structure, process, and outcome indicators that can be used as Level 4 evaluations for the effects of SLEs (Montalvo, 2007). A few examples include how SLEs affect rates of nosocomial infections, such as catheter-associated urinary tract infections, central line catheter-associated blood stream infections, and ventilator-associated pneumonia. Another nurse quality indicator is patient satisfaction. While the Kirkpatrick model indicates that satisfaction surveys represent Level 1 evaluation, this refers specifically to the simulation participant. When the simulation participant takes care of patients and those patients are surveyed about their satisfaction, this represents an outcome of the SLE—Level 4 evaluation!

CONCLUSION

Nursing is a practice-oriented profession requiring effective integration of knowledge, skills, and affect. A SLE designed, delivered, and evaluated according to best practices can credibly and accurately represent the variety and intensity of situations that a nurse will encounter in the clinical setting. SLEs are used extensively in healthcare education as a strategy to challenge the student to practice in a safe environment without risk of harm to the patient. Early research and evaluation of simulation outcomes centers on Kirkpatrick's first two levels: reactions and learning. More recent research has focused on Kirkpatrick's Level 3 (Behaviors) and how SLEs can lead to positive behavioral outcomes. Very recently, physicians have begun to investigate the impact of SLEs on patient outcomes. Nurse researchers have an opportunity and an obligation to study how SLEs effect nurse sensitive patient outcomes and other key indications of the quality of nursing care (Haberfelde et al., 2005; Montalvo, 2007).

REFERENCES

Adamson, K. A., Kardong-Edgren, S., & Willhaus, J. (2013). An updated review of published simulation evaluation instruments. *Clinical Simulation in Nursing*, *9*(9), e393–400. https://doi.org/10.1016/j.ecns.2012.09.004

Aebersold, M., & Tschannen, D. (2013). Simulation in nursing practice: The impact on patient care. *Online Journal of Issues in Nursing*, *18*(2), 6.

Alexander, M., Durham, C. F., Hooper, J. I., Jeffries, P. R., Goldman, N., Kardong-Edgren, S., & Tillman, C. (2015). NCSBN simulation guidelines for pre-licensure nursing programs. *Journal of Nursing Regulation*, *6*(3), 39–42. https://www.ncsbn.org/simulationguidelines_alexander_2015.pdf

Andreatta, P., Saxton, E., Thompson, M., & Annich, G. (2011). Simulation-based mock codes significantly correlate with improved pediatric patient cardiopulmonary arrest survival rates. *Pediatric Critical Care*, *12*(1), 33–38. https://doi.org/10.1097/PCC.0b013e3181e89270

Baillie, L., & Curzio, J. (2009). A survey of first year student nurses' experiences of learning blood pressure measurement. *Nurse Education in Practice*, *9*, 61–71. https://doi.org/10.1016/j.nepr.2008.05.003

Ballard, G., Piper, S., & Stokes, P. (2012). Effect of simulated learning on blood pressure measurement skills. *Nursing Standard*, *27*(8), 43–47. https://doi.org/10.7748/ns.27.8.43.s57

Bambini, D., Washburn, J., & Perkins, R. (2009). Outcomes of clinical simulation for novice nursing students: Communication, confidence, clinical judgment. *Nursing Education Perspectives*, *30*(2), 79–82.

Barleycorn, D., & Lee, G. (2018). How effective is trauma simulation as an educational process for healthcare providers within the trauma networks? A systematic review. *International Emergency Nursing*, *40*, 37–45. https://doi.org/10.1016/j.ienj.2018.03.007

Bearnson, C., & Wiker, K. (2005). Human patient simulators: A new face in baccalaureate nursing education at Brigham Young University. *Journal of Nursing Education*, *44*(9), 421–425. https://doi.org/10.3928/01484834-20050901-07

Bergen, J. S., & Barber, L. A. M. (2019). Student identification and demonstration of caring behaviors during simulated patient experiences. *International Journal for Human Caring*, *23*(3), 221–233. https://doi.org/10.20467/1091-5710.23.3.221

Berkenstadt, H., Haviv, Y., Tuval, A., Shemesh, Y., Megrill, A., & Perry, A. (2008). Improving handoff communications in critical care: Utilizing simulation-based training toward process improvement in managing patient risk. *Chest*, *134*(1), 158–162. https://doi.org/10.1378/chest.08-0914

Brett-Fleegler, M., Rudolph, J., Eppich, W., Monuteaux, M., Gleegler, E., Cheng, A., & Simon, R. (2012). Debriefing assessment for simulation in healthcare: Development and psychometric properties. *Simulation in Healthcare: The Journal of the Society for Simulation in Healthcare*, *7*(5), 288–294. https://doi.org/10.1097/SIH.0b013e3182620228

Brydges, R., Hatala, R., Zendejas, B., Erwin, P., & Cook, D. (2015). Linking simulation-based educational assessments and patient-related outcomes: A systematic review and meta-analysis. *Academic Medicine: Journal of the Association of American Medical Colleges*, *90*(2), 246–256. https://doi.org/10.1097/ACM.0000000000000549

Buckley, T., & Gordon, C. (2010). The effectiveness of high fidelity simulation on medical–surgical registered nurses' ability to recognise and respond to clinical emergencies. *Nurse Education Today*, *31*(7), 716. https://doi.org/10.1016/j.nedt.2010.04.004

Campbell, S. H., & Aredes, N. D. A. (2019). Global interprofessional therapeutic communication scale© (GITCS©): Development and validation. *Clinical Simulation in Nursing*, *34*, 30–42. https://doi.org/10.1016/j.ecns.2019.05.006

Cantrell, M. A., Franklin, A., Leighton, K., & Carlson, A. (2017). The evidence in simulation-based learning experiences in nursing education and practice: An umbrella review. *Clinical Simulation in Nursing, 13*(12), 634–667. https://doi.org/10.1016/j.ecns.2017.08.004

Capella, J., Smith, P., Putnam, G., & Fry, R. (2010). Teamwork training improves the clinical care of trauma patients. *Journal of Surgical Education, 67*(6), 439–443. https://doi.org/10.1016/j.jsurg.2010.06.006

Cioffi, J. (2001). Clinical simulations: Development and validation. *Nurse Education Today, 21*, 477–486. https://doi.org/10.1054/nedt.2001.0584

Colman, N., Patera, A., & Hebbar, K. (2019). Promoting teamwork for rapid response teams through simulation training. *Journal of Continuing Education in Nursing, 50*(11), 523–528. https://doi.org/10.3928/00220124-20191015-09

Cooper, S., Cant, R., Porter, J., Sellick, K., Somers, G., Kinsman, L., & Nestel, D. (2010). Rating medical emergency teamwork performance: Development of the team emergency assessment measure (TEAM). *Resuscitation, 81*(4), 446–452. https://doi.org/10.1016/j.resuscitation.2009.11.027

Cordi, V. L. E., Leighton, K., Ryan-Wenger, N., Doyle, T. J., & Ravert, P. (2012). History of development of the simulation effectiveness tool (SET. *Clinical Simulation in Nursing, 8*(6). https://doi.org/10.1016/j.ecns.2011.12.001

Council for the Accreditation of Healthcare Simulations Programs. (2013). *An informational guide for the 2013 Society for simulation in healthcare accreditation program*. Society for Simulation in Healthcare.

Crowe, S., Ewart, L., & Derman, S. (2018). The impact of simulation-based education on nursing confidence, knowledge and patient outcomes on general medicine units. *Nurse Education in Practice, 29*, 70–75. https://doi.org/10.1016/j.nepr.2017.11.017

Curtis, J., Back, A., Ford, D., Downey, L., Shannon, S., Doorenbos, A., & Engelberg, R. (2013). Effect of communication skills training for residents and nurse practitioners on quality of communication with patients with serious illness: A randomized trial. *JAMA: The Journal of the American Medical Association, 310*(21), 2271–2281. https://doi.org/10.1001/jama.2013.282081

DeBourgh, G. A., & Prion, S. K. (2011). Using simulation to teach prelicensure students to minimize risk and harm. *Clinical Simulation in Nursing, 7*(2), e47–e56. https://doi.org/10.1016/j.ecns.2009.12.009

Decker, S. I., Anderson, M., Boese, T., Epps, C., McCarthy, J., Motola, I., Palaganas, J., Perry, C., Puga, F., & Scolaro, K. (2015). Standards of best practice: Simulation standard VIII: Simulation-enhanced interprofessional education (Sim-IPE). *Clinical Simulation in Nursing, 11*(6), 293–297. https://doi.org/10.1016/j.ecns.2015.03.010

Dillon, P., Moriarty, H., & Lipschik, G. (2018). Using simulation with interprofessional team training to improve RRT/code performance. *Journal of Interprofessional Education & Practice, 11*, 67–72. https://doi.org/10.1016/j.xjep.2018.01.002

Dunnington, R. M., & Farmer, S. R. (2015). Caring behaviors among student nurses interacting in scenario-based high-fidelity human patient simulation. *International Journal for Human Caring, 19*, 44–49. https://doi.org/10.20467/1091-5710-19.4.44

Evaluating Healthcare Simulations. (2020, August 24). *Evaluating simulation*. https://sites.google.com/view/evaluatinghealthcaresimulation/home

Feingold, C. E., Calaluce, M., & Kallen, M. (2004). Computerized patient model and simulated clinical experiences: Evaluation with baccalaureate nursing students. *Journal of Nursing Education*, *43*(4), 156–163. https://doi.org/10.3928/01484834-20040401-03

Ford, D., Seybert, G., Smithburger, A., Kobulinsky, L., Samosky, P., & Kane-Gill, L. (2010). Impact of simulation-based learning on medication error rates in critically ill patients. *Intensive Care Medicine*, *36*(9), 1526–1531. https://doi.org/10.1007/s00134-010-1860-2

Foronda, C. L., Alhusen, J., Budhathoki, C., Lamb, M., Tinsley, K., MacWilliams, B., Daniels, J., Baptiste, D. L., Reese, K. K., & Bauman, E. (2019). A mixed-methods, international, multisite study to develop and validate a measure of nurse-to-physician communication in simulation. *Nursing Education Perspectives*, *36*(6), 383–388. https://doi.org/10.5480/15-1644

Foronda, C. L., Liu, S., & Bauman, E. G. (2013). Evaluation of simulation in undergraduate nurse education: An integrative review. *Clinical Simulation in Nursing*, *9*, e409–e416. https://doi.org/10.1016/j.ecns.2012.11.003

Franklin, A. E., Lieghton, K., Cantrell, M. A., & Rutherford-Hemming, T. (2015). Simulation research for academics: Novice level. *Clinical Simulation in Nursing*, *11*(4), 214–221. https://doi.org/10.1016/j.ecns.2015.001.007

Gerolemou, L., Fidellaga, A., Rose, K., Cooper, S., Venturanza, M., Aqeel, A., Han, Q., Jones, J., Shapiro, J., & Khouli, H. (2014). Simulation-based training for nurses in sterile techniques during central vein catheterization. *American Journal of Critical Care*, *23*(1), 40–48. https://doi.org/10.4037/ajcc2014860

Gibbs, K., Demaria, S., Mckinsey, S., Fede, A., Harrington, A., Hutchison, D., & Goldberg, A. (2018). A novel in situ simulation intervention used to mitigate an outbreak of methicillin-resistant *Staphylococcus aureus* in a neonatal intensive care unit. *The Journal of Pediatrics*, *194*, 22–27.e5. https://doi.org/10.1016/j.jpeds.2017.10.040

Gilbert, M., Prion, S. K., & Haerling, K. A. (2018). Assessing individual teamwork skills in entry-level nurses. *Clinical Simulation in Nursing*, *24*, P9–P13. https://doi.org/10.1016/j.ecns.2018.09.002

Goldenberg, D., Andrusyszyn, M. A., & Iwasiw, C. (2005). The effect of classroom simulation on nursing students' self-efficacy related to health teaching. *Journal of Nursing Education*, *44*(7), 310–314. https://doi.org/10.3928/01484834-20050701-04

Goldshtein, D., Krensky, C., Doshi, S., & Perelman, V. (2020). In situ simulation and its effects on patient outcomes: A systematic review. *BMJ Simulation and Technology Enhanced Learning*, *6*(1), 3–9. https://doi.org/10.1136/bmjstel-2018-000387

Gore, T., Hunt, C. W., Parker, F., & Raines, K. (2011). The effects of simulated clinical experiences on anxiety: Nursing students' perspectives. *Clinical Simulation in Nursing*, *7*(5), 175–180. https://doi.org/10.1016/j.ecns.2010.02.001

Graham, P. L. (2020). Increasing patient and student nurse safety using safe patient handling. *Clinical Simulation in Nursing*, *45*(7), 24–27. https://doi.org/10.1016/j.ecns.2020.01.006

Greenawalt, J. (2014). Report on the NBSBN national simulation study. *International Nursing Association for Clinical Simulation and Learning E-Newsletter*. https://www.inacsl.org/i4a/pages/index.cfm?pageid=3295

Haberfelde, M., Bedecarré, D., & Buffum, M. (2005). Nurse-sensitive patient outcomes: An annotated bibliography. *Journal of Nursing Administration*, *35*(6), 293–299. https://doi.org/10.1097/00005110-200506000-00005

Harvey, E. M., Echols, S. R., Clark, R., & Lee, E. (2014). Comparison of two TeamSTEPPS®Training methods on nurse failure-to-rescue performance. *Clinical Simulation in Nursing*, *10*(2), E57–E64. https://doi.org/10.1016/j.ecns.2013.08.006

Heinrich, B., Rule, A., Grady, M., & Ellis, W. (2002). Nurse anesthesia students' perceptions of the anesthesia patient simulator: A qualitative study. *American Association of Nurse Anesthetists Journal*, *70*(3), 219.

Hwang, W. J., & Kim, J. A. (2020). Development and evaluation of a home-visit simulation scenario for elderly people with diabetes mellitus who live alone. *Journal of Community Health Nursing*, *37*(2), 89–102. https://doi.org/10.1080/07370016.2020.1736399

INACSL. (n.d.-a). *History of the INACSL standards of best practice: Simulation*. https://www.inacsl.org/inacsl-standards-of-best-practice-simulation/history-of-the-inacsl-standards-of-best-practice-simulation/

INACSL. (n.d.-b). *Repository of instruments used in simulation research*. https://www.inacsl.org/resources/repository-of-instruments/

INACSL Board of Directors. (2011). Standards of best practice: Simulation. *Clinical Simulation in Nursing*, *7*(4), S3–S19. https://www.nursingsimulation.org/issue/S1876-1399%2811%29X0005-1

INACSL Standards Committee. (2016). INACSL standards of best practice: Simulation^{SM}: Simulation. *Clinical Simulation in Nursing*, *12*, S5–S50. https://doi.org/10.1016/j.ecns.2016.09.009

INACSL Standards Committee. (2017). INACSL standards of best practice: Simulation^{SM}: Operations. *Clinical Simulation in Nursing*, *13*(12), 681–687. https://doi.org/10.1016/j.ecns.2017.10.005

Jay, M., Schlair, S., Caldwell, R., Kalet, A., Sherman, S., & Gillespie, C. (2010). From the patient's perspective: The impact of training on resident physician's obesity counseling. *Journal of General Internal Medicine*, *25*(5), 415–422. https://doi.org/10.1007/s11606-010-1299-8

Jeffries, P. R., & Rizzolo, M. (2006). *Designing and implementing models for the innovative use of simulation to teach nursing care of ill adults and children: A national multi-site study*. http://www/nln.org/researchgrants/LaerdalReport.pdf

Jeffries, P. R., Rodgers, B., & Adamson, K. (2015). The NLN Jeffries simulation theory. *Nursing Education Perspectives*, *36*(5), 292–293. https://doi.org/10.5480/1536-5026-36.5.292

Justus, T., Wilfong, D., & Daniel, L. (2016). An innovative educational approach to reducing catheter-associated urinary tract infections: A case study. *The Journal of Continuing Education in Nursing*, *47*(10), 473–476. https://doi.org/10.3928/00220124-20160920-09

Kaddoura, M. A. (2010). New graduate nurses' perceptions of the effects of clinical simulation on their critical thinking, learning, and confidence. *The Journal of Continuing Education in Nursing*, *41*(11), 506–516. https://doi.org/10.3928/00220124-20100701-02

Kaplonyi, J., Bowles, K. A., Nestel, D., Kiegaldie, D., Maloney, S., Haines, T., & Williams, C. (2017). Understanding the impact of simulated patients on health care learners' communication skills: A systematic review. *Medical Education*, *51*(12), 1209–1219. https://doi.org/10.1111/medu.13387

Kardong-Edgren, S., Adamson, K. A., & Fitzgerald, C. (2010). A review of currently published evaluation instruments for human patient simulation. *Clinical Simulation in Nursing*, *6*(1), e25–35. https://doi.org/10.1016/jecns.2009.08.004

Karnish, K., Shustack, L., Brogan, L., Capitano, G., & Cunfer, A. (2019). Interprofessional socialization through acute-care simulation. *Radiologic Technology*, *90*(6), 552–562.

Kenny, A. (2002). Online learning: Enhancing nurse education. *Journal of Advanced Nursing*, *38*(2), 127–135. https://doi.org/10.1046/j.1365-2648.2002.02156.x

Kim, L., Lyder, C. H., McNeese-Smith, D., Needleman, J., & Searle Leach, L. (2014). *The effects of simulation-based TeamSTEPPS interprofessional communication and teamwork training on patient and provider outcomes*. ProQuest Dissertations and Theses.

Kinsman, L., Buykx, P., Cant, R., Champion, R., Cooper, S., Endacott, R., & Scholes, J. (2012). The FIRST 2 ACT simulation program improves nursing practice in a rural Australian hospital. *Australian Journal of Rural Health*, *20*(5), 270–274. https://doi.org/10.1111/j.1440-1584.2012.01296.x

Kirkpatrick, A. J., Cantrell, M. A., & Smeltzer, S. C. (2017). Palliative care simulations in undergraduate nursing education: An integrative review. *Clinical Simulation in Nursing*, *13*, 414–431. https://doi.org/10.1016/j.ecns.2017.04.009

Kirkpatrick, A. J., Cantrell, M. A., & Smeltzer, S. C. (2019). Relationships among nursing student palliative care knowledge, experience, self-awareness, and performance: An end-of-life simulation study. *Nurse Education Today*, *73*, 23–30. https://doi.org/10.1016/j.nedt.2018.11.003

Knight, L., Gabhart, J., Earnest, K., Leong, K., Anglemyer, A., & Franzon, D. (2014). Improving code team performance and survival outcomes: Implementation of pediatric resuscitation team training. *Critical Care Medicine*, *42*(2), 243–251. https://doi.org/10.1097/CCM.0b013e3182a6439d

Lapkin, S., Levett-Jones, T., Bellchambers, H., & Fernandez, R. (2010). Effectiveness of patient simulation manikins in teaching clinical reasoning skills to undergraduate nursing students: A systematic review. *Clinical Simulation in Nursing*, *6*(6), e207. https://doi.org/10.1016/j.ecns.2010.05.005

Leighton, K., Foisy-Doll, C., & Gilbert, G. E. (2018). Development and psychometric evaluation of the simulation culture organizational readiness survey. *Nurse Educator*, *43*(5), 251–255. https://doi.org/10.1097/NNE.0000000000000504

Leighton, K., Mudra, V., & Gilbert, G. E. (2018). Development and psychometric evaluation of the facilitator competency rubric. *Nursing Education Perspectives*, *39*(6), E3–E9. https://doi.org/10.1097/01.NEP.0000000000000409

Leighton, K., Ravert, P., Mudra, V., & Macintosh, C. (2015). Updating the simulation effectiveness tool: Item modifications and reevaluation of psychometric properties. *Nursing Education Perpsectives*, *36*(5), 317–323. https://doi.org/10.5480/15-1671

Lewis, K., Ricks, T., Rowin, A., Ndlovu, C., Goldstein, L., & McElvogue, C. (2019). Does simulation training for acute care nurses improve patient safety outcomes: A systematic review to inform evidence-based practice. *Worldviews on Evidence-Based Nursing*, *16*(5), 389–396. https://doi.org/10.1111/wvn.12396

Liaw, S. Y., Wong, L. F., Lim, E. Y. P., Ang, S. B. L., Mujumdar, S., Ho, J. T. Y., & Ang, E. K. (2016). Effectiveness of a web-based simulation in improving nurses' workplace practice with deteriorating ward patients: A pre- and postintervention study. *Journal of Medical Internet Research*, *18*(2), E37. https://doi.org/10.2196/jmir.5294

Lioce, L., Meakim, C. H., Fey, M. K., Chmil, J. V., Mariani, B., & Alinier, G. (2015). Standards of best practice: Simulation standard IX: Simulation design. *Clinical Simulation in Nursing*, *11*(6), 309–315. https://doi.org/10.1016/j.ecns.2015.03.005

Madorin, S., & Iwasiw, C. (1999). The effects of computer-assisted instruction on the self-efficacy of baccalaureate nursing students. *Journal of Nursing Education*, *38*(6), 282–285.

Mariani, B., & Doolen, J. (2016, January). Nursing simulation research: What are the perceived gaps? *Clinical Simulation in Nursing*, *12*(1), 30–36. http://dx.doi.org/10.1016/j.ecns.2015.11.004

McGaghie, W. C., Siddall, V. J., Mazmanian, P. E., & Myers, J. (2009). Lessons for continuing medical education from simulation research in undergraduate and graduate medical education. *Chest*, *135*(3), 62S–68S. https://doi.org/10.1378/chest.08-2521

McNeal, G. J. (2010). Simulation and nursing education. *Association of Black Nursing Faculty Journal*, *21*(4), 78.

Merchant, D. (2012). Does high-fidelity simulation improve clinical outcomes? *Journal for Nurses in Staff Development*, *28*(1), E1–E8. https://doi.org/10.1097/NND.0b013e318240a728

Merritt, L. S. (2020). Preparing nurse practitioner students for virtual visits: An innovative computer-based text-messaging simulation. *Clinical Simulation in Nursing*, *43*(6), 17–20. https://doi.org/10.1016/j.ecns.2020.02.006

Montalvo, I. (2007). The national database of nursing quality indicators®. (NDNQI®). *OJIN: The Online Journal of Issues in Nursing*, *12*(3). Manuscript 2. https://doi.org/10.3912/OJIN.Vol12No03Man02

Moule, P. (2011). Simulation in nurse education: Past, present and future. *Nurse Education Today*, *31*, 645–646. https://doi.org/10.1016/j.nedt.2011.04.005

Murphy, M., Curtis, K., Lam, M., Palmer, C., Hsu, J., & McCloughen, A. (2018). Simulation-based multidisciplinary team training decreases time to critical operations for trauma patients. *Injury, 49*(5), 953–958. https://doi.org/10.1016/j.injury.2018.01.009

Nunes, S., & Harder, N. (2019). Debriefing and palliative care simulation. *Journal of Nursing Education, 58*(10), 569–576. https://doi.org/10.3928/01484834-20190923-03

Nunnink, L., Venkatesh, B., Jones, M., Foot, C., Lucey, M., Corke, C., & Saxena, M. (2014). High-stakes assessment of the non-technical skills of critical care trainees using simulation: Feasibility, acceptability and reliability. *Critical Care and Resuscitation, 16*(1), 6–12.

Palaganas, J. C., Epps, D., & Raemer, D. B. (2014). A history of simulation-enhanced interprofessional education. *Journal of Interprofessional Care, 28*(2), 110–115. https://doi.org/10.3109/13561820.2013.869198

Patterson, M., Geis, G., Lemaster, T., & Wears, R. (2013). Impact of multidisciplinary simulation-based training on patient safety in a paediatric emergency department. *BMJ Quality & Safety, 22*(5), 383–393. https://doi.org/10.1136/bmjqs-2012-000951

Persaud, S., & Thornton, M. (2018). Developing caring behaviors in undergraduate nursing students through simulation. *International Journal for Human Caring, 22*(2), 26–33.8. https://doi.org/10.20467/1091-5710.22.2.26

Peters, V., Harvey, E., Wright, A., Bath, J., Freeman, D., & Collier, B. (2018). Impact of a TeamSTEPPS trauma nurse academy at a level 1 trauma center. *Journal of Emergency Nursing, 44*(1), 19–25. https://doi.org/10.1016/j.jen.2017.05.007

Pollard, C. L., & Wild, C. (2014). Nursing leadership competencies: Low-fidelity simulation as a teaching strategy. *Nurse Education in Practice, 14,* 620–626. https://doi.org/10.1016/j.nepr.2014.06.006

Prakash, V., Koczmara, C., Savage, P., Trip, K., Stewart, J., Mccurdie, T., & Trbovich, P. (2014). Mitigating errors caused by interruptions during medication verification and administration: Interventions in a simulated ambulatory chemotherapy setting. *BMJ Quality & Safety, 23*(11), 884–892. https://doi.org/10.1136/bmjqs-2013-002484

Prion, S.K. (2008a). A practical framework for assessing the impact of clinical simulation experiences in the nursing curriculum. *Clinical Simulation in Nursing Education, 4,* e69–e78. https://doi.org/10.1016/j.ecns.2008.08.002

Prion, S. K. (2008b). Evaluation involved in using simulations. *National League for Nursing.* http://www.sirc4nln.org/dev/mod/resource/view.php?id=38

Prion, S. K., & Adamson, K. A. (2012). The need for rigor in simulation research. *Clinical Simulation in Nursing, 8,* e193. https://doi.org/10.1016/j.ecns.2012.02.005

Prion, S. K., Gilbert, G. E., Adamson, K. A., Kardong-Edgren, S., & Quint, S. (2017). Development and testing of the quint leveled clinical competency tool. *Clinical Simulation in Nursing, 13*(3), 106–115. http://doi.org/10.1016/j.ecns.2016.10.008

Radhakrishnan, K., Roche, J. P., & Cunningham, H. (2007). Measuring clinical practice parameters with human patient simulation: A pilot study. *International Journal of Nursing Education Scholarship, 4*(1), 1–11. https://doi.org/10.2202/1548-923X.1307

Rauen, C. (2004). Simulation as a teaching strategy for nursing education and orientation in cardiac surgery. *Critical Care Nurse, 24*(3), 46–51. https://doi.org/10.4037/ccn2004.24.3.46

Rhodes, M., & Curran, C. (2005). Use of the human patient simulator to teach clinical judgment skills in a baccalaureate nursing program. *CIN Computers, Informatics, Nursing, 23*(5), 256–262. https://doi.org/10.1097/00024665-200509000-00009

Ross, G., & Tuovinen, J. (2001). Deep versus surface learning with multimedia in nursing education. *Computers in Nursing, 19*(5), 213–223.

Sanko, J. S. (2017). Simulation as a teaching technology: A brief history of its use in nursing education. *The Quarterly Review of Distance Education, 18*(2), 77–85.

Sanko, J. S., Shekhter, I., Gattamorta, K. A., & Birnbach, D. J. (2016). Development and psychometric analysis of a tool to evaluate confederates. *Clinical Simulation in Nursing, 12*(11), 475–481. http://dx.doi.org/10.1016/j.ecns.2016.07.006

Schneidereith, T. (2014). Using simulations to identify nursing student behaviors: A longitudinal study of medication administration. *Journal of Nursing Education, 53*(2), 89–92. https://doi.org/10.3928/01484834-20140122-07

Schoening, A. M., Sittner, B. J., & Todd, M. J. (2006). Simulated clinical experience nursing students' perceptions and the educators' role. *Nurse Educator, 31*(6), 253–258. https://doi.org/10.1097/00006223-200611000-00008

Schubert, C. R. (2012). Effect of simulation on nursing knowledge and critical thinking in failure to rescue events. *Journal of Continuing Education in Nursing, 43*(10), 467–471. https://doi.org/10.3928/00220124-20120904-27

Siassakos, D., Hasafa, Z., Sibanda, T., Fox, R., Donald, F., Winter, C., & Draycott, T. (2009). Retrospective cohort study of diagnosis–delivery interval with umbilical cord prolapse: The effect of team training. *BJOG: An International Journal of Obstetrics & Gynaecology, 116*(8), 1089–1096. https://doi.org/10.1111/j.1471-0528.2009.02179.x

Sodhi, K., Singla, M., & Shrivastava, K. (2015). Institutional resuscitation protocols: Do they affect cardiopulmonary resuscitation outcomes? A 6-year study in a single tertiary-care centre. *Journal of Anesthesia, 29*(1), 87–95. https://doi.org/10.1007/s00540-014-1873-z

Stephens, K. P., & Mosser, N. R. (2013). Simulation to improve pediatric patient outcomes: University and hospital collaborative. *Clinical Simulation in Nursing, 9*(7), e243–e247. https://doi.org/10.1016/j.ecns.2011.11.010

Theilen, U., Leonard, P., Jones, P., Ardill, R., Weitz, J., Agrawal, D., & Simpson, D. (2013). Regular in situ simulation training of paediatric medical emergency team improves hospital response to deteriorating patients. *Resuscitation, 84*(2), 218–222. https://doi.org/10.1016/j.resuscitation.2012.06.027

Thomas, E. J., Sexton, J. B., & Helmreich, R. L. (2004). Translating teamwork behaviours from aviation to healthcare: Development of behavioural markers for neonatal resuscitation. *Quality and Safety in Health Care, 13*(Suppl 1), i57–i64. https://doi.org/10.1136/qshc.2004.009811

Todd, M., Manz, K., Hawkins, M., Parsons, M., & Hercinger, M. (2008). The development of a quantitative evaluation tool for simulation in nursing education. *International Journal of Nursing Education Scholarship, 5*(1), article 41. https://doi.org/10.2202/1548-923X.1705

Wolf, L. (2008). The use of human patient simulation in ED triage training can improve nursing confidence and patient outcomes. *Journal of Emergency Nursing, 34*(2), 169. https://doi.org/10.1016/j.jen.2007.11.005

Yudkowsky, R., Luciano, C., Banerjee, P., Schwartz, A., Alaraj, A., Lemole, G., & Frim, D. (2013). Practice on an augmented reality/haptic simulator and library of virtual brains improves residents' ability to perform a ventriculostomy. *Simulation in Healthcare, 8*(1), 25–31. https://doi.org/10.1097/SIH.0b013e3182662c69

CHAPTER 8

Simulation-Based Operations

Crystel L. Farina and Kellie Bryant

ABSTRACT

Simulation pedagogy and the operations of simulation-based experiences have become an integral part of healthcare education. Academic and healthcare institutions constructed simulation centers or dedicated simulation spaces to provide simulation-based experiences for multiple health professions. Architectural designs resemble acute care settings that have the flexibility to change or include virtual reality and enhanced technology. Professional organizations have standards of best practice, credentialing requirements, and accreditation standards that support the need for high-quality, high-fidelity simulation experiences. Within healthcare education, simulation operation has become a specialty in itself that requires knowledge and experience of healthcare, education, and simulation pedagogy (INACSL Standards Committee, 2017). Simulation center administration needs an understanding of personnel management, including standardized patients (SPs), staff, faculty, and learners, as well as knowledge of budgeting, revenue streams, and technology. Personnel with unique skills and knowledge in engineering, healthcare, or information technology are required to support the simulation activities. Resources that manage inventory, supplies, equipment assets, and audiovisual requirements will increase efficiency and enhance fiscal responsibility. Technology assets such as

http://dx.doi.org/10.1891/0739-6686.39.181

high-fidelity human patient simulators can be used to enhance high-quality simulation, while audiovisual and data capturing software can be used for assessment, evaluation, and quality improvement. Simulation operations provides the infrastructure that supports the daily activities of simulation-based education.

SIMULATION-BASED OPERATIONS

Simulation has evolved over time in nursing education and the operations of simulation-based experiences have become an integral part of the process. Academic institutions have invested in the construction of simulation centers to provide simulation-based experiences for multiple health professions. These centers are used as recruiting tools and displays to highlight innovation and state-of-the art technology (Eagle, 2017a; Eagle, 2017b; Ferenc, 2017).

Simulation centers and spaces are also gaining momentum in hospitals and practice settings. Simulation-based learning, in a setting where mistakes are acceptable, creates an opportunity to explore new roles, practice new procedures, pilot-test new protocols, and ensure better patient outcomes (Roussin et al., 2018).

Academic institutions use simulation centers to enhance development of communication, critical thinking, and clinical reasoning skills in health professions and nursing students (Bryant et al., 2020; Lee & Kim 2020). Practice settings rely on simulation activities to provide education on new protocols, new equipment, and safety drills (Bailey & Mixer, 2018: Jones & Potter, 2017; Rutherford-Hemming et al., 2016). This chapter will discuss the operational needs of both academic and practice simulation centers, including strategic planning, personnel, systems management, fiscal resources, systems integration, policies and procedures, and pandemic planning.

Historical Context

Simulation-based experiences have existed for over a century but, in early 2000, standards for the use of simulation in healthcare education began to develop (Harder, 2009). Affinity groups and professional organizations such as Society for Simulation in Healthcare (SSH) and International Nursing Association for Clinical Simulation and Learning (INACSL) began to form. Until standards were first published in 2011 (Ackermann et al., n.d.), simulation activities were often set up, facilitated, reset, and cleaned up by one person, usually a faculty member or lab coordinator (Blodgett et al., 2018).

Connections between simulation-based educational experiences and improvements in patient outcomes were recognized (Stone et al., 2017) alongside the popularity of simulation as a teaching strategy for health professions. This increased the need for dedicated simulation spaces and simulation centers

(Agency for Healthcare Research and Quality, 2015; Barber et al., 2016; Kuiper & Zabriskie, 2012; Seropian et al., 2004). Architectural designs of space became innovative and flexible to accommodate changes in healthcare delivery and technology (Barber et al., 2016; Eagle, 2017a; Eagle, 2017b; Ferenc, 2017; Kuiper & Zabriskie, 2012; Seropian et al., 2004).

Prior to 2017, the INACSL Standards of Best Practice: Simulation^{SM} were primarily focused on the pedagogy and facilitation practices of simulation (INACSL, 2016a, 2016b, 2016c), but questions continued regarding simulation center operations, use of the space, and potential funding (Riley et al., 2019). In 2017, the newest INACSL Standard of Best Practice: Simulation^{SM}: Operations was published, which outlines criteria necessary for a successful simulation program (INACSL Standards Committee, 2017), including strategic planning, personnel, systems management, fiscal resources, systems integration, policies, and procedures.

Strategic Planning

The first step in planning for simulation experiences is a needs assessment, which answers operational questions, determines usage needs, and establishes organizational structure.

Decisions following the needs assessment are imperative for determining allocation of dedicated simulation spaces, including construction of entire buildings, and/or remodeling or expanding current spaces. Strategic planning will guide discussion and provide the path to reach the strategic goals (Byrne et al., 2019; Rosen et al., 2015). Utilizing a theoretical framework or model for strategic planning, such as Appreciative Inquiry or Wilson Centre's Emergent Scholarly model, can guide the efficiency of the strategic planning process (Byrne et al., 2019; He & Oxendine, 2019).

Simulation-specific strategic planning is necessary to determine the mission, vision, and goals for the future (Byrne et al., 2019; INACSL Standards Committee, 2017; Schneidereith et al., 2020). It is an opportunity to (a) brainstorm ideas that support a variety of uses by the simulation center, (b) assist with alignment of resources, and (c) help develop recommended 1-, 3-, and 5-year plans alongside short- and long-term goals (INACSL Standards Committee, 2017). Strategic planning also provides the opportunity to identify and include stakeholders in the process (Jeffs et al., 2019). Every entity that will use the simulation space should have a voice in the strategic planning process to ensure that the simulation center meets the unique needs of each. Having a simulation-specific strategic plan provides the foundational structure for future simulation accreditation and demonstrates to leadership the plan for simulation operations (Committee for

Accreditation of Healthcare Simulation Programs, 2016; INACSL Standards Committee, 2017). Additionally, the strategic plan should include a process for evaluation of simulation events, faculty, leadership, and learning outcomes. Assessment and evaluation plans identify necessary changes and professional development needs for faculty and staff (INACSL Standards Committee, 2017; Rosen et al., 2015; Schneidereith et al., 2020). Lastly, the strategic plan can impact future budgeting, including line items for (a) required professional development of simulation leadership, faculty, and staff and (b) individual or institutional memberships to professional simulation organizations (Eliadis & Verkuyl, 2019: INACSL Standards Committee, 2017; Schneidereith et al., 2020).

Simulation Personnel

One of the most important decisions of a simulation center administrator is focused on the simulation educator. Staffing consumes a major percentage of budgetary funds, therefore decisions that support an ideal simulation team are paramount. Simulation centers often have limited numbers of positions or full-time equivalent (FTE) personnel hours and have to prioritize who should be a part of the team with the goal of adding new roles as the use of the simulation center increases. Although there is no one-size-fits-all approach for staffing, there are three essentials roles for any simulation center: director, technical operations, and simulation educator (Crawford, Baily, et al., 2019). Based on the organizational chart, the director or administrative leadership must determine salaries, job descriptions, and job requirements for each position. Beyond the specific skill set needed for each position, basic qualifications include the ability to learn new technologies, excellent time management skills, problem-solving skills, and an ability to work under pressure (American College of Surgeons, 2013).

One of the first steps toward establishing a simulation program is to hire an experienced director or coordinator (Lazzara et al., 2014). Candidates considered for this position have experience working in a simulation center and the skill set necessary to manage a simulation center including experience with finance, budget oversite, and leadership/managerial roles. The director has knowledge of simulation pedagogy in order to hire high-quality educators and ensure implementation of best practices (Gardner et al., 2018; Lazzara et al., 2014). Additional responsibilities include, but are not limited to, establishing simulation curricula, developing the center's strategic plan, establishing policies and procedures, managing simulation staff, and overseeing fiscal resources. The simulation director will use previous experiences to identify qualified candidates for technical positions (i.e., simulation technicians, simulation operation specialist). Technical operators are key roles for simulation teams and ideal candidates are those with experience working in an information technology and/or a healthcare-related field (Bailey et al., 2015). Simulation relies on the use of rapidly evolving high-fidelity manikins, computer-based software programs, and audiovisual equipment. In a survey of 73 simulation technicians, individuals with an engineering (100%), medical (43.9%), and information technology (40%) backgrounds felt their previous experience prepared them well for their current role (Bailey et al., 2015). Job descriptions can vary but typically include operating simulation equipment and manikins, troubleshooting technical issues, setting up simulation rooms, participating in simulation sessions, collecting simulation center data, communicating with vendors, and performing preventative maintenance of equipment.

Lastly, simulation educators (i.e., simulation faculty or facilitators) develop and facilitate simulation activities. It is essential that simulation facilitators have formal training in best practices of simulation pedagogy, facilitation, design, and debriefing techniques (Beroz et al., 2020; INACSL Standards Committee, 2016a, 2016b, 2016c). Experienced educators ensure standardization of best practices in simulation and delivery of high-quality simulation activities (INACSL Standards Committee, 2016a, 2016b, 2016c). Highly qualified simulation educators create ideal learning environments that engage learners and results in a more positive simulation experience (Gardner et al., 2018). Conversely, inadequately trained simulation staff, lack of administrative support, and insufficient funding are cited as the biggest obstacles to having a successful simulation program (Beroz et al., 2020). Lack of trained simulation staff and administrative support have been shown to negatively affect the quality of simulation activities and can therefore jeopardize the credibility of the simulation center (Beroz et al., 2020; Gardner et al., 2018; Gardner et al., 2018). As the use of simulation increases, additional simulation personnel will help the center flourish. Additional positions include: (a) an operations manager who can oversee ordering of supplies, tracking of expenses, and provide assistance to the director with day-to-day operations, (b) an administrative assistant to perform clerical tasks, (c) simulation researchers to confirm or generate new knowledge, and (d) debriefing facilitators who focus only on facilitating the experiences and debriefing learners after simulation activities.

The use of SP methodology (see Chapter 3) has become increasingly popular as a simulation modality (Smiley, 2019). Smiley (2019), reported that 42.3% of prelicensure nursing programs reported using SP methodology in 2010 compared to 63.2% in 2017. Harold Barrows, founder of one of the first SP programs and originator of the term standardized patient, realized that the use of actors playing the role of a person with an illness or a true patient playing themselves with the illness in a standardized way allowed students to practice the physical, psychological, and emotional aspects of clinical practice (Dickter et al., 2015; Lewis et al., 2017; Rutherford-Hemming et al., 2019; Oh et al., 2015). Compared to human patient simulators, engaging SPs offer students a level of fidelity for learning how to (a) communicate, (b) handle emotional situations, and/or (c) perform physical assessments that exceed what is possible with patient simulators (Oh et al., 2015; Rutherford-Hemming et al., 2019). Implementing an SP program requires additional responsibilities that can impact the simulation staff, such as developing a hiring process, creating SP scenarios, and conducting SP training sessions prior to implementing new scenarios. Before developing an SP program, simulation directors should compare the cost of developing and maintaining a dedicated SP program to the cost of contracting an outside SP agency. Elements to consider include employment of actors versus nonactors, rates of payment, and contract or part-time employment (Dickter et al., 2015). In addition, protocol development will be necessary to protect the safety of the SP, such as clear guidelines on the number of invasive physical examinations and creating a "safe word" that will end the simulation immediately if there is a potential for harm. The Association of Standardized Patient Educators (ASPE) provides guidelines that outline best practices in the use of SP methodology (ASPE, n.d.; Lewis et al., 2017). Centers that have a high volume of SP simulation scenarios should consider hiring a simulation coordinator for scheduling, training, and handling payment of the SPs.

Systems Management

Simulation centers inherently include expensive supplies, equipment, technology, and management of these resources and assets are crucial to efficient and effective operations. A system for managing resources, warranties, preventive maintenance, and equipment operation education are essential to ensure that the simulation center operates smoothly (Nagle et al., 2018). The simulation center administration is responsible for the creation and dissemination of a policy that delineates how the needs of the center are prioritized. This policy will provide guidelines for all requests to ensure that the requirements of learners and other stakeholders are met. This prioritization plan can include an algorithm for decision-making (see Figure 8.1). If two groups request use of the simulation center for the same day and time, a clear decision-making process will reduce conflict. For example, if there is a request for postpartum hemorrhage drills by the obstetrics group and a request for peritoneal dialysis practice from the renal team, the algorithm or decision tree will help determine prioritization.

Equipment is essential to the daily operations of the simulation center. The operating condition of equipment is paramount to the safety of all simulation center end users. Intravenous pumps, beds, defibrillators, carts, computers, cameras,

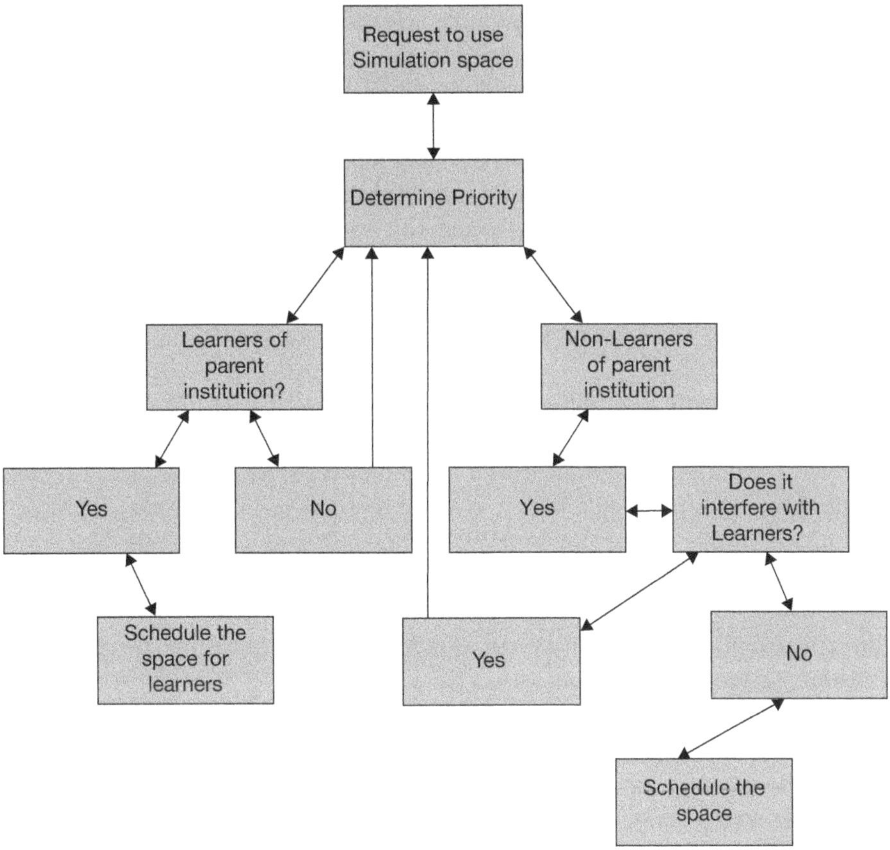

FIGURE 8.1 Simple decision algorithm.
This is an example of a simple decision algorithm. When there are two requests for the simulation space, the priority is always learner's educational needs. When the request is for learner education, the space is scheduled. When the request is not for learner usage, determine if it interferes with learner education. When it is available and does not interfere with learner education, schedule the space.

and recording devices are expensive to maintain and monitor for output errors. Purchasing warranties for new or rebuilt equipment will be necessary to keep it working consistently. When systems fail, there is an impact on the learner and the simulation center; therefore, establishing a consistent plan to maintain reliable equipment and secure extra resources will keep the simulation center operating on schedule (Barber et al., 2016; Eliadis & Verkuyl, 2019; Gardner et al., 2018: INACSL Standards Committee, 2016a: Kuiper & Zabriskie, 2012).

Simulation centers will require basic equipment for specific simulation scenarios to support fidelity and learner expectations (Barber et al., 2016; Eliadis & Verkuyl, 2019; Gardner et al., 2018: INACSL Standards Committee, 2016a:

Kuiper & Zabriskie, 2012). For example, a simulation scenario in an acute care setting loses fidelity if there is no bed, monitor, or intravenous pump. Vendors that specialize in simulation equipment for education are numerous and provide used or refurbished equipment at discounted costs with limited warranties. Lifespans for equipment vary (Table 8.1) and replacement plans should be made at the time of purchase. For example, a refurbished hospital bed usually has a 1-year warranty and will need replacement in 5 to 7 years. If a simulation center has 20 beds, replacing all of them at the same time is costly, but developing a replacement cycle will provide a means to purchase two to four beds every other year. This allows for a regular renewal of updated equipment alongside a budget that supports the plan.

Simulators are one of the costliest assets of a simulation center. Whether low-fidelity manikins for skill training (Laerdal Medical, n.d.; Gaumard Scientific, n.d.) or high-fidelity simulators for scenarios (CAE Healthcare, n.d.; Laerdal Medical n.d.; Gaumard Scientific, n.d.), the cost can range between $1,800.00 and $250,000.00. Technology is developing quickly and it is not possible to get the newest version every time an update is released. When planning for a simulator purchase, review the needs assessment, including the needs of the facility and the usage of all stakeholders. Do not purchase any equipment for the potential of gaining a program that would use a particular high-level function, but instead purchase for the programs currently using the space. For example, undergraduate nursing students should have access to a simulator that allows for assessment and care of the laboring and postpartum patient. Purchasing two moderate-fidelity simulators with laboring, assessment, and postpartum abilities may receive more usage than the simulator that gives birth. Also, consider how the simulator will be used throughout the curriculum and how it can support more than one educational program. For example, if the simulation center serves prelicensure nursing students and midwifery students, a birthing simulator might be the correct purchase. If that same simulator has the ability to be nongravid, then it could support multiple programs and would be worth the higher price. Purchase the simulator that provides the largest range of capabilities and meets the needs of the learner groups. Reach out to the simulation professional groups or simulation colleagues and ask for recommendations prior to purchasing. Ask questions about what works well and areas that are troublesome or complicated for the end users. It would be a costly mistake to purchase a simulator for intubation practice, and learn after the purchase, the oral airway landmarks are not realistic and do not support student learning needs (Eliadis & Verkuyl, 2019).

Depending on the need, task trainers may be appropriate for the learners (Lioce et al., 2020). These are anatomical models used to teach psychomotor skills (Crawford, Huque, et al., 2019; Nicka & Swanson-Biearman, 2019) and some

TABLE 8.1

Estimated Simulation Warranty Recommendations and Replacement Plan

Simulation Equipment	New/Refurbished	Warranties Recommendations	Replacement Plan
High-fidelity simulator	New	Recommend purchase warranty/preventive maintenance for 3–5 years programs to maintain updates. Most manufacturers will continue to provide technology update for life of product marketing. Inquire with sales representative.	7–10 years due to enhanced technology
Moderate-fidelity simulators	New	Recommend warranties/preventive maintenance for minimum 3 years.	10–15 years
Intravenous pumps	New or refurbished	Purchase warranties and preventive maintenance agreements to support updates and recalls.	3–5 years
Hospital beds	Refurbished	Recommend minimum 1-year warranty.	5–7 years
Defibrillators	New or refurbished	Purchase warranties and preventive maintenance agreements to support updates and recalls.	3–5 years
Simulated headwalls	New	Recommend minimum 1-year warranty.	10–15 years
Audiovisual simulation capturing software/hardware	New	Recommend purchase warranty/preventive maintenance for 3–5 years programs to maintain updates. Recommend purchase technical support agreements.	5–7 years

models provide integrated feedback technology to the learner (Butt & Kardong-Edgren, 2018). Because task trainers include less technological hardware, they are typically less expensive than full body simulators and are more durable for repeated practice.

The simulation center will need a procedure in place for cleaning, storing, and maintaining the task trainers. Planning a replacement schedule will also help determine budgetary needs. For example, if an intravenous arm is recommended for up to 300 intravenous attempts and the simulation center has 300 students practicing, multiple arms will need to be purchased and a plan for annual replacements may be necessary. Task trainers are assets to the simulation space and will need maintenance as part of the equipment/asset inventory.

Supplies and consumables are a large percentage of the daily operating budget. Purchasing alliances or group purchasing organizations (GPOs) differ from state to state and can provide access to a catalog of thousands of supplies and a mechanism to decrease prices by leverage bulk purchases (Bruhn et al., 2018). According to Bruhn et al. (2018) greater than 90% of all hospital organizations use GPOs to decrease costs. Universities and colleges have access to GPOs for academic purchases. Additionally, vendors who provide supplies for educational purposes only and not for human use can often be purchased for simulation at a reduced price. For example, Foley catheter insertion kits for education are much more cost-effective for simulation than sterile Foley catheter insertion kits. However, it is vital that these supplies are kept separate from supplies used for real patients—especially in hospital settings (see Chapter 4). Supplies for simulation should be labeled "Not for Human Use" to prevent the accidental use in a direct care setting (Bajaj et al., 2018; Foundation for Healthcare Simulation Safety, n.d.; Schroeder et al., 2015; Torrie et al., 2016). The Foundation for Healthcare Simulation Safety initiative, created to reduce harm to live patients, has products, resources, and references to support healthcare simulation safety.

The enormous amount of equipment and supplies needed for simulation requires storage and inventory management, especially in advance of any expansion or construction (Eliadis & Verkuyl, 2019; Nagle et al., 2018). Ensure that every piece of equipment has a storage space and, if expanding or completing a construction project, ensure that the architects recognize and account for space needed for linen hampers, trash receptacles, bedside tables, intravenous pumps and poles, electronic vital sign monitors, and so on. It is also important to track these supplies and equipment to ensure that items that may have been on loan to other units or learner groups are returned to the facility and receive any required maintenance. Inventory management systems can provide this tracking, as well inventory supplies, establish par levels, reorder alerts, automatic reorders, and track distribution of consumable supplies. Some also have the ability to tabulate usage data that can be applied to future budgets.

Fiscal Resources

Creating a simulation center's budget is one of the most complicated and important tasks required to ensure effective operations and sustainability. That major costs associated with opening simulation centers include construction, consultants, simulation capture systems, audiovisual equipment, and furniture. The next necessity involves planning a yearly operational budget alongside 5-year projections. Dependent upon the parent institution's leadership, the simulation center personnel may have limited input into the annual budget and leadership may base a preestablished amount of funds for the year upon enrollment or donations. Unfortunately, this amount may not be sufficient to operate a simulation program and leaves little funding for improvements. A more accurate allocation of funding is based upon the past year's expenses, predicted future expenses, cost of necessary upgrades and enhancement, upcoming payment of warranties, and the cost of staffing needs for the next fiscal year. Regularly monitoring expenses is necessary to ensure that funds will last the entire fiscal year. In addition, a reserve fund should be established for emergencies, such as the unexpected cost of converting a simulation program to a remote platform due COVID-19. Additionally, centers should anticipate budgeting for newer technologies, such as extended and virtual reality, which can be quite expensive (Ross, 2012).

Simulation equipment, supplies, and warranties consume a large part of a simulation center's budget. Human patient simulator costs can exceed $100,000 and often overlooked are the expenses associated with warranties. The decisions to purchase extended warranties compared to the risk of having to pay for episodic repairs, particularly with older equipment, are essential to maintaining a balanced budget. Options, such as onsite repairs and loaner programs, are available for increased cost. Factors that help determine the value of purchasing a warranty is the availability of trained technicians on staff, frequency of use of the product, warranty cost, and expected lifespan of the product. Disposable supplies are not as expensive as individual items, but can become costly when ordered frequently or in large quantities and should therefore be reused or recycled when possible.

Creating a revenue stream can offset the operational cost of a simulation center. Sources can include:

- Student fees.
- Space rental to television production companies, medical education companies, affiliated hospitals, or universities. Charges for simulation educators

and operation specialist's services can also increase this revenue (Eliadis & Verkuyl, 2019).

- Cardiopulmonary resuscitation (CPR) courses or other continuing education.
- Naming campaigns for the rights to name simulation rooms, the center, and smaller items such as lockers, anatomical models, and simulators.
- Crowdsourced funding targeted to former alumni, past donors, and social media followers.
- Grants.
- Pharmaceutical companies.
- Philanthropic foundations.
- Private donors (Ziv et al., 2006).

Systems Integration

Technology is integral to high-quality, high-fidelity simulation scenarios. However, state-of-the-art technology is not always required to ensure simulation scenarios run smoothly. Prior to purchasing recording equipment, assess available on-site audiovisual recording to ensure it will meet the simulation space needs. Determine the types of equipment needed through thoughtful review of required scenario technology (Box 8.1). Explore commercially available products, including available hardware and software, usability, and functionality. Gather references from other users to inquire about lessons learned.

These questions provide items to ask simulation users, stakeholders of the space, and leadership before making informed purchasing decisions.

System integration requires that simulation activities support the needs and plans of the parent organization (INACSL Standards Committee, 2017; Schneidereith et al., 2020). Having an integrated mission and vision that aligns with that of the parent institution will articulate the offerings of the simulation space and determine how the simulation space will enhance healthcare education (Byrne et al., 2019; Jeffs et al., 2019). Establishing simulation center policies will delineate for the parent organization and end-users processed for prioritizing scheduling, usage, and organizational reporting structures. (Byrne et al., 2019; Committee for Accreditation of Healthcare Simulation Programs, 2016; Jeffs et al., 2019).

Effective integration requires transparent and clear communication with the parent institution and all stakeholders regarding the ways in which the simulation center meets the vision, mission, and goals (Jeffs et al., 2019). Communication also includes assessment and evaluation of learning outcomes and a description of how the evaluation data are used to improve simulation-based experiences (INACSL Standards Committee, 2017).

Box 8.1: Questions to Ask Prior to Purchasing A/V Equipment

- Does the simulation scenario need to be recorded and why?
- What will the recordings be used for?
- Do the recordings need to be in high definition?
- Will the recordings be used to debrief participants?
- Does there need to be technology to provide a voice for the patient/simulator?
- Does there need to be source to communicate with a care provider in the scenario such as a phone or paging system?
- Will participants have access to the recordings remotely?
- Is date in the recordings restricted requiring special security?
- Are there plans to grade the recordings?
- How long will the recordings be stored? When can they be deleted?
- Who will have access to finished products? Is there a way to restrict access?
- Does the facilitator need to have field of vision of the scenario or are they able to view the scenario through the camera only?
- Is there an ability to move camera angles or zoom and retract picture?
- Is there a need for the A/V system to provide other service such as scheduling, notification or learners, inventory management, and grading of simulation scenarios?

The simulation personnel should collaborate in bidirectional initiatives to support the broader outcome of improved patient care, decreased medical errors, and improved healthcare safety through interprofessional experiences, collaborative teams, and dynamic partnerships. Quality indicators and learner evaluation data can be used to continuously support the improvement of simulation-based experiences, healthcare education, and patient outcomes (INACSL Standards Committee, 2017).

Policies and Procedures

Policies and procedures are uniquely developed to meet the specific needs of a simulation center, guide day-to-day operations, and provide the template for decision-making related to simulation activities. They cover topics such as general simulation center information, programs, scheduling, tours, video recording, safety, emergency contingency plans, supplies and equipment, scenario development, learner expectations, and finances. Developing policies and procedures involves a team with input from simulation staff, the institution's administration, and/or legal department. Establishing a simulation advisory group composed of faculty, staff, and learners can assist with policy development. Sample policies and procedures are available from the SSH and are frequently posted on the websites of individual simulation centers (Committee for Accreditation of Healthcare Simulation Programs, 2016).

Determining guidelines for faculty workload in an academic setting is challenging for nursing administration due to the lack of resources or consensus on calculation guidelines (Blodgett et al., 2018). Most programs calculate faculty workload based on FTE, clinical hours, contact hours, and billable hours, which do not take into account time for implementing simulation activities. Educational administrators should consider faculty time required to develop and prepare for simulation activities when allocating FTE to simulation faculty (Blodgett et al., 2018). Simulation centers must also decide whether to hire dedicated simulation educators assigned to teach simulation activities only or utilize faculty that are teaching in other courses.

Oftentimes, simulation facilitators learned how to conduct simulation through self-training, one-on-one mentoring, online training, or external simulation conferences (Nye et al., 2019), and many simulation educators have not received any formal training. In fact, a 2019 study showed that only 64.9% of prelicensure nursing faculty surveyed had formal facilitation training (Smiley, 2019). Resource availability can limit the ability for faculty development through online courses, offsite training (courses and/or conferences), or onsite training with contracted simulation consultants. Therefore, simulation centers should have an established and ongoing faculty development plan for simulation facilitators as part of ongoing, annual budgeting (INASCL Standards Committee, 2016).

Simulation center personnel should also ensure collection of simulation data. Utilization data, including simulation hours, learner visits, generated revenue, and number of simulation sessions offered will guide development of strategic plans and provide the evidence needed for additional resources. Although software programs are available to capture this data, dedicated staff are necessary for data analysis and reporting. Additionally, student feedback data provides assessment information for quality improvements. Data collection is particularly important for centers considering applying for SSH accreditation (Committee for Accreditation of Healthcare Simulation Programs, 2016).

Scheduling is another important component for simulation policy and procedure manuals. The procedure for requesting a simulation session should include a formal request form, approval workflow process, and all necessary information needed to implement the session. Timely review and feedback to the requestor are important in establishing customer service. As noted previously, a published algorithm will assist with prioritizing scheduling decisions. Creating a request form provides standardization and ensures inclusion of necessary information for the approver. Request forms should contain fields for date, time, number of learners, room requested, type of session, necessary equipment/supplies, and level of support staff needed. Policies should have an outlined prioritization and decision algorithm for handling scheduling conflicts, such as prioritizing sessions based on first come, first served; classes that are essential for learners; or prioritizing revenue-producing sessions. The policy should designate one person (usually the director) to make the final decision when dealing with scheduling conflicts.

Pandemic Considerations

The COVID-19 pandemic of 2020 shut down academic institutions and healthcare education programs across the globe. Academic institutions struggled to continue healthcare education while healthcare institutions suspended clinical learning to put all their resources into providing patient care to the 4,748,806 cases of patients infected with the virus (Centers for Disease Control and Prevention, 2020). Hospitals increased their use of simulation, specifically to educate providers on ways to manage COVID-19-positive patients, donning and doffing personal protective equipment, and ventilator management. Academic institutions sought guidance from simulationists to provide opportunities that would continue healthcare education sans onsite clinical learning experiences. Simulation vendors willingly provided trial memberships of virtual simulation experiences and other resources to support the continuance of healthcare education. Professional organizations such as the SSH, INACSL, and National League for Nursing provided simulation resources, educational support to adapt face-to-face simulation to virtual platforms, and webinars on best practices and shared resources.

The COVID-19 pandemic also challenged simulation centers and simulation directors. New policies and procedures to limit the risk of transmission of the virus to students, faculty, and simulation staff were developed. COVID-19 symptom screening, temperature checks, physical distancing, and cleaning protocols became part of daily simulation operations. In the beginning, simulation centers willingly donated personal protective equipment (PPE) to help healthcare providers in need, only to find that they were unable to provide students and personnel the same PPE when academic institutions moved to reopen. Simulation directors became unintended brokers needed to procure valuable PPE. In addition, COVID-19 forced simulation-based education to change the delivery of simulation curricula. Nursing programs had to initiate or increase usage of remote and unfamiliar virtual simulation platforms to maintain continuance of healthcare education. While healthcare education will forever be changed by the COVID-19 pandemic, simulation will continue to be a means to practice clinical decision-making and clinical reasoning to improve patient care outcomes.

CONCLUSION

The COVID-19 pandemic demonstrated that simulation continues to be a valued teaching strategy that can be used to replace inaccessible clinical experiences and, whether in an academic or practice setting, ensuring the standards of best practice for high-quality, high-fidelity simulation is paramount. Knowledge of simulation pedagogy, SPs, personnel, budget, assessment, evaluation, technology, and management systems are quintessential to efficient function. While simulation technology continues to advance, spaces continue to be developed, new knowledge is generated, and simulation operations provide the infrastructure for it all.

REFERENCES

Ackermann, A., Aebersold, M., Carpenter, A., Catron, L., Coggins, R., Dreifuerst, K., Gloe, D., Gonzalez, L., Greenawalt, J., Guhde, J., Guzelaydin, S., Henao, H., Kardong-Edgren, S., Kennedy, K., King, M., LaMar, J., Lambton, J., Lemon, D., Macy, R., & Walker, M. (n.d). *History of INACSL standards of best practice*. INACSL. https://www.inacsl.org/inacsl-standards-of-best-practice-simulation/history-of-the-inacsl-standards-of-best-practice-simulation

Agency for Healthcare Research and Quality. (2015, February). Health care simulation to advance safety: Responding to Ebola and other threats. *AHRQ Issue Brief*. https://www.ahrq.gov/sites/default/files/publications/files/simulation-brief.pdf

American College of Surgeons. (2013). *AEI Director's toolkit: Assembling the pieces for a successful simulation center*. American College of Surgeons: https://www.facs.org/Education/Accreditation/AEI/resources/toolkit

Association of Standardized Patient Educators. (n.d.). *The ASPE standards of best practice*. https://www.aspeducators.org/standards-of-best-practice

Bailey, C., & Mixer, S. (2018). Clinical simulation experiences of newly licensed registered nurses. *Clinical Simulation in Nursing*, *15*, 65–72. https://doi.org/10.1016/j.ecns.2017.11.006

Bailey, R., Taylor, R. G., FitzGerald, M. R., Kerrey, B. T., LeMaster, T., & Geis, G. L. (2015). Defining the simulation technician role: Results of a survey-based study. *Simulation in Healthcare*, *10*(5), 283–287. https://doi.org/10.1097/SIH.0000000000000103

Bajaj, K., Minors, A., Walker, K., Meguerdichian, M., & Patterson, M. (2018). No-go considerations for in situ simulation safety. *Simulation in Healthcare*, *13*, 221–224. https://doi.org/10.1097/SIH.0000000000000301

Barber, J., Eberhardt, A., Kennedy, B., & Kardong-Edgren, S. (2016). Logistical planning and Making the move to a new simulation space. *Clinical Simulation in Nursing, 12*(12), 565–569. https://doi.org/10.1016/j.ecns.2016.08.007

Beroz, S., Schneidereith, T., Farina, C. L., Daniels, A., Dawson, L., Watties-Daniels, D., & Sullivan, N. (2020). A statewide curriculum model for teaching simulation education leaders. *Nurse Educator, 45*(1), 56–60. https://doi.org/10.1097/NNE.0000000000000661

Blodgett, N. P., Blodgett, T., & Kardong-Edgren, S. E. (2018). A proposed model for simulation faculty workload determination. *Clinical Simulation in Nursing, 18*, 20–27. https://doi.org/10.1016/j.ecns.2018.01.003

Bruhn, W., Fracica, E., & Makary, M. (2018). Group purchasing organizations, health care costs, and drug shortages. *Journal of American Medical Association, 320*, 1859–1860. https://doi.org/10.1001/jama.2018.13604

Bryant, K., Aebersold, M., Jeffries, P., & Kardong-Edgren, S. (2020). Innovations in simulation: Nursing leaders' exchange of best practices. *Clinical Simulation in Nursing, 41*, 33–40. https://doi.org/10.1016/j.ecns.2019.09.002

Butt, A., & Kardong-Edgren, S. (2018). Using game-based virtual reality with haptics for skill acquisition. *Clinical Simulation in Nursing, 16*, 25–32. https://doi.org/10.1016/j.ecns.2017.09.010

Byrne, N., Woods, N., Kulasegaram, K., Martimianakis, M., Richardson, L., & Whitehead, C. (2019). Strategic planning in health professions education: Scholarship or management. *Academic Medicine, 94*(10), 1455–1460. https://doi.org/10.1097/ACM.0000000000002852

CAE Healthcare. (n.d.). *CAE HPS: The human patient simulator: The gold standard in patient Simulation*. https://caehealthcare.com/patient-simulation/hps

Centers for Disease Control and Prevention. (2020). Coronavirus disease 2019: CDC is responding to the novel coronavirus outbreak. *Centers for Disease Control and Prevention: CDC 24/7: Saving Lives, Protection People*. https://www.cdc.gov/coronavirus/2019-nCoV/index.html

Committee for Accreditation of Healthcare Simulation Programs. (2016). *Accreditation standards self-study review tool*. Society for Simulation in Healthcare.

Crawford, S., Baily, L., & Monks, S. (2019). *Comprehensive healthcare simulation: Operations, technology, and innovative practice*. Springer Publishing.

Crawford, S., Huque, Y., Austin, D., & Monks, S. (2019). Development and review of the chest tube high-feedback educational simulation trainer (CHEST). *Simulation in Healthcare, 14*(4), 276–279. https://doi.org/10.1097/SIH.0000000000000361

Dickter, D., Stielstra, S., & Lineberry, M. (2015). Interrater reliability of standardized actors versus nonactors in a simulation based assessment of interprofessional collaboration. *Simulation in Healthcare, 10*(4), 249–255. https://doi.org/10.10978SIH.0000000000000094

Eagle, A. (2017a). The reality of designing simulation centers. Health Facilities Management. https://www.hfmmagazine.com/articles/3182-the-reality-of-designing-simulation-center

Eagle, A. (2017b). Principles for efficient simulation center layouts. Health Facilities Management. https://www.hfmmagazine.com/articles/3184-principles-for-efficient-simulation-center-layouts

Ferenc, J. (2017). New high-tech simulation centers provide realistic training. https://hfmmagazine.com/articles/3002-construction-of-new-high-tech-simulation-center s-on-the-upswing

Eliadis, M., & Verkuyl, M. (2019). Balancing the budget in the simulation centre. *Clinical Simulation in Nursing*, *37*, 14–17. https://doi.org/10.1016/j.ecns.2019.06.005

Foundation for Healthcare Simulation Safety. (n.d.). *Incidents: Published reports*. https://he althcaresimulationsafety.org/incidents

Gardner, A., Ritter, E., Dunkin, B., Smink, D., Lau, J., Paige, J., & Gee, D. (2018). Leaders by example: best practices and advice on establishing a state-of-the art surgical simulation center that optimizes available resources. *The American Journal of Surgery*, *215*(2), 259–265. https://doi.org/10.1016/j.amjsurg.2017.11.007

Gaumard Scientific. (n.d.). *Gaumard simulators: Innovating health care for the future*. https://www.gaumard.com/aboutsims.

Harder, N. (2009). Evolution of simulation use in health care education. *Clinical Simulation in Nursing*, *5*, e169–e172. https://doi.org/j.ecns.2009.04.092

He, Y., & Oxendine, S. (2019). Leading positive change in higher education through appreciative inquiry: A phenomenological exploration of the strategic planning process. *Journal of Higher Education Policy and Management*, *41*(2), 219–232. https://doi.org/10.1080/1360080X.2018.1558720

INACSL Standards Committee. (2016a, December). INACSL standards of best practice: Simiulation[SM]: Simulation design. *Clinical Simulation in Nursing*, *12*(S), S5–S12. https://doi.org/10.1016/j.ecns.2016.09.005

INACSL Standards Committee. (2016b, December). INACSL standards of best practice: Simiulation[SM]: Facilitation. *Clinical Simulation in Nursing*, *12*(S), S16–S20. https://doi.org/10.1016/j.ecns.2016.09.007

INACSL Standards Committee. (2016c, December). INACSL standards of best practice: Simulation[SM]: Debriefing. *Clinical Simulation in Nursing*, *12*(S), S21–S25. https://doi.org/10.1016/j.ecns.2016.09.008

INACSL Standards Committee. (2017). INACSL standards of best practice: Simulation[SM]: Operations. *Clinical Simulation in Nursing*, *13*(12), 681–687. https://doi.org/10.1016/j.ecns.2017.10.005

Jeffs, L., Merkley, J., Sinno, M., Thomson, N., Peladeau, N., & Richardson, S. (2019). Engaging stakeholders to co-design an academic practice strategic plan in an integrated health system: The key roles of the nurse executive and planning team. *Nursing Administration Quarterly*, *43*(2), 186–192. https://doi.org/10.1097/NAQ/00000 00000000340

Jones, B., & Potter, C. (2017). Applying best practice in simulation: Critical care response team training. *Clinical Simulation in Nursing*, *13*(9), 442–445. https://doi.org/10.1016/j.ecns.2017.05.009

Kuiper, R., & Zabriskie, A. (2012). Developing a new state of the art simulation learning center. *Clinical Simulation in Nursing*, *8*(9), e437–e442. https://doi.org/10.1016.j.ecns.2011.04.003

Laerdal Medical. (n.d.). *Patient care manikins & trainers*. https://www.laerdal.com/us/products/simulation-training/nursing

Lazzara, E., Benishek, L. E., Dietz, A. S., Salas, E., & Adriansen, D. J. (2014). Eight critical factors in creating and implementing a successful simulation program. *The Joint Commission Journal on Quality and Patient Safety*, *40*(1), 21–29. https://doi.org/10.1016/S1553-7250(14)40003-5

Lee, K., & Kim, E. (2020). Relationship between interprofessional communication and team task performance. *Clinical Simulation in Nursing*, *43*, 44–50. https://doi.org/10.1016/j.ecns.2020.02.002

Lewis, K. L., Bohnert, C. A., Gammon, W. L., Hölzer, H., Lyman, L., Smith, C., & Gliva-McConvey, G. (2017). The association of standardized patient educators (ASPE) standards of best practice. *Advances in Simulation*, *2*(1), 1–8. https://doi.org/10.1186/s41077-017-0043-4

Lioce, L., Lopreiato, J., Downing, D., Chang, T. P., Robertson, J. M., Anderson, M., Diaz, D. A., Spain, A. E., & the Terminology and Concepts Working Group. (2020). *Healthcare simulation dictionary* (2nd ed.). Agency for healthcare Research and Quality; AHRQ Publication No. 20-0019. https://doi.org/10.23970/simulationv2

Nagle, A., Fisher, S., Frazier, S., & McComb, S. (2018). Streamlining a simulation center's inventory management. *Clinical Simulation in Nursing*, *18*, 1–5. https://doi.org/10.1016/j.ecns.2018.01.001

Nicka, A., & Swanson-Biearman, B. (2019). Development of a subcutaneous abscess simulator for incision and drainage. *Clinical Simulation in Nursing*, *37*(C), 40–43. https://doi.org/10.1016/j.ecns.2019.08.001

Nye, C., Campbell, S.., Herbert, S., Short, C., & Thomas, M. (2019). Simulation in advanced practice nursing programs: A North-American survey. *Clinical Simulation in Nursing*, *26*, 33–10. https://doi.org/10.1016/j.ecns.2018.09.005

Oh, P., Jeon, K., & Koh, M. (2015). The effects of simulation-based learning using standardized patients in nursing students: A meta-analysis. *Nurse Education Today*, *35*(5), e6–e15.

Riley, R., Kjaer, C., Naumovski, S., & Straw, B. (2019). Social network analysis of a simulation community. *Simulation in Healthcare*, *14*(2), 71–76. https://doi.org/10.1097/SIH.0000000000000344

Rosen, M., Goeschel, C., Che, X., Fawole, J., Rees, D., Curran, R., Gelinas, L., Martin, J., Kosel, K., Pronovast, P., & Weaver, S. (2015). Simulation in the executive suite: Lessons learned for building patient safety leadership. *Simulation in Healthcare*, *10*(6), 372–377. https://doi.org/10.1097/SIH.0000000000000122

Ross, K. (2012). Practice makes perfect. *Health Facilities Management*, *25*(11), 23–28.

Roussin, C., Larraz, E., Jamieson, K., & Maestre, J. (2018). Psychological safety, self-efficacy, and speaking up in interprofessional health care simulation. *Clinical Simulation in Nursing*, *17*, 38–46. https://doi.org/10.1016/j.ecns.2017.12.002

Rutherford-Hemming, T., Alfes, M., & Breymier, L. (2019). A systemic review of the use of standardized patients as a simulation modality in nursing education. *The Research Journal of the National League of Nursing*, *40*(2), 84–90. https://doi.org/10.1097/01.NEP.0000000000000401

Rutherford-Hemming, T., Lioce, L., Kardong-Edgren, S., Jeffries, P., & Sittner, B. (2016). After the national council of state boards of nursing simulation study – Recommendations next steps. *Clinical Simulation in Nursing*, *12*, 2–7. https://doi.org/10.1016/j.ecns.2015.10.010

Schneidereith, T., Leighton, K., & Foisy-Doll, C. (2020). Operationalizing a simulation program: Practical information for leadership. *Nursing Forum*, *2020*, 1–6. https://doi.org/10.1111/nuf.12463

Schroeder, J., & O'Neal, C. (2015). Practically saline. *Journal of Investigative Medicine High Impact Case Reports*, 1–4. https://doi.org/10.1177/2324709615618980

Seropian, M., Brown, K., Gavilanes, J., & Driggers, B. (2004). An approach to simulation development. *Journal of Nursing Education*, *43*(4), 170–174. https://doi.org/10.3928/01484834-20040401-02

Smiley, R. A. (2019). Survey of simulation use in prelicensure nursing programs: Changes and advancements, 2010–2017. *Journal of Nursing Regulation*, *9*(4), 48–61. https://doi.org/10.1016/S2155-8256(19)30016-X

Stone, J., Bonamico, R., Erturk, E., & Ghazi, A. (2017). Improved surgical outcomes after preoperative rehearsal using 3D printed patient specific simulation for percutaneous nephrolithotomy (PCNL). *The Journal of Urology*, *197*(4S), e807. https://doi.org/10.1016/j.juro.2017.02.1880

Torrie, J., Cumin, D., Sheridan, J., & Merry, A. (2016). Fake and expired medications in simulation-based education: An underappreciated risk to patient safety. *BMJ Quality and Safety*, *25*, 917–920. https://doi.org/10.1136/bmjqs.2015.004793

Ziv, A., Erez, D., Munz, Y., Vardi, A., Barsuk, D., Levine, I., & Berkenstadt, H. (2006). The Israel center for medical simulation: A paradigm for cultural change in medical education. *Academic Medicine*, *81*(12), 1091–1097. https://doi.org/10.1097/01.ACM.0000246756.55626.1b

CHAPTER 9

Professional Development for Simulation Education

Penni I. Watts, Beth Fentress Hallmark, and Sabrina Beroz

ABSTRACT

Professional development in simulation methodologies is essential for implementation of quality, consistent, simulation-based experiences. Evidence demonstrates that participation in comprehensive training positively impacts learner outcomes. There are many benefits to professional development, however, challenges exist requiring thoughtful planning, administrative buy in, and fiscal support. While there are no established guidelines, the literature provides an ongoing consensus related to overall concepts and strategies for training in simulation. We describe a continuum of growth for simulationists, ranging from novice/advanced beginner, competent/proficient, to expert. As a novice, one must conduct a self-assessment of current strengths and create a development plan to advance simulation skills and knowledge. A simulationist should use evidenced-base guidelines, mentorship, and feedback to inform simulation practices. They should be knowledgeable of the standards of best practice, modalities, simulation design, learning theories, and professional integrity. Simulationists must seek ongoing advancement through certification, scholarship, and lifelong learning. This chapter describes the continuum of education and methodologies for the development of simulationists.

http://dx.doi.org/10.1891/0739-6686.39.201

INTRODUCTION

"Traditionally the theory relevant to nursing has been taught in the classroom, in contrast with clinical skills and professional behaviors acquired largely in clinical settings" (Topping et al., 2015, p. 1108). However, research has shown that clinical education is insufficient to meet student learning outcomes and transition to practice (Institute of Medicine, 2011; McNelis et al., 2014). In 2014, a pivotal, longitudinal, multisite study published by The National Council of State Boards of Nursing (NCSBN) demonstrated the effectiveness of replacing up to 50% of "traditional" clinical with simulation (Hayden et al., 2014). During the development of the landmark NCSBN study, the researchers recognized the importance of faculty training and a faculty evaluation plan to "ensure consistent adherence to the standards" (Thomas & Kellegren, 2017, p. 227). The NCSBN subsequently published a set of guidelines (Alexander et al., 2015) for state boards of nursing (BON) to evaluate the readiness of prelicensure programs when using simulation for these substitutions. Notably the guidelines included recommendations for faculty preparation, program preparation, and a set of model rules for nursing programs. However, BON across the United States differ in their educational and preparation requirements for simulationists (Bradley et al., 2019; Rutherford-Hemming et al., 2016). While the guidelines have been provided to the boards by the NCSBN, not all states have adopted these recommendations. Most commonly there is a broad statement about the need for faculty to be "trained in simulation," highlighting the need for more clear direction from the simulation community (Bradley et al., 2019; International Nursing Association for Clinical Simulation and Learning [INACSL] Simulation Regulations Committee, 2020, August; National Council State Boards of Nursing, 2020, August).

In a review of state BON recommendations, Bradley et al. (2019) noted that some "common language was used across the BON, including the need for documented and focused training, maintaining competencies in simulation and debriefing, and participating in ongoing professional development" (p. 23). Simulation training was initially offered by vendors and was often related to the equipment and associated technology (Bogossian et al., 2018; Taibi & Kardong-Edgren, 2014). While this training is imperative, it did not address the pedagogical information that is crucial to the development of simulation professional development (Kardong-Edgren et al., 2012; Waznonis, 2015).

It is essential that those involved in simulation practice gain a foundation in simulation methodologies (Hallmark, 2015; Young et al., 2016). Training may vary for those conducting simulation, however, there are basic evidence-based components necessary to ensure quality simulation experiences (Topping et al.,

2015). While a standard for best practice in faculty development is not yet published, this chapter will outline an overall premise of general literature support for components vital to this process. This chapter will also examine the benefits, challenges, and processes for engaging in professional development. In addition, the essential content and available resources to support the simulationist will be reviewed. Within this chapter the term "simulationist," "faculty," and "educator" will be used interchangeably to reflect the varying titles ascribed to those working in simulation (Downing et al., 2020).

PROFESSIONAL INTEGRITY

One of the primary responsibilities of the simulationist is to practice with professional integrity. According to the INACSL Standard of Best Practice: Simulation^{SM}, the simulationist demonstrates professional integrity and is responsible for learner-centered experiences (INACSL Standards Committee, 2016a, 2018b). This means that ethical behavior and conduct—doing what is right regardless of who is watching—is expected at all times, even when countervailing pressures exist (INACSL Standards Committee, 2016a, 2018b). The Society for Simulation in Healthcare (SSH), in concert with an international working group, developed the Healthcare Simulationist Code of Ethics (Park et al., 2018). This code aims to promote, strengthen, and support an ethical culture among all individuals and organizations engaged in healthcare simulation. The values described in the document include integrity, transparency, mutual respect, professionalism, accountability, and results orientation. The simulationist should demonstrate a compassion for teaching, flexibility, and a professional attitude by combining theory and practice when implementing simulation-based education (Jeffries, 2016).

BENEFITS AND CHALLENGES OF PROFESSIONAL DEVELOPMENT

Professional development is salient to a successful simulation program (Paige et al., 2020; Peterson et al., 2017; Watts et al., 2020). The evidence clearly supports the need for training in simulation methodologies (Nguyen et al., 2011; Rizzolo et al., 2015) to ensure quality, consistent, and impactful experiences for learners. While there are benefits, there are also challenges to integration of simulation due to inadequate faculty development, business plans, or administrative support (Alexander et al., 2015; Page et al., 2020).

Benefits

Following the NCSBN simulation study, schools of nursing recognized the benefits of simulation as a teaching–learning strategy and began substituting simulation for clinical hours (Breymier et al., 2015). However, this often lacked the requisite training, including essential knowledge of the pedagogy necessary to provide consistent standardized simulation learning experiences (Paige et al., 2020; Peterson et al., 2017). The INACSL Standard of Best Practice: Simulation^{SM}: Facilitation requires the facilitator to have the requisite skills and knowledge to effectively conduct simulation as the facilitator has full oversight of the entire simulation experience (INACSL Standards Committee, 2016b). Consequences of not following the standard include poor learner engagement and impaired learning (INACSL Standards Committee, 2016b). Data support the benefits of ongoing development of simulation facilitators that improves educational outcomes for learners (Beroz et al., 2020; Nguyen et al., 2011; Rizzolo et al., 2015). Further benefits of high-quality simulation delivered by knowledgeable facilitators include a safe learning environment that is experiential, collaborative, learner-centered, and interactive (Cheng et al., 2016; Jeffries, 2016). In a statewide survey of simulation practices, benefits of professional development include well-delivered simulation experiences that foster improved critical thinking/clinical judgment, confidence, transition to practice, and consistent experiences (Beroz, 2017; Peterson et al., 2017).

Challenges

Unfortunately, challenges impact the development and limit the effectiveness of simulation as a teaching–learning strategy. Prominent challenges include lack of time and limited resources (Nehring et al., 2013; Thomas & Kellegren, 2017). Nehring et al. (2013) found that costly and time intensive high-fidelity simulation programs impacted efficacy of the program and faculty participation. A survey of healthcare simulation training needs across five large western states identified priority needs for education in debriefing, scenario writing, and curricular integration (Taibi & Kardong-Edgren, 2014). In a mid-Atlantic statewide survey, the top three challenges to simulation-based education were adequate faculty development, space, and equipment (Beroz, 2017).

Workload for those in simulation education varies among institutions. Depending on the setting and workload structure, faculty in academia may have additional workload requirements (i.e., course assignments) that limit available time for simulation teaching. Those facilitating simulations may be a current clinical educator or clinician who receives additional simulation teaching assignments (Blodgett et al., 2018; Diekmann et al., 2018).

Many high-volume simulation programs may have limited staff and educators available for professional development or to orient new simulationists, leaving novice simulationists in situations without adequate training and learners at risk for poor outcomes. Additionally, as nursing programs increase enrollment, the demand for simulation often outweighs the capacity of the program and the number of faculty with simulation expertise (Hallmark, 2015). Faculty workload is further impacted as simulation is integrated into curricula to augment clinical experiences (Blodgett et al., 2018). In a review of the literature, six determinants created a model for simulation faculty workload, including the key factor of faculty preparation for simulation (Blodgett et al., 2018).

Educators who work in simulation fulfill many roles such as administrators, faculty, clinicians, staff, simulation operations, and technical support (Diekmann et al., 2018; Foisy-Doll & Leighton, 2018). At many institutions one person may fulfill all roles, in turn placing a burden on the educator to seek professional development. "Although simulation facilitators may be experts in their fields, they revert to the novice stage as they begin to implement new teaching methods, such as high-fidelity simulation" (Thomas & Kellegren, 2017, pp. 227–228).

While no one organization has outlined specific standards detailing content and delivery, there are several models that can guide professional development. Thomas and Kellegren (2017) and Waxman and Telles (2009) cite Benner's Novice to Expert Theory as a guide for examining faculty development. Beroz et al. (2020) cite multiple theoretical frameworks as guiding principles in the development of faculty development programs. Each of these demonstrates the continuum that exists in the ongoing development of a simulationist. There continues to be robust discussion about the validity of mentoring, online training, number of courses, evaluation, and essential content (Foisy-Doll, & Leighton, 2018; Peterson et al., 2017; Steinert et al., 2016). "The development of formal, validated, and evidence-based curricula for educator training are essential steps to learn [the] use of simulation-based education" (Paige et al., 2020, p. 2).

EVIDENCE-BASED PROCESS FOR PROFESSIONAL DEVELOPMENT

Needs Assessment

Performing a self-assessment of current knowledge and understanding may pinpoint the strengths and gaps that need to be addressed by the simulationist. Several resources have emerged that help facilitate the examination of a simulationist readiness for practice. One such tool is the Facilitator Competency Rubric (FCR; Leighton et al., 2018). The FCR provides a 29-item instrument across five major constructs—preparation, prebriefing, facilitation, debriefing, and evaluation—as measured on a 3-point scale (Leighton et al., 2018). The FCR was developed using the INACSL Standards of Best Practice: Simulation and Benner's Novice to Expert model. Content validity was established, and the content validity index ranged from .75 to 1.0. Interrater reliability ranged from .62 to .90. "The FCR is a valid, reliable tool that can be used for formative or summative evaluation of simulation facilitators. Scores can guide and prioritize faculty development" (Leighton et al., 2018, p. 3.).

Benner published the seminal work *From Novice to Expert* (Benner, 1982) that provided the first structure for nurses' skill acquisition. Benner's model is an adaptation of the Dreyfus and Dreyfus (1980) competency model. The acquisition of knowledge and skills related to simulation pedagogy can be mirrored to Benner's stages: novice, advanced beginner, competent, proficient, and expert. The INACSL Standards help the learner identify areas of needed expertise (Gore & Singh, 2019). The novice simulationist must first begin to have a basic understanding of theoretical underpinnings and simulation modalities, moving through the stages to include expertise in skills such as debriefing, simulation design, learner evaluation, facilitation, ethics, professional values, and educational principles.

Next, the simulation educator should create a development plan based on the FCR self-assessment. The simulationist should perform ongoing assessments to evaluate goal attainment and identify areas for further growth. Figure 9.1 shows a suggested path for gaining knowledge using Benner's Novice to Expert model.

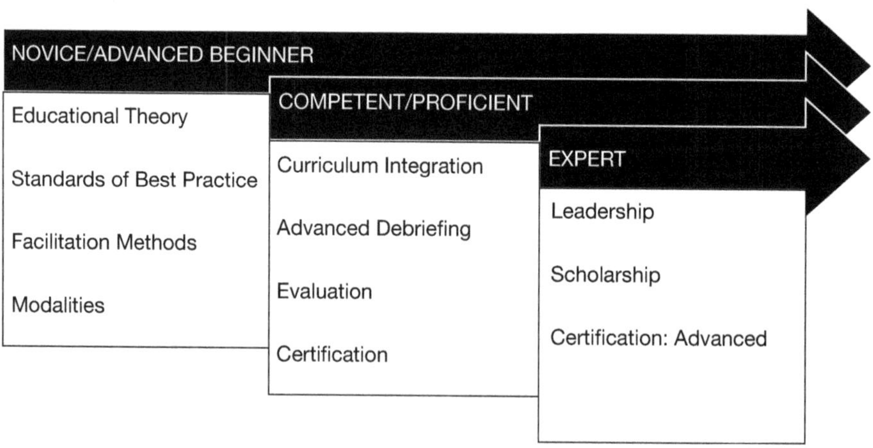

FIGURE 9.1 Suggested path for gaining knowledge.
Source: Adapted from Maryland Clinical Simulation Resource Consortium Curriculum Model for Simulation Education Leaders (Beroz et al., 2020)

Novice/Advanced Beginner

As part of the development plan, there are basic key concepts necessary for becoming a simulationist. At the novice level, educational pedagogy and theories form the foundation for simulation (Thomas & Kellegren, 2017; Waxman, 2009). Bloom's taxonomy and the knowledge and application of learning objectives is key to developing and implementing simulation.

Supporting Theoretical Frameworks

Simulation education is supported by several theories. The two learning theories key to simulation are constructivism and experiential learning. Learning is a process of constructing meaning to make sense of an experience (constructivism), and the knowledge gained from one experience becomes the tool for action in new situations (experiential learning; Bruner, 1961; Dewey, 1938). However, learning resides with the learner and is facilitated by the educator. This is critical to simulation-based education. Kolb (1984) created the learning cycle whereby knowledge is gained through the transformation of experience beginning with a concrete experience (simulation) followed by reflective observation and abstract conceptualization (debriefing) and ending with active experimentation.

Other theories relevant to simulation-based education and important to the development of simulationists include reflective practice and use of adult learning principles. Constructivism and experiential learning support reflective practice in the debriefing process when uncovering taken-for-granted assumptions that drive decision-making (Argyris & Schon, 1997; Dreifuerst, 2015). Training and assessment of debriefing competence are requisite knowledge on debriefing as covered in Chapter 6. Adult learning principles provide educators the tools for understanding how age, maturity, and life experience influence adult learning (Knowles, 1984). "Our field now recognizes the specialized skill set needed among health professional educators in general and simulation educators in particular" (Eppich & Saltzman, 2020, p. 156). All the aforementioned theories work in concert to provide a theoretical framework underpinning the National League for Nursing (NLN) Jeffries Simulation Theory.

The midrange NLN Jeffries Simulation Theory (2016), is essential for professional development. It describes concepts that frame simulation-based education at all levels of nursing preparation. The concepts are context, background, simulation design, simulation experience, the facilitator, the participant, and outcomes. Context surrounds the entire theory guiding the overall purpose of the simulation including the level of evaluation. Background provides context for curriculum alignment and simulation design. The design of the simulation includes outcomes and objectives leveled to the knowledge of the participant including fidelity to support realism. The scenario progression defines expected performance and strategies inherent to prebriefing and debriefing. The simulation experience is characterized as learner-focused, collaborative, experiential, and interactive occurring within an environment of trust. Facilitator and educational strategies describe a dynamic interaction between the facilitator and the participant. It is critical for the facilitator to be knowledgeable in simulation pedagogy and prepared for the experience. The participant brings life experiences and attributes such as age, gender, and self-confidence—all impacting the facilitator–participant relationship. Lastly, outcomes of simulation-based experiences include the participant, patient, and the healthcare system.

Standards of Best Practice for Simulationists

Standards are evidenced-based guidelines for educators, clinicians, and researchers to design, conduct, and evaluate simulation experiences and programs (INACSL Standards Committee, 2016a,2018b; The INACSL Standards Committee, 2017). Standards are foundational and essential to professional development and offer a road map to simulation educators. Outlined below are three sets of standards from simulation-based organizations that support best practices.

The INACSL Standards of Best Practice outline core standards related to key components of simulation, with two standards under development. These standards outline essential elements and criteria for implementing high-quality simulation and can be used conjunctively to learn and develop experiences. Currently there are nine standards that guide practice in simulation and include the following: simulation design, debriefing, participant evaluation, facilitation, professional integrity, outcomes and objectives, operations, sim-enhanced interprofessional education, and the glossary. Simulation educators should immerse themselves in the standards and consider ways to operationalize them. Several sentinel articles laid the groundwork for simulation and are listed in the reference and bibliography associated with each standard. All standards are framed within a common template for consistency and contain criteria and elements for successful implementation. The novice simulationist should seek other references and resources to support development in these areas.

The Association of Standardized Patient Educators (ASPE) focuses on standardized patient (SP) methodology and established standards of best practice intended to be used in conjunction with the INACSL Standards of Best Practice: Simulation (Lewis et al., 2017). The ASPE standards are organized into five domains—safe work environment, case development, SP training, program management, and professional development—informed by five underlying values—safety, quality, professionalism, accountability, and collaboration (Lewis et al., 2017). Table 9.1 shows the alignment across the standards of INACSL and ASPE.

TABLE 9.1
Alignment of ASPE Standards and INACSL Standard of Best Practice: Simulation

ASPE Standard	INACSL Standard of Best Practice
Domain 1: Safe Work Environment	INACSL Standard of Best Practice: Simulation Professional Integrity
Domain 2: Case Development	INACSL Standard of Best Practice: Simulation Design
Domain 3: SP Training	INACSL Standard of Best Practice: Simulation Facilitation and INACSL Standard of Best Practice: Simulation Participant Evaluation
Domain 4: Program Management	INACSL Standard of Best Practice: Simulation Operations
Domain 5: Professional Development	INACSL Standard of Best Practice: Simulation Facilitation and INACSL Standard of Best Practice: Simulation Debriefing

ASPE, Association of Standardized Patient Educators; INACSL, International Nursing Association for Clinical Simulation and Learning.

Another example are the standards of best practice outlined by the Association for Simulated Practice in Healthcare (ASPiH; Purva & Nicklin, 2018). Partnering with Health Education England (HEE), ASPiH designed the Simulation-Based Education in Healthcare: Standards Framework and Guidance (Purva & Nicklin, 2018) as a national set of criteria that combines best practice and evidence related to simulation-based education. Their framework consists of two parts: standards and supporting guidance. ASPiH uses four main themes to organize their standards and includes "faculty, technical personnel, activity, and resources." Their goal was to develop a framework that could be applied in many areas of simulation education and practice ensuring quality and effective simulation delivery.

Simulation Terms

Establishing a common language among simulation practice is essential for a growing simulation science and simulationists must become familiar with the terminology (Haji et al., 2014). In concert with the Agency for Healthcare Research and Quality (AHRQ), SSH published the second edition of the *Simulation Dictionary* (Downing et al., 2020). INACSL has also published a glossary that includes terms that reflect and support the language of the standards of best practice (INACSL Standards Committee, 2016c). While the glossary is intended for the INACSL Standards, efforts are being made to ensure it aligns with the SSH dictionary.

Modalities

Simulation modalities and realism are important to consider when designing a simulation (Lioce et al., 2015). During the design of the simulation, the learning objectives should be examined to ensure that the simulation modality complements the design (INACSL Standards Committee, 2016a). The SSH accreditation requires that applicants demonstrate that they have chosen the appropriate modality. For instance, "a mannequin that does not feature chest tube insertion would not be appropriate when the learning objective includes the procedural skill of chest tube insertion" (Committee for Accreditation of Healthcare Simulation, 2016, p. 5).

Having a working knowledge of simulation modalities is critical to the development of a successful simulation. There are several types of simulation modalities as designed by the *SSH Healthcare Simulation Dictionary* (Downing et al., 2020; Lioce et al., 2015) that should be considered—virtual/augmented reality, screen-based, manikin task trainers, and SPs. Virtual reality is the use of computer technology to create an interactive three-dimensional world with an ocular mask to create spatial presence. Augmented reality is a technology using overlays of digital computer-generated information on real-world objects for the purpose of enhancing the user experience. Screen-based simulation is confined to a computer giving metrics for actions selected when the learner manipulates actions of an avatar. Manikins—high, medium, and low fidelity—represent a human patient with varied capabilities controlled by a simulationist using computers and software. Task trainers offer models representing a part or region of the human body generally used to support procedural skills training. Hybrid modality uses two or more modalities of simulation with the aim of providing a more realistic experience, such as adding a task trainer to a SP experience. Lastly, a SP is a person who portrays a patient, family member, or healthcare provider in order to meet the objectives of the simulation. While there are a variety of simulation modalities, the simulationist must be prepared to carefully select the appropriate modality considering level of the learner, objectives of the simulation, and resources available.

Competent/Proficient

The simulationist that has moved past the advanced beginner stage, then moves along the continuum toward the competent/proficient level with a working knowledge of theories, standards, and modalities. This simulationist generally has approximately 2 years of simulation experience with a recognized need for advancing their knowledge in curricular integration, advanced debriefing, and evaluation (Beroz et al., 2020).

Curricular Integration

Curricular integration is important as the simulationist, in concert with course faculty, must determine where simulation fits best for optimal learner outcomes (Beroz et al., 2020). The simulation objectives should be aligned with course and program outcomes. Use of curricular mapping across the curriculum is helpful to determine appropriate insertion of simulation experiences (Beroz et al., 2020). At this level, simulationists should be familiar with curriculum needs and how to integrate appropriately into the nursing program. Ensuring appropriate scenario design and learning objectives for the level of learners is important when leveling the simulation experience (INACSL Standards Committee, 2016a). Consideration of the complexity of the simulation and the learner's cognitive load are important for the proficient simulationist when designing experiences (Reedy, 2015).

Advanced Debriefing

As a competent/proficient simulationist, debriefing implementation should include beginning application of advanced strategies and management of difficult debriefings (Cheng et al., 2015). According to the INACSL debriefing standard, the simulationist should be able to discern appropriate debriefing techniques effective for a variety of learners ensuring the highest level of learner impact is considered (INACSL Standards Committee, 2016c). Fey et al. (2020) describe the debriefer trajectory as discovery, growth, and maturity. In the growth phase, debriefers move to a "routine" and draw on previous experiences when conducting a debriefing session. Complex or difficult debriefings are managed based upon previous patterns, and ongoing feedback and reflection. (Cheng et al., 2016). See Chapter 6 for more information on debriefing practices.

Evaluation

Evaluation of learners and simulation experiences should occur at all levels. However, at the level of competent/proficient, the simulationist leads the evaluation efforts and mentors others in the simulation program. Each construct of the NLN Jeffries Simulation Theory (Jeffries, 2016) can be aligned with the INACSL Standards of Best Practice: Simulation (INACSL Standards Committee, 2016c) using valid and reliable instruments to measure the construct. The design of the simulation can be evaluated using the Simulation Design Scale or the Simulation Effectiveness Tool-Modified (Leighton et al., 2015; NLN, 2004).

The INACSL Standard of Best Practice: Simulation: Participant Evaluation states that all simulation experiences require evaluation of the participant (INACSL Standards Committee, 2016c). Simulationists formally trained in the evaluation process are imperative to learner success. Potential consequences of not following the participant evaluation standard include inaccurate assessment and poor learning outcomes. There are three levels of participant evaluation: formative, summative, and high stakes. Identifying the level of evaluation is important when designing simulation experiences. Formative evaluation provides feedback toward the achievement of objectives or outcomes. Summative evaluation measures outcomes at a discrete point in time and high stakes refers to an evaluation carrying major implications if unsuccessful. Common instruments to measure participant performance include the Creighton Competency Evaluation Instrument, the Lasater Clinical Judgment Rubric, and the Seattle University Simulation Evaluation Tool (Hayden et al., 2014; Lasater, 2007; Mikasa et al., 2013). It is critical for simulationists to identify desired performance for each simulation scenario and to orient facilitators to the behaviors for consistency across each experience (Gore, & Singh, 2019).

Certification

As simulationists progress along the continuum of development, validating one's basic skills and knowledge in simulation methodologies is demonstrated through certification and program accreditation. The interprofessional organization, SSH, offers both certifications and accreditation in simulation. For a simulationist to be recognized as a Certified Healthcare Simulation Educator (CHSE), applicants must demonstrate expertise in the foundational components outlined as basic domains, including professional values and capabilities, healthcare and simulation knowledge/principles, educational principles applied to simulation, and simulation resources and environments (Society for Simulation in Health, 2018). SSH accreditation is a peer-reviewed program that examines a simulation program's processes and outcomes in assessment, research, teaching/education, and systems integration (SSH, 2020). Specific to both the core standards and standards in teaching/education are details related to "qualified educators." These standards include items such as ensuring annual educator evaluation, professional development, and formal orientation. Accreditation demonstrates that programs meet or exceed these standards, but the term "qualified" is not fully delineated regarding professional development education, except to say that an educational event must be "specific to simulation." This broad definition underscores the need for the simulation community to determine *essential knowledge* for simulation educators.

Expert

An expert simulationist demonstrates expertise in simulation knowledge and provides service, leadership, and scholarship that advances the science of simulation. Novice and competent learners look to experts for guidance and mentorship.

Leadership and Scholarship

Leading the development of education programs and dissemination of scholarly work requires the simulation expert to have a presence at the regional, national, and/or international levels through collaboration, research, and service. Service in professional organizations offers the expert avenues to garner leadership skills through roles such as committee membership, chair positions, or board appointments. The advanced simulationist publishes manuscripts in peer-reviewed journals and engages in endeavors such as peer reviews of abstracts, publications, or grant reviews (SSH, 2020). Conference presentations and webinars disseminate knowledge to all level of simulationists and increase the presence and impact of simulation experts (Cheng, et al. 2015; Thomas & Kellegren, 2017). Lastly, the expert provides foresight into simulation operations, accreditation, and strategic planning. As a leader, the simulationist will coach and mentor others through feedback, observation, ongoing education, and support as needed (Cheng, 2015).

Advanced Certification

The SSH offers an advanced healthcare simulation certification (CHSE-A) for those "who have proven themselves to be advanced educators in their practice in healthcare simulation and serve as mentors and examples to others in the field" (SSH, 2020, p. 1). The biannual application cycle requires that the applicant: (a) has a current CHSE certification, (b) uses healthcare simulation in an educational role, (c) has an earned master's degree or equivalent, (d) demonstrates 5 years of continued simulation education, research, or administration, and (e) demonstrates focused simulation educator expertise in healthcare simulation activities and settings. This distinguished pinnacle of simulation recognizes fewer than 60 individuals worldwide.

ADDITIONAL RESOURCES

There are several organizations that provide professional development surrounding simulation pedagogy. The SSH and the INACSL each host an annual conference filled with robust content (INACSL, 2020; SSH, 2020). Both organizations have mentoring programs, webinars, society journals, and many other training opportunities. The NLN's Center for Innovation in Education Excellence houses the Institute for Simulation and Technology. The Center sponsors webinars, publishes content related to simulation faculty development, releases frequent *Technology Edge Quarterly* (TEQ) blog posts, and provides online training modules for faculty development through the Simulation Innovation and Resource Center (SIRC). In addition, the NLN Leadership Institute for Simulation Educators provides a yearlong program for "participants [to] examine issues related to research in simulation, curricular integration, the role of simulation in interprofessional education, and managing and directing simulation activities within a school of nursing or a service setting" (NLN, 2016). The ASPE has responded to the increased use of SPs in nursing programs and the demand to gain and maintain knowledge of SP methodologies. ASPE hosts an annual conference and webinars to share knowledge aimed at sharing and maintaining best practices for the SP community (ASPE, 2020).

Educational Programs

Ongoing professional development and engaging in lifelong learning is imperative for simulationists (Britton, 2017; Cheng, 2015; Paige et al., 2020). There are many opportunities for continuing and advancing skills in simulation while being immersed in the simulation community. Formal programs have emerged to support those who strive for continual improvement as a simulation educator. Certificate and advanced degree programs now exist to facilitate those wanting a formal degree in simulation (Rho et al., 2016). Fellowship programs are common in many healthcare programs (Ng & Rupple, 2016). SSH and INACSL offer yearlong fellowships or mentoring programs providing a structured approach for professional development. Networking, developing professional relationships, and collaborating with simulationist around the globe enhances one's perspective and broadens understanding of simulation in a variety of arenas. Of note, there are several online learning programs available to those in simulation that tend to be self-paced through learning management system modules (Gantt et al., 2019; Gore & Singh, 2019; Taibi & Kardong-Edgren, 2013). These offer foundational information and, with online availability, can be accessed at any time.

Mentorship has been noted in the literature as an important aspect of professional development, and it is important for the advanced simulationist to consider mentoring the developing simulationist (Peterson et al., 2017). For those seeking mentorship, find a mentor who can be a guide and is willing to provide constructive feedback (Peterson et al., 2017). While receiving feedback in various situations is helpful, a mentor can provide long-term guidance, moral support, and ongoing feedback.

Statewide Consortiums/Alliances

Statewide consortiums and alliances are where educators in academia and practice organize to deliver education, share resources, and/or provide consultation services to stakeholders. Born out of an interest to advance the science of simulation, the main focus of these initiatives is to deliver educational programs or conferences to enhance development of faculty. The Maryland Clinical Simulation Resource Consortium (MCSRC) was created to increase the quality and quantity of simulation across all prelicensure nursing programs and clinical partners throughout the state of Maryland. A statewide curriculum model provided faculty development of simulation educators, and outcomes resulted in the education of hundreds of Maryland faculty who improved simulation practices (Beroz et al., 2020). The Tennessee Simulation Alliance (TNSA) was launched to provide Tennessee nurse educators a central location for communication, collaboration, and sharing of professional development opportunities. Since 2007, the TNSA has hosted 12 annual conferences and provided continuing education in simulation pedagogy. The alliance is funded solely through conference fees and vendor support. The California Simulation Alliance was initially established as the Bay Area Simulation Collaborative (BASC) in 2007. BASC was formed to train and educate nursing faculty and hospital educators on the pedagogy of simulation-based education (Waxman et al., 2011). The collaborative developed a research and evaluation plan that demonstrated the effectiveness of simulation in enhancing the critical thinking skills of nursing students. BASC used Benner's Novice to Expert framework to create a faculty development program for schools of nursing and hospitals (Waxman & Telles, 2009). The funding was leveraged to create regional collaboratives and the California Simulation Alliance (CSA; Waxman, 2016).

CONCLUSION

Professional development is an essential aspect in simulation education. While it comes with challenges, there are enormous benefits for the simulationist, the learner, and organization. Professional development can be compared to Benner's Novice to Expert continuum. While a needs assessment provides a general gauge of current knowledge and skills of the simulationist, the development of an educational pathway moves the learner through basic key components of educating with simulation and beyond. There are foundational concepts and content for a novice, including standards of best practice, ethics, modalities, and simulation design. The key to success is being learner-centered and maintaining an environment of trust throughout the simulation program. Many national and international resources are currently available to the simulationist, such as professional organizations, formal trainings, simulation journals, and conferences. While it is imperative that there is ongoing evaluation and feedback, self-reflection is an integral aspect of professional growth at any level of expertise. As the simulation community works toward a consensus of training and development for simulation education, a continued quest for professional growth, best practice, and evidence will further advance the science and practice of simulation.

REFERENCES

Alexander, M., Durham, C. F., Hooper, J. I., Jeffries, P. R., Goldman, N., Kardong-Edgren, S., & Tillman, C. (2015). NCSBN simulation guidelines for prelicensure nursing programs. *Journal of Nursing Regulation*, *6*(3), 39–42. https://doi.org/10.1016/S2155-8256(15)30783-3

Argyris, C., & Schon, D. (1997). Organizational learning: A theory of action perspective. (77/78), 345–348. https://doi.org/10.2307/40183951

Association of Standardized Patient Educators. (2020). *Resources*. https://www.aspeducators.org/resources

Benner, P. (1982). From novice to expert. *American Journal of Nursing*, *83*(2), 402–407. http://www.jstor.org/stable/3462928

Beroz, S. (2017). A statewide survey of simulation practices using NCSBN simulation guidelines. *Clinical Simulation in Nursing*, *13*(6), 270–277. https://doi.org/10.1016/j.ecns.2017.03.005

Beroz, S., Schneidereith, T., Fraina, C., Daniles, A., Dawson, L., Watties-Daniels, D., & Sullivan, N. (2020). A statewide curriculum model for teaching simulation education leaders. *Nurse Educator*, *45*(1), 56–60. https://doi.org/10.1097/NNE.0000000000000661

Blodgett, N. P., Blodgett, T., & Kardong-Edgren, S. E. (2018). A proposed model for simulation faculty workload determination. *Clinical Simulation in Nursing*, *18*, 20–27. https://doi.org/10.1016/j.ecns.2018.01.003

Bogossian, F., Cooper, S., Kelly, M., Levett-Jones, T., McKenna, L., Slark, J., & Seaton, P. (2018). Best practice in clinical simulation education – are we there yet? A cross-sectional survey of simulation in Australian and New Zealand pre-registration nursing education. *Collegian*, *25*(3), 327–334. https://doi.org/10.1016/j.colegn.2017.09.003

Bradley, C. S., Johnson, B. K., Dreifuerst, K. T., White, P., Conde, S. K., Meakim, C. H., & Childress, R. M. (2019). Regulation of simulation use in United States prelicensure nursing programs. *Clinical Simulation in Nursing*, *33*, 17–25. https://doi.org/10.1016/j.ecns.2019.04.004

Breymier, T. L., Rutherford-Hemming, T., Horsley, T. L., Atz, T., Smith, L. G., Badowski, D., & Connor, K. (2015). Substitution of clinical experience with simulation in prelicensure nursing programs: A national survey in the United States. *Clinical Simulation in Nursing*, *11*(11), 472–478. https://doi.org/10.1016/j.ecns.2015.09.004

Britton, K. L. (2017). *Descriptive comparative study of nursing faculty self-efficacy in the simulation setting (Order No. 10256657)*. Doctoral dissertation, Capella University, ProQuest Dissertations & Theses Global.

Bruner, J. (1961). The act of discovery. *Harvard Educational Review*, *31*, 21–32.

Cheng, A., Grant, V., Dieckmann, P., Arora, S., Robinson, T., & Eppich, W. (2015). Faculty development for simulation programs: Five issues for the future of debriefing training. Simulation in Healthcare, 10(4), 217-222. https://doi: 10.1097/SIH.0000000000000090

Cheng, A., Morse, K., Rudolph, J., Arab, A., Runacles, J., & Eppich, W. (2016). Learner centered debriefing for health care simulation education: Lessons for faculty development. *Society for Simulation in Healthcare: The Journal of the Society for Simulation in Healthcare*, *11*(1), 32–40. https;//doi.org.10.1097/SIH.0000000000000136

Code of Ethics Work Group. (2018). *Healthcare simulationist code of ethics*. https://www.ssih.org/SSH-Resources/Code-of-Ethics

Committee for Accreditation of Healthcare Simulation. (2016). *Teaching/Education accreditation standards*. https://www.ssih.org/Portals/48/Accreditation/CompanionDocuments/Teaching-EducationCompanionDocument.pdf?ver=2016-10-12-160154-983

Dewey, J. (1938). *Experience and education*. MacMillan.

Diekmann, P., Rasmussen, M.B., Issenberg, B., Soreide, E., Oseergaard, E., & Ringsted, C. (2018). Long-term experiences of being simulation educator: A multinational interview study. *Medical Teacher*, *40*(7), 713–720. https://doi.org.10.1080/0142159X.20181471204

Downing, D., Chang, T. P., Robertson, J. M., Anderson, M., & Diaz, D. A. (2020). In L. Lioce (Ed.), *Healthcare simulation dictionary –Second Edition* (2nd ed.). Agency for Healthcare Research and Quality. https://doi.org/10.23970/simulationv2

Dreifuerst, K. T. (2015). Getting started with debriefing for meaningful learning. Clinical Simulation in Nursing, 11(5), 268-275. http://dx.doi.org/10.1016/j.ecns.2015.01.005

Dreyfus, H., & Dreyfus, S. (1980). *A Five-Stage model of the mental activities involved in direct skill acquisition*. Unpublished report supported by the the Air Force of Scientific Research (AFSC), ASAF (Contract F49620-79-C-0063), University of California at Berkeley.

Eppich, W., & Saltzman, M. (2020). Faculty development for mastery learning. In W. D. McGaghie & J. Barsuk (Eds.), *Comprehensive healthcare simulation: Mastery learning in health professions education. Comprehensive healthcare simulation*. Springer Publishing. https://doi.org/10.1007/978-3-030-34811-3_9

Fey, M. K., Auerbach, M., & Szyld, D. (2020). Implementing faculty development programs: Moving from theory to practice. *Simulation in Healthcare*, *15*(1), 5–6. https://doi.org/10.1097/SIH.0000000000000429

Foisy-Doll, C., & Leighton, K. L. (2018). *Simulation champions: Fostering courage, caring and connection* (1st ed.). Wolters Kluwer: Philadelphia.

Gantt, L. T., Robey, W. C., Langston, T., & Bliley, L. (2019). Simulation faculty and staff development: An interprofessional, online approach. *Journal of Interprofessional Education & Practice*, *19*, 1–3. https://doi.org/10.1016/j.xjep.2019.100310

Gore, T., & Singh, O. (2019). Development of a foundations of simulation teaching course for nurse educators. *Nursing Education Perspectives*, *40*, 179–180. https://doi.org/10.1097/01.NEP.0000000000000347

Haji, D., A, F., Hoppe, D. J., Morin, M., Giannoulakis, K., Koh, J., Rojas, D., & Cheung, J. H. (2014). What we call what we do affects how we do it: A new nomenclature for simulation research in medical education. *Advances in Health Sciences Education*, *19*, 273–280. https://doi.org/10.1007/s10459-013-9452-x

Hallmark, B. F. (2015). Faculty development in simulation education. *Nursing Clinics of North America*, *50*(2), 389–397. https://doi.org/10.1016/j.cnur.2015.03.002

Hayden, J. K., Smiley, R. A., Alexander, M., Kardong-Edgren, S., & Jeffries, P. R. (2014). The NCSBN national simulation study: A longitudinal, randomized, controlled study replacing clinical hours with simulation in prelicensure nursing education. *Journal of Regulation Nursing*, *5*(2). https://doi.org/10.1016/S2155-8256(15)300062-4

INACSL Standards Committee. (2016a). INACSL standards of best practice: Simulation^SM: Simulation design. *Clinical Simulation in Nursing*, *12*, S5–S12. https://doi.org/10.1016/j.ecns.2016.09.005INACSL

INACSL Standards Committee. (2016b). INACSL standards of best practice: Simulation^SM: Facilitation. *Clinical Simulation in Nursing*, *12*, S16–S20. https://doi.org/10.1016/j.ecns.2016.09.007

INACSL Standards Committee. (2016c). INACSL standards of best practice: Simulation^SM. *Clinical Simulation in Nursing*, *12*, S5–S47. https://doi.org/10.1016/j.ecns.2016.09.007

INACSL Standards Committee. (2017, December). INASCL standards of best practice: Simulation^SM: Operations. *Clinical Simulation in Nursing*, *13*, 681–687. https://doi.org/10/1016/j.ecns.2017.10.005

INACSL Simulation Regulations Committee. (2020, August). *INACSL regulation map*. https://www.inacsl.org/simulation-regulations/

Institute of Medicine (US) Committee on the Robert Wood Johnson Foundation Initiative on the Future of Nursing, at the Institute of Medicine. (2011). *The future of nursing: Leading change, advancing health*. National Academies Press (US). https://doi.org/10.17226/12956

International Nursing Association for Clinical Simulation and Learning. (2020). *Resources*. https://www.inacsl.org/resources/for-educators/

Jeffries, P. R. (2016). *The NLN Jeffries simulation theory*. Wolters Kluwer.

Kardong, Edgren, S., Wilhaus, J., Bennett. D., & Hayden, J. (2012). Results of the National Council of Stare Boards of Nursing national simulation study survey: Part II. Clinical Simulation in Nursing, 8(4), e117–e123. https://doi.org/10.1016/j.ecns.2012.01.003

Knowles, M. S. (1984). *The adult learner: A neglected species*. Houston.

Kolb, D. (1984). Experiential learning: Experience as the source of learning and development. *Journal of Business Ethics*, Prentice-Hall 1.

Lasater, K. (2007). Clinical judgment development: Using simulation to create an assessment rubric. *Journal of Nursing Education*, *46*(11), 496–503.

Leighton, K., Mudra, V., & Gilbert, G. E. (2018). Development and psychometric evaluation of facilitator competency rubric. *Nursing Education Perspectives*, *39*(6), 3–9. https://doi.org/10.1097/01.NEP.0000000000000409

Leighton, K., Ravert, P., Mudra, V., & Macintosh, C. (2015). Updating the simulation effectiveness tool: Item modifications and reevaluation of psychometric properties. *Nursing Education Perspectives*, *36*(5), 317–323. https://doi.org/10.5480/15-1671

Lewis, K. L., Bohnert, C. A., Gammon, W. L., Holzer, H., Lyman, L., Smith, C., Thompson, T.M., Wallace, A., & Gliva-McConvey, G. (2017). The association of standardized patient educators (ASPE) standards of best practice (SOBP). *Advances in Simulation*, 2(1). https://doi.org/10.1186/s41077-017-0043-4

Lioce, L., Meakim, C. H., Fey, M. K., Chmil, J. V., Mariani, B., & Alinier, G. (2015). Standards of best practice: Simulation standard IX: Simulation design. *Clinical Simulation in Nursing*, *11*(6), 309–315. https://doi.org/10.1016/j.ecns.2015.03.005

McNelis, A. M., Ironside, P. M., Ebright, P. R., Dreifuerst, K. T., Zvonar, S. E., & Conner, S. C. (2014). Learning nursing practice: A multisite, multimethod investigation of clinical education. *Journal of Nursing Regulation*, *4*(4), 30–35. https://doi.org/10.1016/S2155-8256(15)30115-0

Mikasa, A. W., Cicero, T. F., & Adamson, K. A. (2013). Outcome-based evaluation tool to evaluate student performance in high-fidelity simulation. *Clinical Simulation in Nursing*, *9*(9), e361–e367. https://doi.org/10.1016/j.ecns.2012.06.001

National League for Nursing. (2004). *Educational Practices Questionnaire*, 1–2. http://www.nln.org/professional-development-programs/research/tools-and-instruments/descriptions-of-available instruments

National Council State Boards of Nursing. (2020). Leading regulatory excellence. https://www.ncsbn.org/index.htm

Nehring, W., Wexler, T., Hughes, F., & Greenwell, A. (2013). Faculty development for the use of high-fidelity patient simulation: A systematic review. *International Journal of Health Sciences Education*, *1*(1), 1–34.

Ng, G. M., & Rupple, H. (2016). Nursing simulation fellowships: An innovative approach for developing simulation leaders. *Clinical Simulation in Nursing*, *12*(2), 62–68. https://doi.org/10.1016/j.ecns.2015.11.005

Nguyen, D. N., Zierler, B., & Nguyen, H. Q. (2011). A survey of nursing faculty needs for training in use of new technologies for education and practice. *Journal of Nursing Education*, *50*(4), 181–189. https://doi.org/10.3928/01484834-20101130-06

Paige, J. B., Graham, L., & Sittner, B. (2020). Formal training efforts to develop simulation educators. *Simulation in Healthcare: The Journal of the Society for Simulation in Healthcare*, *15*(4), 271–281. https://doi.org/10.1097/sih.0000000000000424

Park, C. S., Murphy, T. F., & the Code of Ethics Working Group. (2018). Healthcare. Simulationist code of ethics. https://www.ssih.org/SSH-Resources/Code-of-Ethics

Peterson, D. T., Watts, P. I., Epps, C. A., & White, M. L. (2017). Simulation faculty development: A tiered approach. *Simulation in Healthcare*, *12*(4), 254–259. https://doi.org/10.1097/SIH.0000000000000225

Purva, M., & Nicklin, J. (2018). ASPiH standards for simulation-based education: Process of consultation, design and implementation. *BMJ Simulation and Technology Enhanced Learning*, *4*(3), 117 LP–125. https://doi.org/10.1136/bmjstel-2017-000232

Reedy, G. B. (2015). Using cognitive load theory to inform simulation design and practice. *Clinical Simulation in Nursing*, *11*(8), 355–360. https://doi.org/10.1016/j.ecns.2015.05.004

Rizzolo, M. A., Kardong-Edgren, S., Oermann, M. H., & Jeffries, P. R. (2015). The national league for nursing project to explore the use of simulation for high-stakes assessment: Process, outcomes, and recommendations. *Nursing Education Perspectives*, *36*, 299+. https://link.gale.com/apps/doc/A429736140/AONE?u=tel_a_belmont&sid=AONE&xid=e8bd91cd

Rho, S. Y., Kim, M. K., & Tandkawanich, T. (2016). Survey of outcomes in a faculty development program on simulation pedagogy. *Nursing and Health Science*, *18*, 210–215. https://doi.org/10.1111.nhs/12254

Rutherford-Hemming, T., Lioce, L., Kardong-Edgren, S., Jeffries, P. R., & Sittner, B. (2016). After the national council of state boards of nursing simulation study-Recommendations and next steps. *Clinical Simulation in Nursing*, *12*(1), 2–7. https://doi.org/10.1016/j.ecns.2015.10.010

Society for Simulation in Health. (2018). *Certified healthcare simulation educator examination blueprint, 2018 version examination blueprint*. https://www.ssih.org/Portals/48/Certification/CHSE_Docs/CHSE_Examination_Blueprint.pdf

Society for Simulation in Healthcare (2016). SSH Accreditation of Healthcare Simulation Programs. https://www.ssih.org/Credentialing/Accreditation

Steinert, Y., Mann, K., Anderson, B., Barnett, B. M., Ceneno, A., Naismith, L., Prideaux, D., Spencer, J., Tullo, E., Viggiano, T., Ward, H., & Dolmans, D. (2016). A systematic review of faculty development initiatives designed to enhance teaching effectiveness: A 10-year update: BEME Guide No. 40. *Medical Teacher*, *38*(8), 769–786. https://doi.org/10.1080/0142159X.2016.1181851

Taibi, D. M., & Kardong-Edgren, S. (2013). Health career educator training in simulation: A survey and web site development. *Clinical Simulation in Nursing*, *10*(1), e47–e52. https://doi.org/10.1016/j.ecns.2013.05.013

Thomas, C. M., & Kellegren, M. (2017). Benner's novice to expert model-an application for simulation facilitators. *Nursing Science Quarterly*, *30*(3), 227–234. https://doi.org/10.1177/0894318417708410

Topping, A., Bøje, R. B., Rekola, L., Hartvigsen, T., Prescott, S., Bland, A., & Hannula, L. (2015). Towards identifying nurse educator competencies required for simulation-based learning: A systemised rapid review and synthesis. *Nurse Education Today*, *35*(11), 1108–1113. https://doi.org/10.1016/j.nedt.2015.06.003

Waznonis, A. (2015). Simulation debriefing practices in traditional baccalaureate nursing programs: National survey results. Clinical Simulation in Nursing, 11(2), 110-119. https://doi.org/10.1016/j.ecns.2014.10.002

Watts, P., Peterson, T., Brown, M., White, T., Epps, C., & White, M. (2020). Faculty reflections on effective strategies utilized to implement simulation-enhanced IPE for future health care providers. Clinical Simulation in Nursing, 44, 22-29. https://doi.org/10.1016/j.ecns.2020.03.005

Waxman, K. (2016). Sustaining a statewide simulation alliance. *Clinical Simulation in Nursing*, *12*(10), 448–452. https://doi.org/10.1016/j.ecns.2016.07.001

Waxman, K. T., Nichols, A. A., O'Leary-Kelley, C., & Miller, M. (2011). The evolution of a statewide network: the bay area simulation collaborative. *Simulation in Healthcare Journal of the Society for Simulation in Healthcare*, 6(6), 345. https://doi.org/10.1097/SIH.0b013e31822eaccc

Waxman, K. T., & Telles, C. L. (2009). The use of Benner's framework in high-fidelity simulation faculty development: The bay area simulation collaborative model. *Clinical Simulation in Nursing*, 5(6), e231–e235. https://doi.org/10.1016/j.ecns.2009.06.001

Young, S. R., Kim, M. K., & Tangkawanich, T. (2016). Survey of outcome sin a faculty development program on simulation pedagogy. *Nursing and Health Sciences*, *18*(1), 210–215. https://doi.org/10.111.nhs.12254

Part IV

Technologies in Simulation

CHAPTER 10

Virtual and Augmented Realities in Nursing Education: State of the Science

Michelle Aebersold and Dawne-Marie Dunbar

ABSTRACT

The use of simulation in nursing education is an integrated part of the curriculum and has demonstrated the benefit for learning in nursing students at all levels. The next stage in simulation-based learning will utilize the wide variety of new technologies that are currently available, including virtual and augmented reality. The use of these new technologies brings with it a need for standard definitions, evaluation of its impact on learning, and new opportunities for research. Efforts are underway to standardized definitions and publish early findings on research using these new technologies. There are many opportunities available for nursing educators to create a new era of simulation-based learning methodologies by incorporating virtual and augmented realities in their curriculum. The state of the science is showing promising outcomes and commercial products are maturing.

The utilization of these new technologies should be approached in the same way as other learning methodologies as many new ideas and ways of learning are emerging in this area. It will be critical for nursing educators and faculty to determine the optimal ways to utilize them.

http://dx.doi.org/10.1891/0739-6686.39.225

The contemporary period of manikin-based simulation began in the early 1990s (Aebersold, 2016). This is when the ability for nursing schools to purchase higher fidelity manikins increased due to affordability and relative ease of use. Early publications in nursing focused on how to use this type of simulation in nursing education (Haskvitz & Koop, 2004; Hyland & Hawkins, 2009; Rauen, 2001; Scherer et al., 2003). Currently, manikin-based simulation is well-integrated into most, if not all, prelicensure nursing education programs. During the 2000s, work in virtual reality (VR) began. VR is defined as a technology-based representation of a real-world environment. Early articles in nursing focused on the use of computer-based VR environments or worlds such as Second Life (Linden Labs), which is an open-access virtual environment (Aebersold et al., 2012; Caylor et al., 2015; Hansen, 2008; Irwin & Coutts, 2015; Schmidt & Stewart, 2010; Tiffany & Hoglund, 2014). Other articles focused on the creation and use of VR environments or worlds that were built by the users or colleges/universities (Beedasy & Ramloll, 2010; Nelson et al., 2005). Often these purpose-built environments never moved beyond their original home. It was also during this time that exploration and small pilot studies were conducted in health science education using early virtual and augmented reality (AR) devices (Chaballout et al., 2016; Goodwin et al., 2014). In the 1990s, some companies began moving this work into entertainment and healthcare and eventually into education. However, the full range of VR and AR technology did not really take off until there were affordable, commercially available devices (Robinson & Delenko, n.d.) Now, through use of extended reality (XR), there is a growing interest in a new set of technologies to increase the diversity of learning methods in both prelicensure and graduate nursing programs ("Augmented reality" 2019; Maddox, 2018; Patel, 2019). Briefly, XR (explained in detail later) is an overarching term to encompass several types of technology. This technology provides more opportunities for practice as well as multidisciplinary and interprofessional learning that spans geographical boundaries. This chapter will focus on the state of the science in XR, challenges that currently exist, and practical information to enhance and grow simulation programs.

OVERVIEW OF VIRTUAL REALITIES

Definitions/Taxonomy

Currently, there is no single, consistently used definition of VR or AR across nursing or health science education. The *Healthcare Simulation Dictionary*, first published in 2016, was an early attempt to create a common taxonomy in healthcare simulation (Lopreiato, 2016). The second edition of the dictionary (Lioce et al., 2020) included terms such as virtual reality (VR), virtual reality simulation (VRS), augmented reality (AR), and mixed reality (MR). However, the term XR is only present within the MR definition. Many XR educators, authors, and researchers tend to define the terms they are using (Cant, et al., 2019); however, identifying common elements across these definitions is recommended to create a consistent taxonomy needed to move the science forward. The term XR, or extended reality, is becoming widely used as an umbrella term to group the various forms of alternate realities, such as VR, AR, MR, and others. **VR** is often described as a technologically generated representation of a three-dimensional (3D) environment. There are four important elements, including virtual world (context, rules), immersion (sense of being present), sensory feedback (visual, haptic feedback), and interactivity (responsiveness to user input; Makhkamova et al., 2020). Other terms found in the literature include virtual environment (Kardong-Edgren et al., 2019; Lopreiato, 2016), VRSs (Kardong-Edgren et al., 2019; Lopreiato, 2016), immersive virtual reality (Bailenson, 2018; Bailenson et al., 2008), and computer-generated virtual reality (Kardong-Edgren et al., 2019; Kilmon et al., 2010). **AR** has a more stable definition. AR projects digitally created content into the user's environment (Azuma, 1997; Lopreiato, 2016). **MR** blends the user's world with digital content in such a way that the environments can interact with each other (Nebeling et al., 2020). The extended reality safety initiative (XRSI) has provided a definition of XR, which could become a key term moving forward:

> **XR** is a fusion of all the realities—including AR, VR, and MR—which consists of technology-mediated experiences enabled via a wide spectrum of hardware and software, including sensory interfaces, applications, and infrastructures. XR is often referred to as immersive video content, enhanced media experiences, as well as interactive and multidimensional human experiences. (Lioce et al., 2020, p. 20)

The various features and hardware of several different types of XR technologies including VR, AR, and MR are included in Table 10.1 and provide the reader with a current review of the hardware used in XR today. This is an everchanging area and new products will continue to be developed.

CURRENT USES OF XR TECHNOLOGIES IN NURSING

VRS and computer-based simulation are often used interchangeably. The features of this type of simulation involve the use of computer-generated simulations that mimic real-life situations. The interactions usually involve a keyboard and a mouse to interact with the various components in the simulation.

TABLE 10.1

Features of Extended Reality

Category	Description	Hardware
Virtual reality systems	Fully immersed in environment, 360-degree view, uses hand controllers to fully interact with virtual world, can pick up and interact with objects, move in all directions, can hear, talk, both single and multiplayer. Can track actions in the environment including hand movements, object selection, and eye tracking. Can provide robust learning analytics.	Oculus Rift and Rift-S Oculus Quest (https://www.oculus.com/) HTC Cosmos and Pro series (https://www.vive.com/us/product/) PlayStation VR (https://www.playstation.com/en-us/explore/playstation-vr/) These systems require varying degrees of computing power, and head-mounted displays may be tethered to the computer or be wireless.
Augmented reality/mixed reality	Overlays digital computer-generated information and/or images onto objects or into the real world to augment one's perception of the real world. The technology involves the use of a head-mounted display through which the user sees the digital images. The user communicates with the device and the objects through hand gestures, handheld devices, voice commands, and/or head movement. Interactions with the system can be tracked as well as eye-tracking mechanisms.	Microsoft HoloLens 2 (https://www.microsoft.com/en-us/hololens) Magic Leap 1 (https://www.magicleap.com/en-us)
Augmented reality	Uses mobile devices such as smartphones and tablets (IOS/Android) to project a digital object/image into the real world. The object is manipulated through controls on the mobile app. Field of view is limited to the forward-facing lens of the phone's camera.	

VRS, as defined in the SSH Healthcare Dictionary:

> Simulations that use a variety of immersive, highly visual, 3D characteristics to replicate real-life situations and/or healthcare procedures; virtual reality simulation is distinguished from computer-based simulation in that it generally incorporates physical or other interfaces such as a computer keyboard, a mouse, speech and voice recognition, motion sensors, or haptic devices. (ASSH; Lioce et al., 2020, p. 54)

According to an article in *HealthTech*, 65% of nursing schools use some type of virtual simulation and other adaptive digital learning methods (Lea, 2020). An article published in *Clinical Simulation in Nursing* demonstrated that students who used VRS to learn how to place a urinary catheter spent more time on practice and demonstrated competency at the same rate as those who practiced in the lab (Butt et al., 2018). Another study using a tablet-based program to teach nurses how to insert a nasogastric tube demonstrated that those trained using the anatomy-augmented program demonstrated higher competency that those trained using traditional methods. When surveyed, 86% of the students in the study rated the program as "superior" or "far superior" to other training methods (Aebersold et al., 2018).

The following examples of VRS are currently commercially available:

- **Sentinel U.** This product includes a variety of community settings in which nursing students can engage in activities such as a community windshield survey, home assessment, delegation, and patient priority decisions. (https://www.sentinelu.com/)
- **vSim** (Laerdal and Wolters Kluwer). These are a variety of nursing simulations with medical-surgical, pediatrics, maternity, fundamentals, health assessment, geriatrics, mental health, and pharmacology content. Students practice assessment, prioritization, and patient care delivery when working through the scenarios. (http://nursingeducation.lww.com/our-solutions/clinical-simulation/vsim-for-nursing.html)
- **Shadow Health.** These contain modules in health assessment (basic and advanced), pharmacology, leadership, mental health, and gerontology and allow students to practice communication skills with patients who have a variety of backgrounds. (https://www.shadowhealth.com/)

Other VRS programs use video clips to create branching case stories in which nursing students progress through scenarios by viewing clips and then selecting best options (Verkuyl et al., 2019). This type of simulation was developed using a gaming methodology and supports decision-making skills.

Immersive virtual reality, sometimes referred to as IVR or just VR, refers to immersive virtual reality programs that make use of head-mounted displays to create an entirely virtual environment in which the learner is immersed (Bailenson et al., 2008).

Currently available commercial applications for IVR/VR include:

- **Acadicus** (Arch Virtual). A completely immersive program that has a variety of simulation content available and also allows the user to create some of their own content. The simulations can be single or multiplayer. (https://acadicus.com/)
- **SimX**. This provides immersive virtual simulations that work with currently available VR systems such as HTC Vive or Oculus Quest. (https://www.simxar.com/)
- **Oxford Medical Simulation.** These are immersive scenarios for nursing that are either single or multiplayer. (http://oxfordmedicalsimulation.com/)

WHERE TO BEGIN

Reasons to consider implementation of a VRS platform are varied and can be unique to the educational setting. A review of the literature reveals that VRS provides an immersive experience that improves student-learning outcomes and enhances skill performance (Aebersold et al., 2020; Foronda et al., 2020). VRS can offer the opportunity for interaction between multiple disciplines depending on the platform design and can be cost-effective over time (Farra et al., 2019) when compared to repeated live simulation exercises over a 3-year period. Common barriers to experiential learning can be addressed through VRS, including limited time, large numbers of learners, faculty resistance, and difficulty covering the entire curriculum (Verkuyl et al., 2016; Wurdinger & Allison, 2017).

Evidence-based/peer-reviewed VRS scenarios are commercially available and can bridge the gaps between theory and practice. Simulation allows for the practice of complex procedures, clinical decision-making, and patient safety (Berndt, 2014; Shearer, 2013). The ability to repeat a scenario and providing unbiased learner feedback is achievable using VR platforms. VRS could prove to be a valuable tool for distance learning when clinical placements are limited or nonexistent. Many state nursing boards allowed VRS to replace traditional clinical hours during the recent COVID-19 pandemic, thus allowing nursing students to continue to progress and in some cases to graduate on time. The economic and professional impact of VRS has yet to reach its full potential.

Several factors should be considered when vetting the feasibility of investing in and implementing VRS platforms. The International Nursing Association for Clinical Simulation and Learning (INACSL), Standards of Best

Practice^{SM}: Simulation Glossary points to the importance of recognizing key aspects of VRS (INACSL Standards Committee, 2016). Those include the skill level(s) of the targeted learners (including the level and comfort of technology utilization) and a review of learning objectives to provide a baseline for comparing VR products and their ease of curricular integration (INACSL Standards Committee, 2016). Identification of knowledge and skill development goals provides guidance for the VR features of each platform. For example, if the development of psychomotor skills required to perform advanced or basic lifesaving skills is the goal, then a VR product that provides for haptic feedback would be important. Alternatively, if more cognitive-based simulations that focus on clinical judgment or interprofessional team communication is a desired goal, then haptic feedback features are not necessary. VR platform-available content should be reviewed for each vendor. Researching available VRS cases is important and Table 10.2 provides a list of questions that can aid vendor selection.

Institutional information technology (IT) input is crucial during the vetting process. A thorough understanding of institutional IT policies, cybersecurity including Federal Student Records Privacy Act (FERPA) compliance, firewall, and current hardware capabilities are needed when comparing system requirements and performance of each VR platform that will impact the end-user experience. The additional purchase or upgrade of hardware may influence overall cost-to-benefit ratios. Defining pricing structures including pay per case/session, per-student subscription, or institutional license options is necessary for budgetary planning and sustainability. Other fiscal factors include the cost to administer each VR platform, including faculty/staff time and the need to create new physical spaces (VR Lab) to house and secure hardware.

Creating Inclusive Buy-In

VRS platforms are an engaging educational tool for teaching high-level skills in a low-stakes environment, but many faculty have limited if any experience with VR technology resulting in a resistance to consider integration into existing curricula (Foronda & Bauman, 2014). Creating inclusive buy-in from all stakeholders can be the most important factor to successful implementation and return on investment (ROI; Al-Ghareeb & Cooper, 2016; Harder et al., 2013; Hollema, 2015). Researching and trying all available products is an essential first step. Initial impressions are important for faculty and learners, so the speed with which the participant becomes immersed in the VRS and the comfort of wearing any equipment (headset, controller) can ultimately contribute to supporting VRS. Look for platforms that provide content/cases that already align with existing course outcomes, program objectives, competencies, or projects in development. Demonstrating how a VRS program can immediately impact learners

TABLE 10.2
Questions to Ask Vendors

Question	Rationale
What is the level of difficulty of the cases and can they be modified or adjusted?	This helps faculty decide if the cases are at the appropriate level and how easy it is to level up or level down the scenarios.
Can the faculty develop new cases and how is that accomplished?	This helps the faculty determine if new cases can be added and how difficult that might be.
Are cases peer reviewed? How often are they reviewed and updated to reflect changes in practice?	This is important to ensure the accuracy of the scenarios and to make sure they do not become unusable because of practice changes.
What are the delivery options for the cases? Can they be run on a regular computer used by most students? Do they require special equipment like an Oculus or HTC head-mounted display?	This will determine what equipment is needed and how much flexibility you have for the learners.
What learning analytics are available and how easy are they to access?	This will allow faculty to evaluate how well students are performing.
What safeguards are in place to ensure security and fidelity of the product to avoid improper use by students and/or faculty?	This will allow faculty to determine how prevalent misuse like cheating is occurring.

using the current curriculum will set the stage for acceptance and justification for funding.

Once one or two VRS platforms have been identified, designing a pilot study and collecting stakeholder feedback should be completed (INACSL Standards Committee, 2016). Faculty, learners, IT/simulation staff, and administrators should be invited to participate in a guided VRS demonstration. Vendors can provide initial training and suggest the best cases and strategies to support individualized demonstrations for a variety of stakeholders. Provide stakeholders with a targeted literature review of VRS to include effects on learning outcomes, ROI, and cost ratio compared to other forms of simulation and effects on resource management (staff time, space, scheduling conflicts). Collection of data during the survey should include (a) participant feedback regarding the physical comfort of using VR (headset or screen-based), (b) the ease of navigating virtual patient encounters (virtual room, equipment, environment), and (c) how partnering with the VR technology is envisioned for current and/or future learners (Jensen & Konradsen, 2017). Individual surveys and small focus groups are possible options for data collection.

Once a VR platform is selected, identifying start-up and long-term funding is necessary. Start-up needs may include the purchase of hardware (computers, headsets, controllers), creation or refurbishing of a dedicated physical space (VRS lab), and supplies to clean and care for the equipment (headphone covers, disinfectant wipes; Dyer et al., 2018; Occulus Rift VR, LLC., 2016; Ydo, 2020). Many VR platforms may require a service/payment contract, so allowing time for the proper institutional review, negotiation, and approvals is also a consideration. Long-term funding is required to support the agreed-upon pricing structure (pay-per-use, student subscription, or institutional license) and sources can include yearly operating budgets; capital improvement budgets; cost sharing between academic programs, institutional research, and development funds; donations; and grants. A favorable ROI with a VRS program is rooted in a multi-year plan.

Comparison to Other Learning Methods

Reviews of the literature support the use of traditional manikin-based simulation for the development and retention of students' critical thinking, nursing knowledge, clinical skill performance, and self-confidence (Aebersold et al., 2018; Cant & Cooper, 2017; Foronda et al., 2020). Limited work on VRS's impact on learning as compared to other instructional methods is currently available. Although several articles describe the intervention of VRS as having improved student-learning outcomes, more evidence-based research is needed to firmly establish VRS as a proven method of teaching, and VRS standards of best practices need to be developed (Foronda et al., 2020). An advantage of VRS is the ability to immerse students in realistic environments that can be challenging to replicate in the traditional simulation and laboratory settings (Berg & Steinsbekk, 2020; Farra et al., 2015) and allowing for greater diversity in learning. Foronda et al. (2020) noted that VRS resulted in achievement of learning outcomes when compared to similar manikin-based simulation and improved psychomotor skill after a VRS intervention. Students performed clinical skills more quickly after participating in VRS when compared to other traditional methods like skills lab sessions (Farra et al., 2015; Leflore et al., 2012). In a 2016 study of nursing students' phlebotomy skills following VRS or traditional simulation, no significant difference between methods was shown (William et al., 2016). Several studies have been published examining student's perceptions of VRS's impact on learning. A study by Gerdprasert et al. (2011) noted that self-directed study using VRS was perceived by students to be more beneficial than reading from textbooks. Overall, the literature reflects mixed and sometimes conflicting findings (Berg & Steinsbekk, 2020; Smith et al., 2018; Foronda et al., 2020). Two studies examined retention of knowledge and skills over time and showed no significant differences between VR and other traditional learning methods (Fernández Alemán et al., 2011; Liaw et al., 2014). Variances in duration, level of learner, and even the discrepancies in the definition of VRS throughout the literature indicates the need for more evaluation of objective data using quantitative methods (Foronda et al., 2020).

IMPLEMENTATION CASE STUDY

One VR company contracted with a mid-sized private university in the northeast United States to provide VRS for two prelicensure nursing cohorts, including a 4-year traditional and an 18-month accelerated bachelor degree program. The nursing programs identified critical thinking, clinical decision-making, and patient safety as the foci of VRS. The university chose a VRS platform that uses a headset and handheld controller that could also be used remotely by the learner on a personal computer. A pilot study with individually guided 30-minute sessions was completed with faculty, simulation center professional staff, IT staff, students, and administration. Data regarding ease of use, level of engagement, and headset comfort were collected and evaluated and used to direct changes to the implementation plan. Funding was secured through a cost-sharing agreement between the simulation center, nursing program, dean's office, and internal university research development funds. A small work group formed by the simulation center director and nursing faculty reviewed the nursing curriculum, identified individual course outcomes, reviewed the VRS case scenarios, and aligned both high-fidelity and new VRS sessions to course outcomes. The simulation center director and professional staff were responsible for VRS platform maintenance, policy and procedure creation, faculty training, and student orientation sessions. The course faculty were responsible for syllabi inclusion and student learning evaluation criteria. Implementation was specific to each nursing course and students completed VRS sessions individually or in small groups, both remotely (via home computer) and in the newly created VR lab (via immersive headsets). Debriefing was conducted in person by faculty or through the student's written reflections. Institutional review board approval was secured to study student perceptions of the impact on learning.

Lessons learned and student evaluations guided revision of the implementation plan for the following semester. Flexibility was key as several time management issues became apparent. A staggered introduction to VRS for each individual cohort, not all students at once, proved to be less stressful for faculty and staff. Planning open VR lab times that did not interfere with scheduled didactic classes and allowing for flexible online scheduling were changes introduced the following semester. The simulation center's schedule was expanded to provide additional time to showcase the VRS technology to prospective students, faculty in other health professions programs, the board of trustees, and community partners. Students reported that VRS positively impacted their perceived learning and noted that the ability to repeat scenarios was helpful when applying new knowledge. The ability for students to complete VRS remotely became especially impactful with the sudden closure of the university campus and transition to online learning due to the COVID-19 pandemic.

EVIDENCE

As XR technologies are adopted for use in nursing education, research on these educational methodologies is important. The use of appropriate pedagogical frameworks should be used to guide the implementation of XR-based educational strategies (Pomerantz, 2019). Many of the frameworks currently used in manikin-based simulation education are very relevant to this work. Kolb's (2014) experiential learning cycle can serve as a sound framework in using XR-based simulations in education as well as Ericsson's (2008) Deliberate Practice framework. Both of these identify the importance of practice, feedback, and repeating what is gained (Aebersold, 2018). It is important to develop a method for debriefing in XR, particularly when the learners are not on site. Verkuyl et al. (2020) evaluated different types of debriefing in VR, including self-debriefing and group debriefing. Self-debriefing can be completed using a written format guided by questions from the faculty. This can be followed at a later time by a facilitated group debrief where learners can share their reflections. Self-debriefing can be useful in many situations including VRS and team-based learning (Oikawa et al., 2016; Verkuyl et al., 2018).

In addition to frameworks that guide the implementation of XR technologies, it is also important to use sound pedagogical theories to develop XR simulations. To support this process, it is beneficial to look at the literature for development techniques used for serious games, educational games, computer-based or immersive games. There are foundational guides in this area including work by Clark Aldrich (2009). This can be combined with health science educational pedagogies such as Miller's (1990) pyramid, Knowles's adult learning theory (Clapper, 2010), and social constructivism (McLeod, 2019), to name just a few.

Most importantly, when developing XR simulations, make sure to use a theory-guided approach for development, implementation, debriefing, and evaluation. This will ensure an optimal experience for all learners. As with all new technologies, it is also important to ask the learners to give feedback on the technology itself to help guide future work to improve and match technologies with the right simulation scenarios.

State of the Science in XR

Studies have been done in nursing, healthcare, and other industries that can be used to guide faculty and educators interested in utilizing XR technologies. Although there have been advances in the technologies themselves, much of what was learned still applies. In the *Journal of Medical Internet Research*, a systematic review and meta-analysis was published on VR in health professions education (Kyaw et al., 2019). The meta-analysis of eight articles found that VR slightly improves the postintervention knowledge score compared to traditional learning, and a meta-analysis of four studies found improvement in cognitive scores. Although many of the studies included nonimmersive VR, this is still a strong trend in nursing education. Another systematic review analyzed the impact of VR on nontechnical skills. The studies reviewed included those that used screen-based VR simulators and virtual worlds. Overall findings showed that VR was an acceptable method for nontechnical skills training and most of the studies were scenario-centered (Bracq et al., 2019). In the area of AR, a scoping review was published to determine the current research on AR in nursing (Wüller et al., 2019). Many of the studies reviewed used tablet-based AR or smart glasses. Findings indicated that the current focus has been on evaluating the technology in pilot studies and future studies should look at longer term evaluations (Wüller et al., 2019).

Nursing and healthcare education are just beginning to look at best options for using these new technologies. It will be helpful to look at other areas such as aviation, military, engineering, and marketing to identify relevant cases. Some of the pioneering work in immersive VR comes from communications, care of patients with post-traumatic stress disorders, and pain management (Bailenson, 2018; Marcus, n.d.).

CONCLUSIONS

XR technologies have emerged into nursing, medicine, and other health professions' education. The recent pandemic has highlighted the increased need for virtual options. The research is beginning to demonstrate the ability of XR to provide quality education and training and has some advantages that can be leveraged (Aebersold et al., 2020; Bailenson et al., 2008). Although XR will not replace the need for in-person and manikin-based simulation, in the next 3 to 5 years, the authors believe that it will become an integral part of that education (Bryant et al., 2020). Now is the time for nursing faculty, educators, and leaders to be part of the design and use of these incredibly versatile tools.

Why Every Nursing Curriculum Should be Using XR

Nurse educators engaged in curriculum design and implementation are increasingly challenged to consider a greater diversity of learning technologies that support experiential learning (Berg & Steinsbekk, 2020; Pomerantz, 2019). These technologies should be engaging and immerse learners in opportunities that support the practice of higher level clinical decision-making and psychomotor skill competency. VRS is experiential in nature and provides a pedagogical bridge between didactic learning and clinical practice, which is the embodiment of the immersion level of learning (Charles et al., 2010). This chapter provides the background, current uses, and compelling evidence of the effectiveness VRS has on education as a strategic technology to facilitate meaningful learning for both prelicensure and graduate nursing programs. VRS is offered in varied platforms that range from screen-based branching logic cases that can be facilitated on student's personal devices to VR and AR products that require special hardware like headsets and controllers. The beauty of VRS technology is the potential for flexible applications that are scalable and can be adopted with a wide range of resources.

REFERENCES

Aebersold, M. (2016). The history of simulation and its impact on the future. *AACN Advanced Critical Care*, 27(1), 56–61. http://dx.doi.org/10.4037/aacnacc2016436

Aebersold, M. (2018, April 3). Simulation-based learning: No longer a novelty in undergraduate education. *OJIN: The Online Journal of Issues in Nursing*, 23(2). http://dx.doi.org/10.3912/OJIN.Vol23No02PPT39

Aebersold, M., Rasmussen, J., & Mulrenin, T. (2020). Virtual Everest: Immersive virtual reality can improve the simulation experience. *Clinical Simulation in Nursing, 38*, 1–4. https://doi.org/10.1016/j.ecns.2019.09.004

Aebersold, M., Tschannen, D., Stephens, M., Anderson, P., & Lei, X. (2012). Second life®: A new strategy in educating nursing students. *Clinical Simulation in Nursing*, 8(9), e469–e475. http://dx.doi.org/10.1016/j.ecns.2011.05.002

Aebersold, M., Voepel-Lewis, T., Cherara, L., Weber, M., Khouri, C., Levine, R., & Tait, A. R. (2018). Interactive anatomy-augmented virtual simulation training. *Clinical Simulation in Nursing, 15*, 34–41. http://dx.doi.org/10.1016/j.ecns.2017.09.008

Al-Ghareeb, A., & Cooper, S. J. (2016). Barriers and enablers to the use of high-fidelity patient simulation manikins in nurse education: An integrative review. *Nurse Education Today*, 36, 281–286. http://dx.doi.org/10.1016/j.nedt.2015.08.005

Anders Ericsson, K. (2008). Deliberate practice and acquisition of expert performance: A general overview. *Academic Emergency Medicine*, *15*(11), 988–994. https://doi.org/10.1111/j.1553-2712.2008.00227.x

Augmented Reality in Healthcare will be Revolutionary: 9 Examples. (2008, February 18). *The medical futurist*. https://medicalfuturist.com/augmented-reality-in-healthcare-will-be-revolutionary/

Azuma, R. T. (1997). A survey of augmented reality. *Presence*, *6*, 355–385. https://doi.org/10.1162/pres.1997.6.4.355

Aldrich, C. (2009). The complete guide to simulations and serious games: How the most valuable content will be created in the age beyond Gutenberg to Google. *John Wiley & Sons*.

Bailenson, J. (2018). *Experience on demand: What virtual reality is, how it works, and what it can do*. WW Norton & Company.

Bailenson, J. N., Yee, N., Blascovich, J., Beall, A. C., Lundblad, N., & Jin, M. (2008). The use of immersive virtual reality in the learning sciences: Digital transformations of teachers, students, and social context. *The Journal of the Learning Sciences*, *17*(1), 102–141. https://doi.org/10.1080/10508400701793141

Beedasy, J., & Ramloll, R. (2010). Lessons learned from a pandemic influenza triage exercise in a 3D interactive multiuser virtual learning environment—Play2Train. *Journal of Emergency Management*, *8*(4), 53. https://doi.org/10.5055/jem.2010.0026

Berg, H., & Steinsbekk, A. (2020). Is individual practice in an immersive and interactive virtual reality application non-inferior to practicing with traditional equipment in learning systematic clinical observation? A randomized controlled trial. *BMC Medical Education*. 20, 1–10. https://doi.org/10.1186/s12909-020-0n.d.-7

Berndt, J. (2014). Patient safety and simulation in prelicensure nursing education: An integrative review. *Teaching and Learning in Nursing*, *9*, 16–22. https://doi.org/10.1016/j.teln.2013.09.001

Bracq, M. S., Michinov, E., & Jannin, P. (2019). Virtual reality simulation in nontechnical skills training for healthcare professionals: A systematic review. *Simulation in Healthcare: The Journal of the Society for Simulation in Healthcare*, *14*(3), 188–194. http://dx.doi.org/10.1097/SIH.0000000000000347

Bryant, K., Aebersold, M. L., Jeffries, P. R., & Kardong-Edgren, S. (2020). Innovations in simulation: Nursing leaders' exchange of best practices. *Clinical Simulation in Nursing*, *41*, 33–40. https://doi.org/10.1016/j.ecns.2019.09.002

Butt, A. L., Kardong-Edgren, S., & Ellertson, A. (2018). Using game-based virtual reality with haptics for skill acquisition. *Clinical Simulation in Nursing*, *16*, 25–32. http://dx.doi.org/10.1016/j.ecns.2017.09.010

Cant, R. P., & Cooper, S. J. (2017). Use of simulation-based learning in undergraduate nurse education: An umbrella systematic review. *Nurse Education Today*, *49*, 63–71.

Cant, R., Cooper, S., Sussex, R., & Bogossian, F. (2019). What's in a name? Clarifying the nomenclature of virtual simulation. *Clinical Simulation in Nursing*, *27*(2), 26–30. http://dx.doi.org/10.1016/j.ecns.2018.11.003

Caylor, S., Aebersold, M., Lapham, J., & Carlson, E. (2015). The use of virtual simulation and a modified TeamSTEPPS™ training for multiprofessional education. *Clinical Simulation in Nursing*, *11*(3), 163–171. https://doi.org/10.1016/j.ecns.2014.12.003

Chaballout, B., Molloy, M., Vaughn, J., Brisson Iii, R., & Shaw, R. (2016). Feasibility of augmented reality in clinical simulations: Using Google glass with manikins. *JMIR Medical Education*, 2(1), e2. https://doi.org/10.2196/mededu.5159

Charles, G., Bainbridge, L., & Gilbert, J. (2010). The University of British Columbia model of interprofessional education. *Journal of Interprofessional Care*, 24(1), 9–18. http://dx.doi.org/10.3109/13561820903294549

Clapper, T. C. (2010). Beyond Knowles: What those conducting simulation need to know about adult learning theory. *Clinical Simulation in Nursing*, 6(1), e7–e14. https://doi.org/10.1016/j.ecns.2009.07.003

Dyer, E., Swartzlander, B., & Gugliucci, M. R. (2018). Using virtual reality in medical education to teach empathy. *Journal of the Medical Library Association*, *106*(4), 498–500. https://doi.org/10.5195/jmla.2018.518

Farra, S. L., Gneuhs, M., Hodgson, E., Kawosa, B., Miller, E. T., Simon, A., Timm, N., & Hausfeld, J. (2019). Comparative cost of virtual reality training and live exercises for training hospital workers for evacuation. *CIN: Computers, Informatics, Nursing*, *37*(9), 446–454. https://doi.org/10.1097/CIN.0000000000000540

Farra, S. L., Smith, S., Gillespie, G. L., Nicely, S., Ulrich, D. L., Hodgson, E., & French, D. (2015). Decontamination training. *Advanced Emergency Nursing Journal*, *37*(2), 125–133. http://dx.doi.org/10.1097/TME.0000000000000059

Fernández Alemán, J. L., Carrillo de Gea, J. M., & Rodríguez Mondéjar, J. J. (2011). Effects of competitive computer-assisted learning versus conventional teaching methods on the acquisition and retention of knowledge in medical surgical nursing students. *Nurse Education Today*, *31*(8), 866–871. http://dx.doi.org/10.1016/j.nedt.2010.12.026

Foronda, C. L., & Bauman, E. B. (2014). Strategies to incorporate virtual simulation in nurse education. *Clinical Simulation in Nursing*, *10*(1), 412–418. http://dx.doi.org/10.1016/j.ecns.2014.03.005

Foronda, C. L., Fernandez-Burgos, M., Nadeau, C., Kelley, C. N., & Henry, M. N. (2020). Virtual simulation in nursing education: A systematic review spanning 1996 to 2018. *Simulation in Healthcare: The Journal of the Society for Simulation in Healthcare*, *15*(1), 46–54. http://dx.doi.org/10.1097/SIH.0000000000000411

Gerdprasert, S., Pruksacheva, T., Panijpan, B., & Ruenwongsa, P. (2011). An interactive web-based learning unit to facilitate and improve intrapartum nursing care of nursing students. *Nurse Education Today*, *31*(5), 531–535. http://dx.doi.org/10.1016/j.nedt.2010.10.008

Goodwin, J., Elkattah, R. A., & Olsen, M. (2014). Wearable technology in obstetrical emergency simulation: A pilot study. *International Journal of Health Sciences Education*, 2(2), 3.

Haskvitz, L. M., & Koop, E. C. (2004). Students struggling in clinical? A new role for the patient simulator. *Journal of Nursing Education, 43*(4), 181–184.

Hansen, M. (2008). Versatile, immersive, creative and dynamic virtual 3-D healthcare learning environments: A review of the literature. *Journal of Medical Internet Research, 10*(3), e26. https://doi.org/10.2196/jmir.1051

Harder, B. N., Ross, C. J. M., & Paul, P. (2013). Instructor comfort level in high-fidelity simulation. *Nurse Education Today*, *33*, 1242–1245. http://dx.doi.org/10.1016/j.nedt.2012.09.003

Hollema, C. (2015). Faculty development in high fidelity clinical simulation. *International Journal of Nursing Didactics*, *5*(9), 1–5. http://dx.doi.org/10.15520/ijnd.2015.05.09.110.01-05

Hyland, J. R., & Hawkins, M. C. (2009). High-fidelity human simulation in nursing education: A review of literature and guide for implementation. *Teaching and Learning in Nursing, 4*(1), 14–21.

INACSL Standards Committee. (2016, December). INACSL standards of best practice: Simulation[SM] Simulation glossary. *Clinical Simulation in Nursing*, *12*(S), S39–S47. https://doi.org/10.1016/j.ecns.2016.09.012

Irwin, P., & Coutts, R. (2015). A systematic review of the experience of using Second Life in the education of undergraduate nurses. *Journal of Nursing Education*, *54*(10), 572–577. https://doi.org/10.3928/01484834-20150916-05

Jensen, L., & Konradsen, F. (2017). A review of the use of virtual reality head-mounted displays in education and training. *Education and Information Technologies*, 1–15. https://doi.org/10.1007/s10639-017-9676-0

Kardong-Edgren, S. S., Farra, S. L., Alinier, G., & Young, H. M. (2019). A call to unify definitions of virtual reality. *Clinical Simulation in Nursing*, *31*, 28–34. https://doi.org/10.1016/j.ecns.2019.02.006

Kilmon, C. A., Brown, L., Ghosh, S., & Mikitiuk, A. (2010). Immersive virtual reality simulations in nursing education. *Nursing Education Perspectives*, *31*(5), 314–317.

Kolb, D. A. (2014). *Experiential learning: Experience as the source of learning and development*. FT press.

Kyaw, B. M., Saxena, N., Posadzki, P., Vseteckova, J., Nikolaou, C. K., George, P. P., ... & Car, L. T. (2019). Virtual reality for health professions education: systematic review and meta-analysis by the digital health education collaboration. *Journal of medical Internet research, 21*(1), e12959.

Lea, M. (2020). *How virtual training is set to change nursing education*. https://healthtechmagazine.net/article/2020/05/how-virtual-training-set-change-nursing-education

Leflore, J. L., Anderson, M., Zielke, M. A., Nelson, K. A., Thomas, P. E., Hardee, G., & John, L. D. (2012). Can a virtual patient trainer teach student nurses how to save lives—Teaching nursing students about pediatric respiratory diseases. *Simulation in Healthcare: Journal of the Society for Simulation in Healthcare*, *7*(1), 10–17. http://dx.doi.org/10.1097/SIH.0b013e31823652de

Liaw, S. Y., Chan, S. W., Chen, F., Hooi, S. C., & Siau, C. (2014). Comparison of virtual patient simulation with manikin-based simulation for improving clinical performances in assessing and managing clinical deterioration: Randomized controlled trial. *Journal of Medical Internet Research*, *16*(9), e214. http://dx.doi.org/10.2196/jmir.3322

Lioce, L., Lopreiato, J., Downing, D., Chang, T. P., Robertson, J. M., Anderson, M., Diaz, D. A., & Spain, A. E. (2020). *Healthcare simulation dictionary–Second edition*. Agency for Healthcare Research and Quality. https://doi.org/10.23970/simulationv2

Lopreiato, J. O. (2016). *Healthcare simulation dictionary*. Agency for Healthcare Research and Quality.

Maddox, T., & Fitzpatrick, T. (2019). The promise of virtual reality in health-care education and training: It's all in the neuroscience. *Digital Medicine, 5*(4), 133.

Makhkamova, A., Exner, J. P., Greff, T., & Werth, D. (2020). Towards a taxonomy of virtual reality usage in education: A systematic review. In *Augmented reality and virtual reality* (pp. 283–296). Springer Publishing. https://link.springer.com/book/10.1007/978-3-030-37869-1

Marcus, J. (n.d.). *Virtual reality in pediatrics*. https://www.chla.org/virtual-reality-pediatrics

McLeod, S. (2019). Constructivism as a theory for teaching and learning. *Simply Psychology*.Retrieved from https://www.simplypsychology.org/constructivism.html

Miller, G. E. (1990). The assessment of clinical skills/competence/performance. *Academic Medicine*, *65*(9), S63–S67. https://doi.org/10.1097/00001888-199009000-00045

Nebeling, M., Speicher, M., Wang, X., Rajaram, S., Hall, B. D., Xie, Z., & Sun, Y. (2020, April). *MRAT: The mixed reality analytics toolkit*. Proceedings of the 2020 CHI Conference on Human Factors in Computing Systems, Association for Computing Machinery Digital library. pp. 1–12.

Nelson, L., Sadler, L., & Surtees, G. (2005). Bringing problem based learning to life using virtual reality. *Nurse Education in Practice*, *5*(2), 103–108. https://doi.org/10.1016/j.nepr.2004.05.001

Occulus Rift VR, LLC. (2016). *Occulus rift: Overview*. www3.occulus.com/en-us/rift/

Oikawa, S., Berg, B., Turban, J., Vincent, D., Mandai, Y., & Birkmire-Peters, D. (2016). Self-debriefing vs instructor debriefing in a pre-internship simulation curriculum: Night on call. *Hawai'i Journal of Medicine & Public Health*, *75*(5), 127. https://www.ncbi.nlm.nih.gov/pmc/articles/PMC4872264/

Patel, R. (2019, July 16). *A new reality in clinical care: how XR could transform healthcare*. Inside Digital Health. https://www.idigitalhealth.com/news/new-reality-clinical-care-xr-transform-healthcare

Pomerantz, J. (2019, October). *XR for teaching and learning: Year 2 of the EDUCAUSE/HP campus of the future project. ECAR research report*. EDUCAUSE. https://library.educause.edu/-/media/files/library/2019/10/2019hpxr.pdf?la=en&hash=306474918AA2F101DDDCABD59E4366AD7244D572

Rauen, C. A. (2001). Using simulation to teach critical thinking skills: You can't just throw the book at them. *Critical Care Nursing Clinics of North America, 13*(1), 93–103.

Robinson, A., & Delenko, M. (n.d.). *Voices from a virtual past*. https://www.theverge.com/a/virtual-reality

Schmidt, B., & Stewart, S. (2010). Implementing the virtual world of Second Life into community nursing theory and clinical courses. *Nurse Educator*, *35*(2), 74–78. https://doi.org/10.1097/NNE.0b013e3181ced999

Scherer, Y. K., Bruce, S. A., Graves, B. T., & Erdley, W. S. (2003). Acute care nurse practitioner education: Enhancing performance through the use of clinical simulation. *AACN Advanced Critical Care, 14*(3), 331–341.

Shearer, J. E. (2013). High-fidelity simulation and safety: An integrative review. *Journal of Nursing Education*, *52*(1), 39–45. http://dx.doi.org/10.3928/01484834-20121121-01

Smith, S., Farra, S., Ulrich, D., Hodgson, E., Nicely, S., & Mickle, A. (2018). Effectiveness of two varying levels of virtual reality simulation. *Nursing Education Perspectives*, *39*(6), E10–E15. https://doi.org/10.1097/01.NEP.0000000000000369

Tiffany, J., & Hoglund, B. A. (2014). Teaching/learning in second life: Perspectives of future nurse-educators. *Clinical Simulation in Nursing*, *10*(1), e19–e24. http://dx.doi.org/10.1016/j.ecns.2013.06.006

Verkuyl, M., Atack, L., Mastrilli, P., & Romaniuk, D. (2016). Virtual gaming to develop students' pediatric nursing skills: A usability test. *Nurse Education Today*, *46*, 81–85. https://doi.org/10.1016/j.nedt.2016.08.024

Verkuyl, M., Atack, L., McCulloch, T., Liu, L., Betts, L., Lapum, J. L., Hughes, M., Mastrilli, P., & Romaniuk, D. (2018). Comparison of debriefing methods after a virtual simulation: An experiment. *Clinical Simulation in Nursing*, *19*(6), 1–7. https://doi.org/10.1016/j.ecns.2018.03.002

Verkuyl, M., Lapum, J. L., St-Amant, O., Hughes, M., Romaniuk, D., & Mastrilli, P. (2019). Designing virtual gaming simulations. *Clinical Simulation in Nursing*, *32*(7), 8–12. https://doi.org/10.1016/j.ecns.2019.03.008

Verkuyl, M., St-Amant, O., Hughes, M., Lapum, J. L., & McCulloch, T. (2020). Combining self-debriefing and group debriefing in simulation. *Clinical Simulation in Nursing*, *39*(2), 41–44. https://doi.org/10.1016/j.ecns.2019.11.001

William, A., Vidal, V., & John, P. (2016). Traditional instruction versus virtual reality simulation: A comparative study of phlebotomy training among nursing students in Kuwait. *Journal of Education and Practice*, *7*(9), 18–25. https://eric.ed.gov/?id=EJ1095814

Wüller, H., Behrens, J., Garthaus, M., Marquard, S., & Remmers, H. (2019). A scoping review of augmented reality in nursing. *BMC Nursing*, *18*(1), 19. http://dx.doi.org/10.1186/s12912-019-0342-2

Wurdinger, S., & Allison, P. (2017). Faculty perceptions and use of experiential learning in higher education. *Journal of E-Learning and Knowledge Society*, *13*(1). https://www.learntechlib.org/p/188130/

Ydo, E. (2020). *VR hygiene and safety: Everything you need to know*. https://www.linkedin.com/pulse/vr-hygiene-safety-everything-you-need-know-evelien-ydo/?trackingId=FlSyfsBJSj2xwRYgzcvSKQ%3D%3D

CHAPTER 11

Three-Dimensional Printing: Collaborative Nurse-Led Research

Lori Lioce, Kimberly Budisalich, and Darlene A. Showalter

ABSTRACT

Though three-dimensional (3D) printing is often touted as cutting-edge technology, it actually made its appearance in the 1980s. Since then, this technology has made significant progress from its humble origins of layering polymers to create simple structures to the more sophisticated printing with elements such as metals used to create complex structures for aircraft. This technology has advanced and been finely tuned largely in thanks to the engineering profession. The variance within the printers, software, and printing material allows for broad application beyond engineering and manufacturing. Healthcare and academic applications are beginning to get traction. The National Institutes of Health has established a platform for sharing 3D ideas to support biotechnology and modeling for healthcare. It makes sense that nursing programs would, minimally, utilize 3D printers to enrich their institutional simulation laboratory and to manufacture specialty materials for training students in a cost-efficient manner. Opportunities to collaborate with other academic departments and community partners in the development and production of timely and effective solutions to pressing healthcare needs enriches student learning, nursing programs, and their graduates. Faculty buy-in and purposeful integration throughout the curriculum are vital variables

http://dx.doi.org/10.1891/0739-6686.39.243

associated with the successful implementation of 3D printing in a nursing program. Additional benefits include opportunities for publications, presentation of papers, and interprofessional collaboration.

INTRODUCTION

This chapter presents the basic and thoughtful application of three-dimensional (3D) printing in healthcare education and research. The authors review the advantages and disadvantages of 3D printing, implications for research and education, and application within community and interdisciplinary collaborations. The chapter concludes with an education integration exemplar as a "how-to" guide with applications for advance practice nursing education.

3D printing, also known as additive manufacturing, has the appearance of a very modern technology, but is actually around 30 years old. In the early 1980s, rapid prototyping was developed by Charles W. Hull. In its beginnings, 3D printing started out as an idea of using photopolymers to create a cross-sectional slice in a model to build it up in layers (Stuart, 2014). This led to the creation of stereolithography (SLA), which translates digital code into an actual object, usually made into plastic from photopolymers heated by a ultraviolet (UV) laser beam. In 1986, Hull was granted a patent for the first 3D printing technology using SLA Hatch & Shaw (2019). SLA 3D printers are based on photopolymerization, which uses a laser to harden an ultraviolet sensitive resin, layer by layer. Huge gains were made for inventors who could now easily create complex designs and parts using this technology.

In the second decade of the technology, huge leaps in the medical field were made with the creation of a working miniature kidney, a prosthetic leg, and a blood vessel that was printed with human cells (Shahrubudin et al., 2019; Sharma & Goel, 2019). This time, 3D printing's history also included the launch of open-sourced 3D printing. Open-sourced printers and software are the product of creative and open collaboration without associated intellectual property boundaries. Contributors on such platforms embrace four principles: right to see, use, modify, and redistribute (Depoorter, 2013). The Open Source Hardware Association, Public Lab, and Wevolver are just a few of the many organizations that provide platforms for open-sourced printer and software specifications. With present-day 3D printing technology, printers are no longer limited to just printing with plastic. Printing with metals such as gold and silver, printing an entire aircraft, and printing the body of an ecological car can all be accomplished with 3D printing (Goldberg, 2014). Diversity of materials allows for varied applications. Cement and ceramics can also be used in 3D printing to create structures (Ngo et al.,

2018). The 3D printing process builds a 3D object from a computer-aided design (CAD) model by successively adding material layer by layer (Lioce et al., 2020).

FOUNDATIONS OF 3D PRINTING

3D printing machines work by printing virtual designs with special filament to create a 3D product. The filament is heated, then expelled through the extruder in thin layers onto the heated printer bed (Coakley & Hurt, 2016). The smoothness of the finished product depends on the resolution and settings of the printer; the thinner the layers, the smoother the end product. Print time varies on the speed of the printer, design, and quality of the print, which can be changed in the settings of the slicer software (Sharma & Goel, 2019).

Types of Printers

There are a variety of printer choices available for both the novice personal user and the business professional. When choosing a printer, it is important to look at the features offered and determine which features are important for its intended use. The complexity of the hardware and software should be considered, especially for the beginning novice. Software compatibility with slicer software options is also important, especially for the industry-standard software known as Cura. The quality of the print is essential if the desired end product is to have a fine, smooth surface. The connection capability of the printer is also a valuable assessment point as some printers are not equipped to send print files via Wi-Fi. If so, a printer connected with universal serial bus (USB) cables or secure digital (SD) card is needed. If a larger project is planned, a printer with a large enough surface area and print volume should be utilized. A printer with a heated bed improves adhesion to the bed, helps reduce warping, and can use a variety of filament types since some filaments will shrink as they cool. Compatibility with filament types is also an important consideration as some companies require their exclusive brand use of filament (Brewster, 2020).

Specifications and Cost

The 3D printer most familiar to the authors is the Monoprice MP10 mini. This printer has an open design, is easy to set up, and is an excellent, inexpensive option for the novice user. The average cost for this printer starts at $299 and includes assisted bed leveling, reachable magnetic extruder, touchscreen, and a useful print function that resumes printing in the event of a power interruption. The print bed is heated, removeable, and has a flexible plate that allows for easy removal of the finished print. The print quality is good, although not as smooth and detailed as some of the higher end printers (Monoprice, 2020).

Although the Monoprice MP10 is a great, affordable option for 3D printing, the Prusa i3 MK3S has more features, offers a higher quality and more detailed print, and is an excellent option for the novice as well as the more advanced user. Reviewers report the Prusa to be quieter than most 3D printers, small enough to fit on a desk, and easy to set up. It can be purchased for self-assembly and also has parts that can be purchased for printer repair by more advanced users. Purchasing the build-it-yourself kit from the company will save about $250, with the preassembled printer starting at $1,000. The Prusa also comes with a heated, removable bed that allows for easy removal of prints. This printer is compatible with all open-source software and a large variety of filament types; however, it works best with polylactic acid (PLA) and acrylonitrile butadiene styrene (ABS). The open design will cause chemicals to be released when using certain filaments, such as ABS, and should only be used with a closed-design printer and good ventilation. This printer is targeted toward the 3D enthusiast and therefore lacks professional features, such as dual extrusion, touch screen, or Wi-Fi capabilities (Brewster, 2020; 3D HUBS, 2020).

The Makerbot Replicator Plus is designed for the educator and offers special packages to enhance the learning experience for teachers and students. The price of this printer starts at $2,000 and, although it does have some additional features marketed toward educators, it does not have a heated bed. The print software is user-friendly, although it lacks the ability for customization of various settings. This could also be considered a plus for those who want simplicity to print with minimal options. Makerbot Replicator Plus has connectivity via Wi-Fi, USB, and Ethernet. Unfortunately, only Makerbot filament is compatible and it does not have a heated bed; therefore, the only filament option is Makerbot PLA. The Makerbot produces a good quality print and there is a camera and liquid crystal display (LCD) to allow for easy control and monitoring of the printer (3D HUBS, 2020; Makerbot, 2020a).

The Ultimaker 3 is an exceptional 3D printer for educational and commercial settings (Ultimaker, 2020). The user-friendly click-and-print design creates high-quality prints and utilizes Cura software to provide step-by-step assistance through the printing process. However, the exceptional print quality results in a slower print time. Print files can be sent wirelessly via Wi-Fi, which can be convenient when sharing in a large facility. This printer also has the capability of connecting via USB. The built-in camera and Cura software allow for live viewing during the printing process. Ultimaker 3 is capable of printing from a large selection of different types of material, from PLA to higher strength plastics, and supports filaments from other manufactures. The printer has an open enclosure, with access during printing, that can present a safety hazard to younger users. Starting at approximately $3,500, the Ultimaker 3 is more expensive than the others but offers additional features, including a touch screen, auto bed leveling, and access to a large library with educational resources (3D HUBS, 2020).

Slicer Software

Slicer software is required once the 3D model is created and ready for print. The model will usually be in an standard triangle language (STL) file, and the slicer software prepares the model for printing by breaking it down or "slicing" the model into thin layers, then producing a G-code file with specific instructions for the 3D printer (Gigante, 2019). According to experts, the 3D printing software directly affects the quality of the final print (Gigante, 2019; Simplify 3D, 2020).

Free, open-source slicer software is available online from Ultimaker (2020), as well as others that can be purchased (Gigante, 2019). When choosing a slicer software, consider cost, ease of use, software compatibility, and customizable print settings. Cura is one of the industry's most popular slicer software. Developed by Ultimaker, Cura is a free and open-source slicer software that is compatible with Windows, Mac, and Linux operating systems. Cura offers beginners the ability to prepare prints quickly and easily, while still offering advanced users the ability to customize settings for additional refinement. There are adjustment tools available to assist with moving and scaling the print model. Cura works with several different file formats including STL, X3D, 3MF, OBJ, as well as some image file formats (Gigante, 2019; Ultimaker Cura, 2020).

Repetier-Host is also a free and open-source slicer software that is compatible with Mac, Windows, and Linux operating systems. This software provides support for several different slicers and is capable of printing multiple models simultaneously, saving time when needing to print multiple parts. This software is easy to use for the beginner, but also allows for full control for the more advanced user that includes multicolor preview prior to printing. Repetier-Server allows access and control of the printer through a browser from any location accessible by a Mac, PC, tablet, or smartphone. A webcam can also be used to view a live printing or record a video to share (Gigante, 2019; Repetier, n.d.).

Simplify 3D is a slicer software developed for the professional user. Over a hundred different 3D printer models are supported and the software is compatible with Mac, Windows, and Linux systems. Issues can be identified prior to starting the print with a preprint simulation. An animated view of the print is provided as the extruder lays out each thin layer of filament. This software costs approximately $150 for one lifetime license and comes with expert support and professional resources to enhance print quality. Discounts are available for students and teachers (Simplify 3D, 2020).

Design Programs

When choosing a 3D modeling software for printing, consider cost, file support, operating compatibility, and simplicity of use. Design programs are essential for creating 3D printing models and various tools can offer design customization. CAD is the most commonly used software to create models for 3D printing. Computer-aided manufacturing (CAM) programs are used to prepare a design for manufacturing, and computer-aided engineering (CAE) programs analyze and simulate a product. CAD programs can be used independently; however, CAD is required for both CAE and CAM software since a design model is required to perform analysis or manufacturing (Huckstepp, 2020).

There are several different file formats used for 3D printing. STL (stereolithography), also known as standard triangle language is the most popular and was the first file format, which was developed by Chuck Hull in 1987. STL files provide the surface geometry of a 3D model but are unable to store information on color or material. OBJ (Object) file format, developed by Wavefront Technologies, can be used when wanting color or appearance stored. Scalable Vector Graphics (SVG) is a 2D graphic file that can be converted to a STL file for 3D printing (Chakravorty, 2019).

TinkerCAD is a user-friendly 3D design and modeling software that is great for the beginner. Created by Autodesk, this web-based browser is free and does not require download. TinkerCAD is compatible with both Windows and Mac systems. Design models can be a simple shape or more detailed through additional shapes and grouping. Once the 3D model is created, it is ready to print with the software-supported STL file. TinkerCAD offers an assortment of free, online design tools and has the ability to import STL, OBJ, and SVG files. Other features include online cloud storage, laser cutting, and simple click-to-print 3D files (Gigante, 2019; Tinkercad Autodesk, 2020).

Fusion 360 is a 3D cloud-based modeling software combining CAD, CAM, and CAE to design, engineer, and manufacture with an all-in-one platform. Fusion 360 is one of many software programs developed by Autodesk that can be used by the novice user as well as the experienced engineer. The software requires an annual subscription of up to $500 a year, but educators and students are eligible for free access to this and several other software offered by Autodesk. Fusion 360 is compatible with both Mac and Windows operating systems. Fusion 360 allows several prototypes to be created at the same time during the design process as not to limit the user. Other features include electronics and simulation tools to create layouts, test designs, assure accuracy through creation of full 3D models from a 2D drawing, and improve quality of the finished product (Autodesk, 2020).

FreeCAD (n.d.) offers an open-source 3D software developed to design real-life projects of all sizes. The software is easily customizable and is compatible with Mac, Windows, and Linux systems and numerous file types, including SVG, STL, Drawing Exchange Format (DXF), OBJ, and many others. FreeCAD was designed for everyone, from novice student users to the experienced engineer. This software is free, although contributions to update designs, fix bugs, or add new features are welcomed. Active community developers provide software updates and support (FreeCAD, n.d.).

Filaments

The most common filaments used in 3D printing are made from plastic. PLA is one of the most frequently used due to its low cost, accuracy, and usability. PLA is firm and durable, with minimal flexibility and is one of the easiest to work with. If a stronger material is needed to withstand a higher stress load, then ABS is a better choice. ABS material shrinks as it cools and should be kept warm as it prints. This material, therefore, works best with a heated bed with an enclosed chamber. Due to toxic fumes, ABS should only be used with an enclosed system printer with good ventilation. There are over 16 different types of filaments that can be used for different projects (see Table 11.1) and users should always confirm filament compatibility with specific 3D printers (Pinshape Blog, 2015).

TABLE 11.1

Filament Type, Quality, and Use for Simulation

Filament Type	Quality	Use for Simulation
PLA	Hard/most commonly used	Vein finder, splints, mask holder
Flexible/ TPU	Flexible/stretch/bend	Trachea, toenail
ABS	Hard/highly durable—able to withstand stress	Moving and replacement parts, electronic housing
HIPS	Durable/lightweight/dissolvable	Used for support structures—paired with ABS
PVA	Durable/dissolvable	Used for support structures—paired with PLA

RESOURCES

Establishing an open-source mechanism to collaborate, share innovations, sustain projects, and support expanded 3D solutions through feedback is vital (Ventola, 2014, p. 706). An example is the Model Exchange and Development of Nursing and Engineering Technologies also known as MED NET (Systems Management and Production [SMAP] Center, 2020). MED NET was developed after 2 years of transformative collaboration between nursing faculty at The University of Alabama, Huntsville (UAH) College of Nursing (CoN)'s Learning and Technology Resource Center (LTRC) and the engineering staff from UAH Systems Management and Production (SMAP) Center. This collaboration developed and produced models to enhance nursing education and classroom training. The SMAP Center utilized undergraduate engineers to consult, develop, fine-tune, and create physical models using 3D printing and injection molding. The partnership resulted in significant cost savings as the SMAP Center supported design and creation costs within student projects. This also allowed for further improvements of models and trainers by customizing products to meet the needs of the CoN program objectives (Micheck, 2018).The interprofessional collaborations yielded additional unanticipated benefits. Faculty and staff noticed enhanced communication skills throughout the project development due to the natural process of increased communication to revise prototypes. This enhanced communication increased confidence in project collaboration and has been added as a collaborative objective of the projects to prepare students for the workforce upon graduation. The SMAP UAH collaboration led to expanded external community collaborations to included school safety in late 2019 through a joint project with a local county school system to provide active shooter emergency response training for over 150 educators, administrators, school nurses, and staff. Multiple items were 3D printed for this collaboration, including wounds, shields, and fake weapons, to provide the training. The community impact led to a critical annual review and quality improvement of their emergency plans (SMAP Center, 2020). This led to sharing 3D files for their high school lab to provide items for teaching in their primary and secondary education programs.

MakerBot's Thingiverse boasts the largest community in the world of 3D printing and uploads of roughly 1.9 million models. The community welcomes beginners by giving them a platform in which to create their own designs, rework others' designs, or create their own mod template using Thingiverse's app, Customizer. The primary focus of MakerBot's Thingiverse is the discovery, design, and sharing of 3D printable models through a Creative Commons license that allows anyone to use or customize the design. This license allows a wide variety of creativity and mixing of all types of designs ranging from basic desk paperweights to functional engineering models to high-level medical applications (Makerbot Thingiverse, 2020).

The NIH 3D Print Exchange through the National Institutes of Health (NIH) offers a platform for anyone to discover, share, create, and learn about creating and customizing biomedical 3D models (National Institute of Health, 2020). The 3D print exchange is a collection of highly accurate models ranging from fully functional prosthetic designs to protein and macromolecule structures that are already in ready-to-print formats. An open license can be applied that permits others to share or modify designs, allowing for more collaboration among the community. NIH has five categories of models: medical and anatomical; labware and devices; small molecules; proteins, macromolecules, and viruses; and bacteria, cell, tissue, organism. NIH's creation page utilizes web-based tools that will automatically turn molecular or medical imaging data into scientifically accurate 3D printable model files. Video tutorials on creating custom molecular models in an open source software can be found on the NIH's learning page. These seek to encourage learning and increase the number of accurate models in the biomedical world (National Institute of Health, 2020).

Embodi3d was created by Dr. Mike Itagaki, MD, MBA, to provide affordable resources that allow for training prior to challenging procedures (Embodi3D, n.d.). While seeking a way to practice for an extremely dangerous surgery, Dr. Itagaki spent hundreds of hours exploring the growing idea of 3D printing and its applications in medicine. He used 3D printing to create an exact replica of his patient's artery and used this to practice and perfect an upcoming surgery. Dr. Itagaki discovered the value of 3D printing in the medical world and founded the biomedical 3D printing community. Here, numerous, affordable, ready-to-print 3D medical models, created from patients' medical scans, are available for purchase. Printed models can also be requested and shipped. Custom models for medical devices or procedure training can be requested or created from computed tomography (CT) scans using their exclusive tool, Democratiz3D. An online community with forums, tutorials, and blogs about medical 3D printing is also available (Embodi3D, n.d).

ADVANTAGES AND DISADVANTAGES

There are many reasons to create and incorporate 3D printing in education and clinical training. Research has found there are learner benefits, industry benefits, cost savings improvement, and increased access to clinical training (Garcia et al., 2018; Greenhalgh, 2016). They also promote collaboration and problem-solving skills.

3D printing has been incorporated in primary and secondary education, providing learners with a more advanced introduction to this technology (Ford

& Minshall, 2017). It is up to those in higher education to embrace new technology and incorporate innovative practice solutions into curricula. Producing practitioners who are not completely reliant on healthcare systems, reimbursable equipment, and third-party reimbursement for effective solutions and affordable, accessible durable medical supplies (i.e., custom splints) will expand access and improve quality of care.

Learners benefit from exposure to technology, innovation, enhanced "collaboration and speaking skills" (EdTech, 2019), communication skills, and critical thinking development (Elsworthy, 2014). Studies show 3D printing and working with 3D objects engages multiple learning styles, increases use and understanding of math and science, exploring trial and error, teaching technical fabrication, and promoting science and technology education (EdTech, 2019; National Association for Education of Young Children, 2002; Walrack, 2016). The use of active learning strategies has become even more important with the increase in online learning. There is an expansive network of curricular integration support and manufacturers, such as an educator's guidebook offered by Makerbot (2020b).

Considerations should be made for obtaining faculty/staff buy-in, planning for initial costs, designating space, and developing a resident expert as well as engaging students in mentored research to promote creativity and patient-centered solutions (Lioce et al., 2020). Short- and long-range plans for continued integration that include special interest groups, and project mentors, are crucial so scholarly posters and papers can help advance the science and dissemination of improved models (Hatch & Shaw, 2019).

After several years of collaboration, the SMAP Center at UAH donated a Monoprice MP10 Mini 3D printer to UAH CoN (see Figure 11.1). This provides the resources that allow for expanded research and printed projects. Additionally, CoN has further expanded utilization of 3D printing through creation of new designs and introduction of this novel technology to other nursing faculty.

Orientation, Training, and Installation

Before receipt of the 3D printer, a small CoN team met for training with the engineering and 3D printing teams from the SMAP Center. Through the 4-hour, hands-on training, the CoN team learned, step by step, how to program and 3D print. The training session included Cura software download and setup, online file searching, and printer naming conventions. After completing the training, the engineering team delivered the 3D printer to the CoN and completed the initial setup. The printer was leveled and PLA filament was installed. The team at the SMAP Center continues to provide support by phone, e-mail, and on site as needed. The CoN team operationalized and refined an internal step-by-step procedure to post for open collaboration within the CoN and LTRC (see Table 11.2).

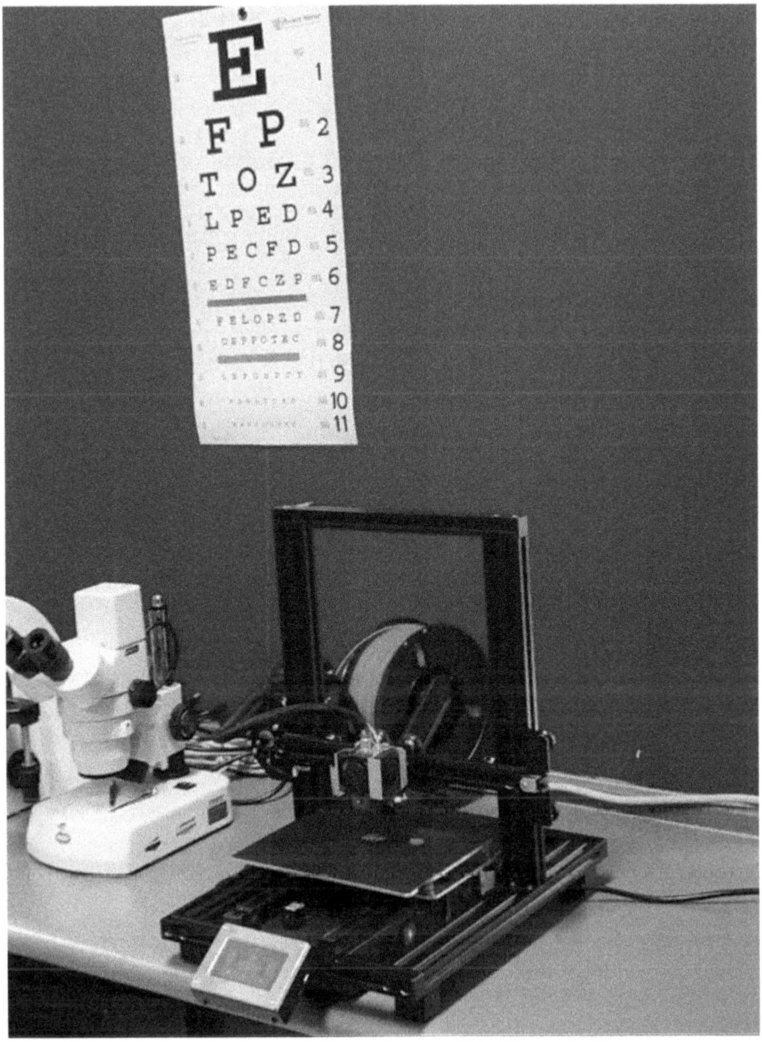

FIGURE 11.1 Monoprice 3D printer.
Source: Used with permission from UAH College of Nursing Learning & Technology Resource Center, Dr. Lori Lioce.

TABLE 11.2

3-D Printing Process

The slicer program (Cura) must be downloaded onto the computer you will be using with your 3D Printer.

A. Download Cura software on your Windows computer

1. The Cura program for Windows is located on the microSD card provided
2. Put the microSD card from the printer into the adapter provided and insert the card into the computer
3. Double click "Ultimaker Cura 3.3.1" on the SD card
4. "Welcome to the Ultimaker Cura 3.3.1 Setup Wizard" will appear
5. Click "Next"
6. Click "I Agree"
7. Click "Install"
8. If Microsoft License Agreement appears, click, "Agree" and "Install"
9. Once it says completed, click "close"

B. After Installation

a. Open Cura 3.3.1
b. Disclaimer by Ultimaker
c. Click "I understand" and "Agree"
d. In the top-right corner, click the drop-down menu
e. Select "Add Printer"
f. Select "Other"
g. Scroll down to Monoprice MP10 mini
h. Select "Add Printer"
i. Exit out of any updates
j. This will now be the default printer when you open Cura

C. Selecting Model to Print

a. Go to www.thingiverse.com
  i. Search "keychain"
  ii. Scroll down until you find this file
  iii. Click on picture
  iv. Select "Thing Files" (located below the picture)
  v. Double click on the file ending with .stl
    1. This printer will only work with .stl file

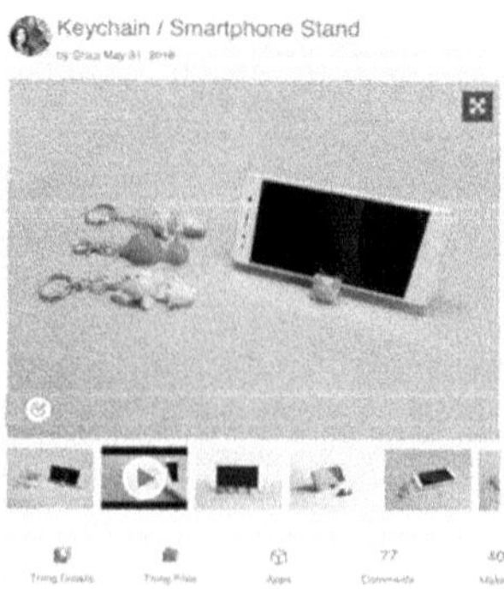

TABLE 11.2
3-D Printing Process (Continued)

b. File will be saved to the "Download Folder"

c. Loading a Model into Cura

   i. Open Cura
   ii. Place miniSD card with adapter in computer
   iii. Select "File Folder Icon" in top-left corner
   iv. Select "Downloads"
   v. Double-click on your file
   vi. Select "Slice" — located at bottom right of Screen "Prepare"
   vii. Once slicing is complete, you will see the time to print (1 hr 14 min)
      1. You can adjust size if wanted – this will affect print time
   viii. Select "Save File to Removable Disk" – located in the bottom-right corner
   ix. Select "Eject" once the file has been saved
      1. Now it is safe to remove SD card

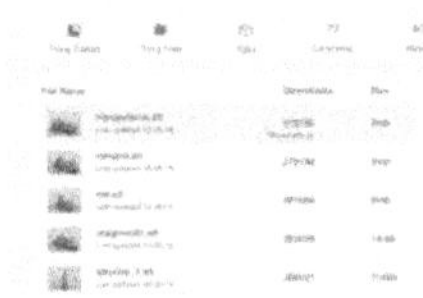

Pen

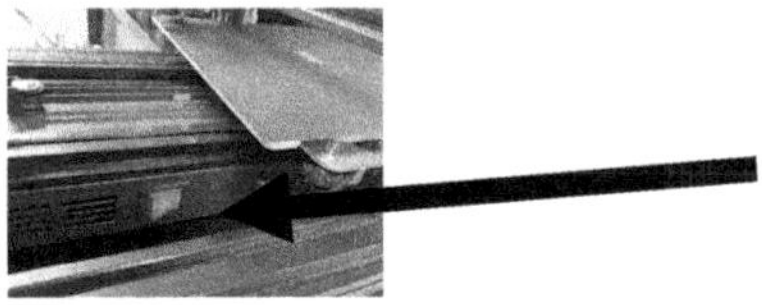

D. Printing

   i. Turn on Printer

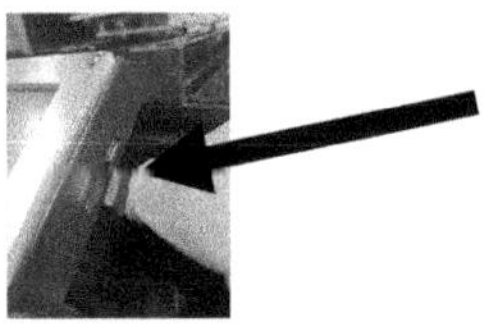

a. Insert mini SD card into printer
b. Select "Preheat"

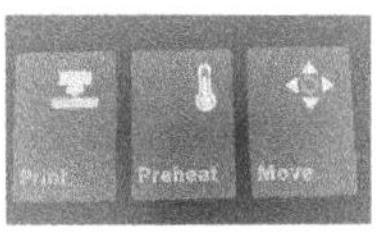

(*Continued*)

TABLE 11.2

3-D Printing Process (Continued)

1. Nozzle – Set to 210°
2. Bed – Set to 65°
3. Once Nozzle is preheated go to "Move"

E. Prepare Filament and Extractor

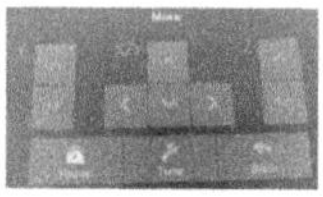

1. Press and hold E ⇑ — This will clean filament from nozzle
2. Home Printer
3. Select "Tune," then "Auto Leveling"
   a. (May need if moved)
4. Return to Main Menu by selecting "Back"
5. Select "Print"
6. Select your file to print (Printing will begin once preheating is complete)

F. How to Change Filament Color

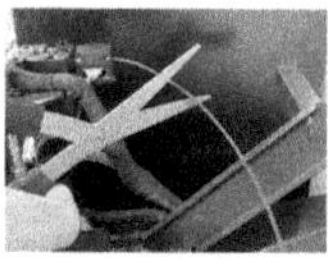

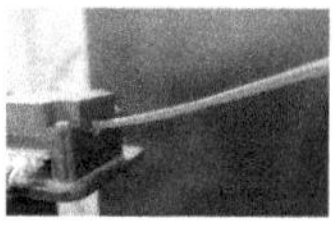

1. Select "Preheat"
2. Nozzle — Set to 210°
3. Cut filament to be removed
4. Once Nozzle is preheated go to "Move"
5. Press and hold E ⇑ — This is to remove Filament
6. Insert filament you wish to use then press and hold E ⇓ (until new filament color comes out of the extruder).

Source: Used with permission from UAH College of Nursing Learning & Technology Resource Center, Dr. Lori Lioce.

COMMUNITY INTEGRATION

Over the past 3 years, the authors, faculty, and LTRC staff from the CoN have collaborated with the SMAP Center to develop multiple medical models and task trainers to support active immersive learning for nursing students and assist engineering students and interns with project development and communication skills. These models allow students to practice for a fraction of the price of purchasing these anatomical or task training models. For example, anatomical heart models were printed for cardiac lectures, tracheostomy task trainers for procedural and dressing changes, and digit task trainers for onychectomies.

When the COVID-19 pandemic hit the United States, the SMAP Center and the CoN recognized the community's need for medical supplies and personal protective equipment (PPE). The SMAP engineering staff began 3D printing face shields and surgical mask straps. Intubation boxes were manufactured with a 3D printer. These were distributed to frontline healthcare workers. MED NET provided scalable, free, platforms that allowed technical schools to implement projects in local learning centers and care for their own communities. Products from their labs provided resources such as face shields for teachers and staff to safely return to schools.

As a part of a community service project, the SMAP Center donated 16 3D printers to schools in the local school district. They provided similar training and installation to the faculty and staff in the school district and continue to provide support as needed.

RELEVANCE TO NURSE PRACTITIONER EDUCATION

Simulated learning allows students to practice in a safe environment before entering the clinic or hospital setting. Simulation also allows students to learn from mistakes and build confidence in their clinical and procedure skills, as well as enhance critical thinking (Hatch, 2019). The technological advancements, including 3D printing, offer a unique opportunity to enhance simulation for nurse practitioner (NP) education. 3D printing can model structural, anatomical differences of various disease processes that create a more realistic experience. 3D printing can also enhance clinical skills and procedural training for the NP student at a reduced cost.

There are challenges to overcome to successfully integrate 3D printing into nursing education. Faculty buy-in is critical to the success of implementing change and adopting new teaching strategies. A significant amount of time and resources are needed to incorporate the new technology into the curriculum (Hatch & Shaw, 2019). Additionally, as 3D printing technology continues to grow, the education of healthcare professionals will need to include novel applications of this technology to ensure healthcare professionals are prepared to competently care for patients (Maryville University, 2020).

Examples of 3D Applications in Advanced Practice Nursing Education

3D printing can offer myriad training solutions such as (a) cricothyrotomy trainer, (b) vein finder, (c) onychectomy (toenail removal) trainer, (d) customized wrist splints/braces, (e) injection pad trainer, (f) face shields for healthcare workers, (g) mask holders, (h) intubation box, (i) mechanical vent (MIT, El Paso Texas, UAH with NASA Cubic), (j) I & D suture pads, (k) wound tattoos, and (l) placenta. Some of these examples are further explained in detail below.

Cricothyrotomy is the surgical procedure in which an incision is made through the skin and cricothyroid membrane to establish a patient's airway during certain life-threatening situations (Barak et al., 2019). 3D units were printed using biodegradable thermoplastic and nontoxic PLA filament as task trainers for this procedure.

The 3D-printed vein finder consists of a battery-powered circuit with multiple red LEDs with a wavelength between 620 and 680 nm. Light at this wavelength will penetrate skin, fatty tissue, and oxygenated blood, but will not penetrate deoxygenated blood. This results in darkened veins that can be used for intravenous and central venous line insertion. The vein finder was printed using PLA filament.

Onychectomy is a surgical procedure in which part or all of a fingernail or toenail is removed. The digit units were printed using PLA filament.

The wrist splints/braces were printed flat with open shapes in various sizes for use by patients of all ages. They were then thermoformed to soften the material and custom-fitted on the wrist. The wrist splints/braces were printed with PLA.

The 3D-printed injection pad trainer simulates tissue layers representing epidermis, dermis, fat, and muscle layers. The pad is used for simulating intradermal, intramuscular, and subcutaneous injections. Each skin layer is made differently to simulate thickness, texture, and color. Layers of skin were made with a PLA filament and thermoplastic polyurethane (TPU) filament.

The nursing faculty were actively involved throughout the 3D printing process to ensure the desired texture, elasticity, density, strength, color, and realism. The 3D-printed training devices have been embedded into simulations and are being used to provide nursing students with much needed hands-on experiences, allowing students to practice specific skills at a lower cost in a safe setting. The multidisciplinary collaborative research has been a rich learning experience for all involved. Each of these projects have been presented by students and faculty and submitted to engineering and nursing conferences.

SUMMARY

Though 3D printing experienced its humble beginnings as stereolithography, it has since made a significant impact across much of the manufacturing, healthcare, transportation, and engineering professions. This technology is now readily accessible and no longer cost prohibitive. Open-source websites offer the user opportunities to collaborate in the continued development and application of the software and provide crucial pointers submitted by users. This innovative tool is essential in promoting creative thinking and in the development of solutions for complex problems. Advance practice nurses are perfectly poised to learn how to design structures and operate 3D printers to manufacture time-sensitive equipment. Implementation of simulations where these skills might be utilized in a nursing curriculum is likely to yield a well-rounded provider able to not only diagnose and identify a need, but also design and produce a solution in real time. 3D printing continues to unfold as a technology with myriad applications. Nurses must remain curious, even visionary, exploring methods to deliver educational and skill training opportunities through the implementation of cutting-edge technology.

ACKNOWLEDGMENTS

Thank you to Dr. Marsha Howell Adams, dean, The University of Alabama, Huntsville (UAH) College of Nursing, for her support of our individual research visions, personal scholarship, and her belief in interprofessional collaboration. To Dr. Gary Maddux, director of the Systems Management and Production (SMAP) Center, for his leadership and belief in providing resources and a lasting sustainable model to support our community and support of teaching and learning. To Norven Goddard, research scientist, UAH SMAP Center, for valuing interprofessional collaboration from the moment we met, for his professional curiosity, and his follow through! To Ishella Fogle for her inspiration, support, and management of projects and to Bernard Schroer for his inspirational writing and documentation of the collaborative achievements. To Caroline Ursprung, Jarvee Liles, Luke Forkum, Marquis Myler, Andrew Couch, Garrett George, Shelby Tull, Dominick Lioce, Sydney Gunter, Makenzie Fogle, Lauren Fogle, Glenda Scott, and Andrew Budisalich, our UAH students, for their collaboration in mentored research and collaboration for biomedical research and 3D printing projects.

REFERENCES

Autodesk. (2020). *Fusion 360 integrated CAD, CAM, and CAE software*. https://www.autodesk.com/products/fusion-360/overview

Barak, M., Leiser, Y., & Kluger, Y. (2019). Airway management in trauma patients. In P. Aseni, L. De Carlis, A. Mazzola, & A. Grande (Eds.), *Operative techniques and recent advances in acute care and emergency surgery* (p. 146). Springer Publishing.

Brewster, S. (2020). *The best 3D printer*. https://www.nytimes.com/wirecutter/reviews/best-home-3d-printer/

Chakravorty, D. (2019). *The most common 3D file formats*. https://all3dp.com/3d-file-format-3d-files-3d-printer-3d-cad-vrml-stl-obj/#stl

Coakley, M., & Hurt, D. (2016). 3-D printing in the laboratory: Maximized time and funds with customized and open-sourced labware. *Journal of Laboratory Automation*, *21*(4), 489–495. https://doi.org/10.1177/2211068216649578

3D HUBS. (2020). *Best 3D printer guide 2019*. https://www.3dhubs.com/best-3d-printer-guide/#original-prusa-i3-mk3s

Depoorter, G. (2013). La communauté du logiciel libre. Espace contemporain de reconfiguration des luttes? In B. Frère (Ed.), *Résister au quotidian* (pp. 133–160). Presses de Sciences Po.

EdTech. (2019). *The resurgence of 3D printers in modern learning environments*. https://edtechmagazine.com/k12/article/2019/06/resurgence-3d-printers-modern-learning-environments-perfcon

Elsworthy, C. (2014). *3D Printing can inspire collaboration and innovation in many academic subject areas*. https://www.emergingedtech.com/2014/09/3d-printing-inspires-collaboration-innovation-many-academic-subjects/

Embodi3D. (n.d.). *About us*. https://www.embodi3d.com/about-us/

Ford, S., & Minshall, T. (2017). *Invited review article: Where and how3D printing in teaching and education*. https://www.researchgate.net/publication/320617391_Invited_review_article_Where_andhow_3D_printing_is_used_in_teaching_and_education

FreeCAD. (n.d.). *FreeCAD your own 3D parametric modeler*. https://www.freecadweb.org/

Garcia, J., Yang, Z., Mongrain, R., Leask, R., & Lachapelle, K. (2018). 3D printing materials and their use in medical education: A review of current technology and trends for the future. *BMJ Simulation and Technology Enhanced Learning*, 4(1), 27–40. https://stel.bmj.com/content/bmjstel/4/1/27.full.pdf

Gigante, M. (2019). 8 best free 3D printing software to try in 2019. *Learning Hub*. https://learn.g2.com/free-3d-printing-software

Goldberg, D. (2014). The history of 3D printing. *Product Design & Development*. https://elib.uah.edu/login?url=https://search-proquest-com.elib.uah.edu/docview/1611001471?accountid=14476

Greenhalgh, S. (2016). The effects of 3D printing in design thinking and design education. *Journal of Engineering, Design and Technology*, *14*(4), 752–769. https://doi.org/10.1108/JEDT-02-2014-0005

Hatch, N., & Shaw, R. (2019). *3D printing: The future of nursing and clinical education*. https://medtechboston.medstro.com/blog/2019/01/18/3d-printing-the-future-of-nursing-and-clinical-education/

Huckstepp, A. (2020). *3D printing software overview*. https://www.engineeringclicks.com/3d-printing-software-overview/

Lioce, L., Maddux, G., Goddard, N., Fogle, I., Fogle, M., Gunter, S., & Schroer, B. (2020). *Application of 3D printing in the development of training simulation for nursing students*. The International Workshop on Innovative Simulation for Healthcare (IWISH). 32nd European Modeling & Simulation Symposium, Athens, Greece.

Makerbot. (2020a). *Educators guidebook for 3d printing in the classroom*. https://www.makerbot.com/education/3d-printing-guidebook/

Makerbot. (2020b). *The classroom 3D printer solution*. https://www.makerbot.com/3d-printers/replicator-educators-edition/

Makerbot Thingiverse. (2020). *About thingiverse*. https://www.thingiverse.com/about

Maryville University. (2020). *How 3D printing could revolutionize the field of nursing*. https://online.maryville.edu/blog/how-3d-printing-could-revolutionize-the-field-of-nursing/

Micheck, K. (2018). *Educators turn to 3D printing to train nursing students*. https://www.healthleadersmedia.com/nursing/educators-turn-3d-printing-train-nursing-students

Monoprice. (2020). *MP10 mini 3D printer*. https://www.monoprice.com/product?p_id=34438

National Association for Education of Young Children. (2002). Early childhood mathematics. *Promoting Good beginnings*. https://www.naeyc.org/sites/default/files/globally-shared/downloads/PDFs/resources/position-statements/psmath.pdf

National Institute of Health. (2020). *NIH 3D print exchange*. https://3dprint.nih.gov

Ngo, T., Kashani, A., Imbalzano, G., Nguyen, K., & Hui, D. (2018). Additive manufacturing (3D printing): A review of materials, methods, applications and challenges. *Composites Part B: Engineering*, *143*, 172–196. https://doi.org/10.1016/j.compositesb.2018.02.012

Pinshape Blog. (2015). *3D filament guide: Popular 3D printing filaments*. https://pinshape.com/blog/popular-3d-printing-filaments-3d-printer-filament-types/

Repetier. (n.d.). *Repetier-Host overview*. Retrieved from https://www.repetier.com

Shahrubudin, N., Lee, T. C., & Ramlan, R. (2019). An overview on 3D printing technology: Technological, materials, and applications. *Procedia Manufacturing*, *35*, 1286–1296. https://doi.org/10.1016/j.promfg.2019.06.089

Sharma, S., & Goel, S. (2019). 3D printing and its future in the medical world. *Journal of Medical Research and Innovation*, *3*(1). https://doi.org/10.15419/jmri.141

Simplify 3D. (2020). *Amazing features*. https://www.simplify3d.com/software/features/

SMAP Center. (2020). *Model exchange and development of nursing and engineering technologies (MEDNET)*. https://mednet.uah.edu/home.

Stuart, N. (2014, July 14). Ten minutes with the inventor of 3D printing. *The Engineer (Online)*. https://www.theengineer.co.uk/ten-minutes-with the inventor-of-3d-printing/

Tinkercad Autodesk. (2020). *From mind to design in minutes*. https://www.tinkercad.com/

Ultimaker Cura. (2020). *Cura slicer software free download*. https://ultimaker.com/software/ultimaker-cura

Ventola, C. (2014). Medical applications for 3D printing: Current and projected uses. *Pharmacy and Therapeutics*, *39*(10), 704–711. https://www.ncbi.nlm.nih.gov/pmc/articles/PMC4189697/#__ffn_sectitle

Walrack, J. (2016). *6 different ways 3D printing improves education at all levels*. https://blog.zmorph3d.com/6-ways-3d-printing-improves-education-levels/

Index

www.ingramcontent.com/pod-product-compliance
Ingram Content Group UK Ltd.
Pitfield, Milton Keynes, MK11 3LW, UK
UKHW021845100926
8556IPUK00019B/1059